HIV, RESURGENT INFECTIONS AND POPULATION CHANGE IN AFRICA

T0140520

International Studies in Population

Volume 6

The International Union for the Scientific Study of Population (IUSSP)

The IUSSP is an international association of researchers, teachers, policy makers and others from diverse disciplines set up to advance the field of demography and promote scientific exchange. It also seeks to foster relations between persons engaged in the study of demography and population trends in all countries of the world and to disseminate knowledge about their determinants and consequences. The members of the IUSSP scientific group responsible for this book were chosen for their scientific expertise. This book was reviewed by a group other than the authors. While the IUSSP endeavors to assure the accuracy and objectivity of its scientific work, the conclusions and interpretations in IUSSP publications are those of the authors.

International Studies in Population (ISIP) is the outcome of an agreement concluded by IUSSP and Springer in 2004. The joint series covers the broad range of work carried out by IUSSP and includes material presented at seminars organized by the IUSSP. The scientific directions of the IUSSP are set by the IUSSP Council elected by the membership and composed of:

John Cleland (UK), President
Peter McDonald (Australia), Vice-President
Nico Van Nimwegen (Netherlands), Secretary General and Treasurer

Elizabeth Annan-Yao (Ivory Coast)
Graziella Caselli (Italy)
John Casterline (USA)
Maria Coleta de Oliveira (Brazil)
Thomas Kingston Le Grand (Canada)

Hoda Rashad (Egypt)
Catherine Rollet (France)
Yasuhiko Saito (Japan)
Zeba Sathar (Pakistan)
Zeng Yi (China)

For other titles published in this series, go to
www.springer.com/series/6944

HIV, Resurgent Infections and Population Change in Africa

Edited by

MICHEL CARAËL

Social Sciences Faculty,
Free University of Brussels, Brussels, Belgium

and

JUDITH R. GLYNN

London School of Hygiene and Tropical Medicine,
London, UK

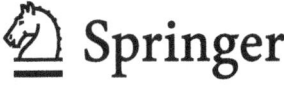 Springer

Editors
Michel Caraël
Free University of Brussels
Pleinlaan 2
1050 Bruxelles
Belgium
caraelm@yahoo.fr

Judith Glynn
London School of Hygiene and
  Tropical Medicine (LSHTM)
Keppel Street
London WC1E 7HT
United Kingdom
judith.glynn@lshtm.ac.uk

ISBN: 978-1-4020-6173-8   e-ISBN: 978-1-4020-6174-5

Library of Congress Control Number: 2008932951

Printed on acid-free paper

9 8 7 6 5 4 3 2 1

springer.com

CONTENTS

PREFACE

MICHEL CARAËL
JUDITH R. GLYNN

The time has come to close the book on infectious diseases.
(United States Surgeon General, 1967)

Forty years ago, the age-old battle against infectious diseases as a major threat to human health was believed close to being won. This followed spectacular improvements in public health measures, such as sanitation, the advent of antibiotics, and insecticides. In addition, with the biotechnology revolution and the discovery of vaccines that helped to eradicate smallpox and control poliomyelitis, measles, diphtheria and other killer diseases, hope was raised that tuberculosis and malaria vaccines would soon follow.

However, by the late twentieth century, the increase of emerging and re-emerging infectious diseases was evident in both low and high income countries. About 30 new infectious diseases have been identified in the last few decades, and some of them have received considerable media and public attention, such as Legionnaires' disease, hepatitis C, bovine spongiform encephalopathy and new variant Creutzfeldt-Jakob disease, viral haemorrhagic fevers such as Ebola, and, most recently, severe acute respiratory syndrome (SARS). The re-emergence of H5N1 influenza A virus is a current and real threat. Among the "new" diseases, and most importantly, the Human Immunodeficiency Virus (HIV) epidemic, with 40 million persons infected and 25 million deaths since its first description, presents one of the most significant health, societal and security challenges facing the global community. By 2002, HIV/AIDS had become the leading cause of death among both women and men aged 15 to 59 years, causing one in every seven deaths in this age-group globally. The interaction of HIV/AIDS with tuberculosis, malaria and bacterial infections have increased HIV-related morbidity and mortality; and in turn, the HIV pandemic has brought about devastating increases in tuberculosis.

In addition to new pathogens, "old" diseases persist, and in some cases have re-emerged or grown increasingly resistant to conventional treatment, showing the limits of modern medicine and of a pharmaceutical development system driven by the diseases of the North.

As 40 years ago, the leading causes of death among children under five are still pneumonia, diarrhoea, malaria, and measles; but AIDS has now appeared on the list of causes of childhood deaths in sub-Saharan Africa. Nutritional insecurity and malnutrition—the underlying cause of more than half of the deaths occurring among children—has also increased, partly because of the impact of adult AIDS mortality and morbidity on nutrition in the most affected countries. Most infectious diseases are increasingly driven by, and contribute to, factors that also create malnutrition—in particular, poverty, emergencies and inequalities.

Infectious diseases are still responsible for approximately 25% of global mortality—but for an estimated 53% of all deaths in sub-Saharan Africa—and for more than 60% of deaths in children aged younger than 5 years. Sub-Saharan Africa suffers disproportionately from infectious diseases partly because of poverty and under-development, but also because of the continuous erosion of the public health infra-structure in most countries: Health delivery systems are generally under-staffed and over-burdened.

The emergence and resurgence of infectious diseases reflect macro changes or inten-sification of trends that have occurred throughout history, in both global economy and human ecology: increasing poverty in large segments of the world popula-tion, resulting in high rural-to-urban migration and high-density peri-urban slums; increasing long-distance mobility due to globalization, trade and tourism; the social disruptions of war, conflict, and insecurity; and, increasingly, intense human–animal interactions and changes in the way that food is processed and distributed. Global-ization continues, and there is little doubt that societal, technological, and environ-mental factors will continue to provoke a dramatic increase in infectious diseases worldwide.

This evolution and the profound impact of AIDS on social institutions in Southern and Eastern Africa have triggered renewed interest in infectious diseases—largely driven by concerns about national and international security—under the label "new health threats". The creation of the Global Fund to fight AIDS, Tuberculosis and Malaria and several other global initiatives for vaccines and for improved surveil-lance show that mechanisms for innovative, global efforts to control infectious dis-eases are emerging.

Understanding the population impact and the dynamics of infectious diseases in the most affected region is critical to efforts to reduce the morbidity and mortality of such infections, and for decisions on where to use limited resources in the fight against infections. This book on '*HIV, Resurgent Infections and Population Change in Africa*', by offering a demographic and epidemiological perspective on emerging and re-emerging infections in sub-Saharan Africa, aims to contribute to these efforts.

THE AUTHORS

Joseph Brunet-Jailly. Laboratoire Population Environnement Développement - UMR 151, Université-de Provence. Institut de Recherche pour le Developpement, Paris. 213 rue Lafayette, 75780-Paris cedex 10, France. joseph.brunet-jailly@wanadoo.fr

Michel Caraël. Faculté des Sciences Sociales, Université Libre de Bruxelles, 50 avenue F D Roosevelt, B-1050 Brussels, Belgium. caraelm@yahoo.fr

Sabada Dube. Department of Infectious Disease Epidemiology, Imperial College London, St Mary's Campus, Norfolk Place, London W2 1PG, UK. s.dube@imperial.ac.uk

Geoffrey P Garnett. Department of Infectious Disease Epidemiology, Imperial College London, St Mary's Campus, Norfolk Place, London W2 1PG, UK. g.garnett@imperial.ac.uk

Andrew Karanja Githeko. Kenya Medical Research Institute, Centre for Vector Biology and Control Research, Climate and Human Health Research Unit, PO Box 1578, Kisumu 40100, Kenya. agitheko@kisian.mimcom.net

Judith R Glynn. Department of Epidemiology and Population Health, London School of Hygiene and Tropical Medicine, Keppel St, London WC1E 7HT, UK. judith.glynn@lshtm.ac.uk

Nicholas C Grassly. Department of Infectious Disease Epidemiology, Imperial College London, St Mary's Campus, Norfolk Place, London W2 1PG, UK. n.grassly@imperial.ac.uk

Simon Gregson. Department of Infectious Disease Epidemiology, Imperial College London, St Mary's Campus, Norfolk Place, London W2 1PG, UK. s.gregson@imperial.ac.uk

Richard Lalou. Laboratoire Population Environnement Développement - UMR 151, Université-de Provence. Institut de Recherches pour le Développement, Centre de Hann, BP 1386, CP 18524, Dakar, Sénégal. richard.lalou@ird.sn

David A Leon. Department of Epidemiology and Population Health, London School of Hygiene and Tropical Medicine, Keppel St, London WC1E 7HT, UK. david.leon@lshtm.ac.uk

James JC Lewis. Department of Epidemiology and Population Health, London School of Hygiene and Tropical Medicine, Keppel St, London WC1E 7HT, UK. james.lewis@lshtm.ac.uk

AD McNaghten. CDC Zimbabwe and Centers for Disease Control & Prevention, 1600 Clifton Rd, Atlanta, GA 30333, USA. aom5@cdc.gov

France Meslé. Research Unit, Population and Development, Institut National d'Etudes Démographiques (INED), 133 Boulevard Davout, 75980 Paris cedex 20, France. mesle@ined.fr

Jean-Paul Moatti. INSERM Research Unit 379 (Social Sciences Applied to Medical Innovation), University of the Mediterranean, 232 Boulevard de Sainte Marguerite, 13273 Marseille cedex 9, France. moatti@marseille.inserm.fr

Kath Moser. Department of Epidemiology and Population Health, London School of Hygiene and Tropical Medicine, Keppel St, London WC1E 7HT, UK. kathmoser83@hotmail.com

Owen Mugurungi. Ministry of Health & Child Welfare, Mkwati Building, 4th Street, Harare, Zimbabwe. atp.director@africaonline.co.zw

Victor Piché. Département de démographie, Université de Montréal, CP 6028, Succursale Centre-Ville Montréal, Québec H3C 3J7, Canada. victor.piche@umontreal.ca

Gilles Pison. Institut National d'Etudes Démographiques (INED), 133 Boulevard Davout,75980 Paris cedex 20, France. pison@ined.fr

Vladimir M Shkolnikov. Laboratory for Demographic Data, Max Planck Institute for Demographic Research, Konrad-Zuse-Str, 1 D-18057 Rostock, Germany. shkolnikov@demogr.mpg.de

Emma Slaymaker. Centre for Population Studies, London School of Hygiene and Tropical Medicine, 49-51 Bedford Square, London WC1B 3DP, UK. emma.slaymaker@lshtm.ac.uk

Ian M Timæus. Centre for Population Studies, London School of Hygiene and Tropical Medicine, 49-51 Bedford Square, London WC1B 3DP, UK. ian.timaeus@lshtm.ac.uk

Bruno Ventelou. GREQAM-CNRS and Regional Centre for Disease Control (ORS-PACA). INSERM Research Unit 379 (Social Sciences Applied to Medical Innovation), University of the Mediterranean, 232 Boulevard de Sainte Marguerite, 13273 Marseille cedex 9, France. ventelou@marseille.inserm.fr

Florence Waïtzenegger. Consultant in Demography, waitzf@ hotmail.com

Dominique Waltisperger. Research Unit, Population and Development, Institut National d'Etudes Démographiques (INED), 133 Boulevard Davout, 75980 Paris cedex 20, France. d_waltis@club-internet.fr

Basia Zaba. Centre for Population Studies, London School of Hygiene and Tropical Medicine, 49-51 Bedford Square, London WC1B 3DP, UK. basia.zaba@lshtm.ac.uk

INTRODUCTION

FRANCE MESLÉ
Research Unit, Population and Development,
Institut National d'Etudes Démographiques (INED), Paris, France

VLADIMIR M. SHKOLNIKOV
Laboratory for Demographic Data, Max Planck Institute
for Demographic Research, Rostock, Germany

In the early 1970s, Omran (1971) [1] defined the concept of the epidemiologic transition in order to characterize trends in mortality patterns in the world. For him, the decrease in infectious mortality is the driving force of the epidemiologic transition. Societies go from the "age of pestilence and famine" to the age of "degenerative and man-made diseases", thanks to the recession of pandemics.

The theory was conceived at a time when progress in health seemed to run out of steam in Western countries. It was assumed that life expectancy would soon reach a limit that could not be overstepped. Very rapidly Omran's theory was undermined by the dramatic decrease in mortality from circulatory diseases, and this decrease produced new gains in life expectancy, especially at advanced ages, in most industrialized countries. To fit the new situation several authors, including Omran himself, proposed an extension of the theory by adding a fourth or even a fifth stage to Omran's first three ages [2, 3, 4, 5, 6]. Others enlarged the concept and suggested that Omran's epidemiologic transition could itself be a first stage in the broader process of health transition [7, 8].

This new step in health transition did not benefit all people equally. Inside the most favoured national populations, some groups (women, highly-educated, married) took greater advantage of health achievements, which resulted in a widening gap between population segments. From the mid-sixties onwards, Central and Eastern European countries were not successful in their fight against degenerative and man-made diseases, and life expectancy stopped increasing and even sometimes decreased in that part of Europe.

A number of developing countries followed the way opened up by the first-industrialized countries. Benefiting from technologies and tools developed in the latter, they experienced a rapid decline in mortality after World War II, mainly related to the decrease of infectious diseases. This progress, however, was not universal: some countries, especially in sub-Saharan Africa, were unable to control infectious diseases and could not catch up.

1

M. Caraël and J.R. Glynn (eds.), HIV, Resurgent Infections and Population Change in Africa, 1–8.
© Springer Science + Business Media B.V. 2008

In the year 2000, the International Union for the Scientific Study of Population (IUSSP) launched a new Scientific Committee on Emerging Health Threats, which was mandated to contribute to a better understanding of these failures of health transition. Why were some populations at a national or sub-national level deviating from the "normal" path of health transition? Were these deviations questioning the theory itself? Was it possible to forecast future mortality trends? Would all countries finally converge towards an insuperable threshold or would divergence and convergence continue to alternate according to the speed of diffusion of health progress?

The first Seminar of the Scientific Committee on Emerging Health Threats held in June 2002 jointly with the Max Planck Institute for Demographic Research was devoted to the determinants of diverging trends with a special focus on industrialized countries. The seminar was organized around two main issues: the divergence between Eastern and Western European countries during the last three decades of the 20th century, and the widening gap between different population groups inside countries. A selection of papers presented at this seminar was published in a special collection of *Demographic Research* [9].

In Central and Eastern Europe, particularly among the less fortunate classes of the population, the people were unable to cope with the increase of degenerative and man-made diseases as described by Omran. In Western countries, and especially for more favoured segments of the population, trends were reversed, thanks to the implementation of health policies consisting of reinforced prevention, widespread screening, new therapeutics and improved efficiency of emergency units, the Communist regimes, which relied almost exclusively on the centralized administration of modern health care, were not successful in the struggle against degenerative diseases. Indeed, these new health policies required financial means for long-term care of people with serious diseases requiring costly therapy, widespread use of sophisticated technical equipment, creation of a dense network of emergency medical services, etc., but the means were unavailable. The new policies also required changes in individual behaviour and the active participation of citizens in the management of their own health care, which could be more rapidly achieved among better-educated populations, having easy access to all sources of information. In recent years, health care progress has resumed in most Central European countries, and in particular there has been a decrease in cardiovascular mortality. This recent improvement shows that a significant trend reversal can occur rapidly even in the case of chronic diseases.

Another priority of the IUSSP Scientific Committee on Emerging Health Threats was to contribute to a better understanding of the reasons why sub-Saharan Africa was lagging so much behind the other regions of the world. Most African countries were not able to control infectious diseases and were still far from achieving the epidemiologic transition, as defined by Omran. Not only the emergence of AIDS but also the resurgence of well-known infectious diseases like tuberculosis or malaria in these countries resulted in very poor health conditions. At present, the region faces a combination of endemic poverty and fragile health care systems with a variety of unfavourable epidemiological, behavioural, and environmental patterns.

The second seminar of the Scientific Committee on Emerging Health Threats was entitled *HIV, Resurgent Infections, and Population Changes in Africa*: it was aimed at facilitating studies of relationships between population, development, and resurgent infectious disease in Africa. Particular attention was paid to conditions leading to the spread of disease and the impact of disease on demographic and socioeconomic trends.

The seminar was held from 12 to 14 February 2004 in Ouagadougou, Burkina Faso. It included ten sessions and twenty-six presentations of research reports. The papers gave new information on the current burden of infectious diseases and on major trends in mortality due to infections, as well as on the major determinants of infectious disease spread, such as mobility and urbanization, governance, health care systems, poverty and social exclusion. The impact of environmental changes (climate or agricultural systems) was also examined. Finally the impact of infectious diseases on mortality and on more general population trends were discussed.

After the seminar, participants were invited to submit their final papers for possible publication in a collective work. The initial selection of papers was performed by a committee consisting of M. Caraël, F. Meslé, V. Shkolnikov, and I. Timæus. All further editorial work on the manuscripts and exchanges with their authors were performed by the editors—Michel Caraël and Judith Glynn.

The book which resulted is divided into two parts. The first is entitled "Trends and Diseases" and consists of six chapters devoted to changes in mortality trends worldwide. They describe the major components and determinants of mortality and infectious diseases in Sub-Saharan Africa.

The first chapter, by K. Moser, D.A. Leon and V.M. Shkolnikov, introduces a Gini-type dispersion measure of mortality for analysis of changes in the amount of inter-country diversity according to life expectancy for all countries of the world with a population size exceeding one million. This shows that the long-term global trend towards convergence to a lower mortality has reversed since the late 1980s. This unfavourable upturn is largely attributable to rising adult-age mortality in Sub-Saharan Africa and (to a lesser extent) in the former Soviet Union and several other countries. At the same time, infant mortality continues to decrease in most countries. The analysis suggests that adult mortality should be given greater emphasis as a global health priority than is the case with the Millenium Development Goals.

The next chapter, by G.P. Garnett and J.J.C. Lewis, describes a mathematical model of the spread of infectious disease in populations. The potential for spread is determined by the duration of infectiousness, the contact rate, and the likelihood of transmission if there is contact. Depending on certain conditions, the number of risky contacts may either increase with population density or be constant. Population growth has three major consequences for infectious disease: growing populations in poor urban areas increase contact rates, facilitating epidemics; the sheer scale of cities provides more opportunities for a disease to persist with a ready supply of susceptible people; the conditions associated with increase in travel and migration can turn epidemics into pandemics. Population growth combined with young, poorly resourced communities is a key factor affecting global health. Better housing and medical care, but also slowing population growth due to demographic transition, can help tackle the problem.

The decline in child (under five) mortality has slowed down significantly in Sub-Saharan Africa over the last 15 years. After reviewing this trend in countries of the region, G. Pison examines in his chapter the components and determinants of this adverse trend in Senegal, a country little affected by AIDS, but with stabilization in child mortality closely resembling that for the whole region. His study is based on reliable mortality data from three demographic surveillance sites in rural Senegal. In all of them, under-five mortality remained at about the same high level since the mid-1980s. Analysis of causes of death and of medical facilities suggests that this stagnation could be mainly caused by malaria, in a new epidemiological situation created by spreading resistance to chloroquine, and by the inability of local health facilities to ensure the provision of vaccinations and other basic health services.

The chapter by A. Githeko discusses the complex relationship between climate change and malaria. Climate change includes gradual change in mean temperature and other meteorological parameters, but also strong shorter-term weather fluctuations such as heavy rainfall, floods, unusually warm periods, and droughts. Some weather anomalies are associated with periodical El Niño events. Impacts of climate change on malaria are determined by dependence of the disease transmission on vector density, duration of malaria parasite maturation, and the immunity level of exposed populations. The study provides examples of malaria outbreaks associated with weather anomalies. It emphasizes the particular vulnerability of populations living in highland areas in Kenya, Rwanda, Madagascar and other African countries characterized by low background prevalence of disease and low immunity. Such populations experience high morbidity and mortality in periods of anomalously warm and humid seasons.

The chapter by D. Waltisperger and F. Meslé investigates an important health crisis in Madagascar, including striking famine-related mortality from 1984 to 1988. The study uses the register of deaths in Antanarivo in 1976–2001 and benefits from the unusual (for the region) availability of cause-of-death data. The socio-economic situation in Madagascar continuously deteriorated between 1976 and the early 1990s. From 1976 to 1988 mortality was increasing and in the 1980s poorly managed economic reforms resulted in severe food shortages and extremely high mortality. A recovery during the 1990s led to a return to the 1976 mortality level in 2000. Changes in general mortality were largely driven by nutritional deficiencies, and infectious and respiratory diseases. The findings suggest that progress in the fight against infectious disease is unlikely to be sustained if the economic situation does not make it possible to provide the population with adequate supplies of food.

Which health interventions should be applied in order to reduce the heavy burden of health problems in low-resource settings of the region? J. Brunet-Jailly argues in his chapter that the choice of health strategies should be based strictly on a cost-effectiveness approach. As the available funds are very restricted, not all effective interventions can be carried out. Only the most effective of them should be chosen, otherwise a portion of the scarce resources will be wasted by using them inefficiently. In order to make an evaluation, the disability adjusted life years saved (DALY) are used as a health outcome for the purpose of comparing monetary costs of health intervention alternatives. This "best buy" framework leads to the conclusion that for HIV/AIDS the most effective intervention is prevention, whereas the highly active antiretroviral therapy of HIV (HAART) for adults is least cost effective.

The second part of the book is devoted to HIV/AIDS. Its seven chapters assess mortality and the economic impacts of the disease; they also examine various factors affecting the epidemics in different parts of Sub-Saharan Africa and discuss opportunities for HIV/AIDS prevention. The studies emphasise the enormous scale of the health challenge, the extreme complexity of the epidemic's causal mechanisms, and the great difficulties but also some potential opportunities for efficient interventions.

The second part opens with a review of the evidence about risk factors and opportunities for prevention of HIV in young adults by M. Caraël and J. Glynn. Young adults are not only the group with the highest HIV incidence but also the key target group for interventions. The study divides HIV factors into three groups: contextual, proximate, and biological factors. The contextual group includes poverty, urbanization and growth of slums, migration and separation of partners, political crises and armed conflicts, and gender inequality. These factors generally aggravate health conditions and influence the proximate (behavioural) determinants. These include: early sexual debut, sex with multiple partners, commercial and transactional sex, sexual abuse, sex between young girls and much older men, and early marriage of young women. The third group of biological factors has potential for the modification of risks conditioned by the proximate behavioural factors. The probability of acquiring HIV via sexual intercourse is elevated for those with other sexually transmitted infections and may be higher for young girls than for older women. Circumcision of men is associated with a lower risk of acquiring HIV. The spread and dynamics of the epidemics depend on the interplay of the three groups of factors. Existing HIV control programmes target mostly the group of proximate factors. So far, few interventions with proven efficacy have been made available to the majority of young people in need of them.

In Africa, the vast majority of new HIV cases are attributable to heterosexual contacts. This suggests that not only is the behaviour of individuals important, but also the similarity or dissimilarity of behaviour patterns between partners within couples. Much HIV infection is acquired within marriage: either because an infected person marries an uninfected one or because, in marriage where both spouses are initially uninfected, one partner gets infected outside the marriage and passes on the infection. The chapter by E. Slaymaker and B. Zaba makes this important point and addresses it by analysing the Zambian Demographic and Health Survey data sets of 1996 and 2001–2002. Between the two surveys married couples became more similar to each other with lower proportions of both men and women having had sex before age 15. The proportion of married couples in which men had been married before increased. In 2001, in only 3% of couples had both partners tested for HIV. The fact that HIV prevalence and mortality has remained stable between 1996 and

2001, while there was a substantial decline in unsafe behaviours among individuals, suggests that patterns of HIV transmission could have changed.

The chapter by R. Lalou, V. Piché and F. Waïtzenegger uses data from a survey on "Mobility and STI/AIDS in Senegal" for an in-depth analysis of pathways connecting migration with spread of HIV. Associations of migration status with knowledge, perceptions, and actual risk behaviours are examined. The study detects a difference between behaviours of international and internal migrants. The former perceive "others" or "foreigners" as a source of danger. Therefore they use condoms more often when staying abroad and use them less frequently than non-migrants after coming back to their original community. The internal migrants perceive infection risk to be related to sexual encounter and use condoms more often than non-migrants. These findings suggest the importance of socio-cultural variability in shaping behavioural patterns.

The chapter on HIV in Zimbabwe by O. Mugurungi, S. Gregson and colleagues is a case-study presenting an overview of the HIV epidemic in Zimbabwe. Zimbabwe is one of the most economically developed African countries, but also among those hardest hit by AIDS. Because of the disease, mortality of adults has increased by about 2.5-fold between the late 1980s and the mid-1990s. About 25% of the adult population are estimated to be HIV positive. HIV prevalence in rural areas is higher than in other African countries, perhaps because of intensive economic migration to the countryside for agricultural work, with no family accommodation for labour migrants. HIV is associated with other sexually transmitted infections and risky sexual behaviours such as multiple-partners and extra-marital sex. Odds of being infected are higher in non co-resident marriages and for individuals with a higher number of sex partners during the last year. Some evidence suggests that HIV prevalence has begun to decrease since the mid-1990s especially in younger age groups. The high level of economic and human capital in Zimbabwe helps to increase knowledge and awareness and to intensify HIV prevention activities.

Part of the total health burden caused by HIV/AIDS is related to a higher risk of acquiring other infections in people with suppressed immune status. The onward transmission of these infections further increases the population burden of disease. The chapter by J. Glynn is a synthesis of previous studies linking HIV with TB. Since the early 1980s TB notification rates have doubled in Africa. The risk of TB among people with HIV is 4–10 times higher than among people with no HIV. The proportion of TB directly attributable to HIV is conservatively estimated at 31%. Antiretroviral therapy is likely to have a limited impact on reduction of TB incidence in the population.

Throughout Africa, routine statistical systems fail to report reliable information about mortality and its changes. Therefore, "windows of clarity" produced by localized demographic surveillance sites are of great importance. The chapter by I. Timæus examines patterns of adult-age mortality on the basis of data from three surveillance sites in South Africa, Zimbabwe, and Namibia. Principal component analysis applied to mortality–age schedules identifies two components responsible for the background mortality curve and for the excess mortality at adult ages.

Comparison of these components between pre-AIDS and with-AIDS periods suggests that the second component reflects mortality from HIV/AIDS. Modelling of AIDS mortality–age distributions could allow the development of a simple system for approximate description of a range of African mortality schedules.

The final chapter by JP. Moatti and B. Vantelou applies a novel approach to estimation of the economic impact of AIDS. The existing low estimates of its economic impact originate from models looking at AIDS as an exogenous shock. These projections consider that HIV-related deaths reduce both total income and also the number of people between whom this income must be divided. This approach is at odds with the evident economic impact of HIV seen both at the micro and at the sectorial level and ignores phenomena that have been highlighted in recent years. Individuals with poor health are generally less productive. HIV-positive individuals without appropriate treatment would tend to behave differently and their ability to make savings and investments would be low. Numerous households taking care of sick persons or orphans would experience higher consumption of capital and its lower accumulation. Poor health and early death lead to wasted investment in human capital and decrease the productivity resulting from a better education. The proposed model of economic development describes inter-relationships between economic capital, labour, human capital, and public productive spending. Its application to a number of African countries leads to closer estimates of the present and future GDP losses.

This book is a collection of interesting high-quality studies. They provide important information about ideas and methods in the research area, and reveal key health and population processes and their causal mechanisms. The book includes synthetic studies and more specific investigations of situations in particular countries and population groups. All the studies presented in this book are accessible to non-specialists with a basic knowledge of demography, health and statistics. We hope that the book will be useful to researchers and students in a variety of academic fields such as public health, epidemiology, medicine, demography, economics and other social sciences.

References

1. Omran, A. R., (1971). The epidemiologic transition: A theory of the epidemiology of population change. *Milbank Memorial Fund Quarterly, 49*, 509–538

2. Olshansky, J. & Ault, B., (1986). The fourth stage of the epidemiologic transition: The age of delayed degenerative diseases. *The Milbank Quarterly, 64*, 355–391

3. Omran, A., (1983). The epidemiologic transition theory: A preliminary update *Journal of Tropical Pediatrics, 29*, 305–316

4. Omran, A. R., (1998). The epidemiologic transition theory revisited thirty years later. *World Health Statistics Quarterly/Rapport trimestriel de statistiques sanitaires, 51*, 99–119. (Historical epidemiology: Mortality decline, and old and new transitions in health, special number edited by Odile Frank)

5. Rogers, R. G., & Hackenberg, R., (1987). Extending epidemiologic transition theory, *Social Biology, 34*, 234–243

6. Olshansky, S. J., Carnes, B. A., Rogers, R. G., & Smith, L. (1998). Emerging infectious diseases: The fifth stage of the epidemiologic transition?. *World Health Statistics Quarterly/Rapport trimestriel de*

statistiques sanitaires, *51*, 207–217. (Historical epidemiology: Mortality decline, and old and new transitions in health, special number edited by Odile Frank)

7. Frenk, J., Bobadilla, J. L., Stern, C., Frejka, T. & Lozano, R., (1991). Elements for a theory of the health transition, *Health Transition Review*, *1*, 21–38

8. Vallin, J. & Meslé, F., (2004). Convergences and divergences in mortality. A new approach to health transition. *Demographic Research*, 12–43. (Special Collection 2. Determinants of Diverging Trends in Mortality). Retrieved from http://www.demographic-research.org/special/2/default.htm

Part I

Trends and Diseases

CHAPTER 1. WORLD MORTALITY 1950–2000: DIVERGENCE REPLACES CONVERGENCE FROM THE LATE 1980s

KATH MOSER
Department of Epidemiology and Population Health, London School of Hygiene and Tropical Medicine, London, UK

VLADIMIR M. SHKOLNIKOV
Laboratory for Demographic Data, Max Planck Institute for Demographic Research, Rostock, Germany

DAVID A. LEON
Department of Epidemiology and Population Health, London School of Hygiene and Tropical Medicine, London, UK

Abstract. The objective of this chapter is to investigate to what extent worldwide improvements in mortality over the past 50 years have been accompanied by convergence in the mortality experience of the world's population. A novel approach to the objective measurement of global mortality convergence is adopted. The global mortality distribution at a point in time is quantified using a Dispersion Measure of Mortality (DMM). Trends in the DMM indicate global mortality convergence and divergence. The analysis uses United Nations data for 1950–2000 for all 152 countries with populations of at least 1 million in 2000 (99.7% of the world's population in 2000). The DMM for life expectancy at birth declined until the late 1980s but has since increased, signalling a shift from global convergence to divergence in life expectancy at birth. In contrast, the DMM for infant mortality indicates continued convergence since 1950. The switch in the late 1980s from the global convergence of life expectancy at birth to divergence indicates that progress in reducing mortality differences between many populations is now more than offset by the scale of reversals in adult mortality in others. Global progress needs to be judged on whether mortality convergence can be re-established and indeed accelerated.

* This chapter appeared in the Bulletin of the World Health Organization and is reprinted with their permission. Moser K, Shkolnikov V, Leon DA. World mortality 1950–2000: divergence replaces convergence from the late 1980s. Bulletin of the World Health Organization 2005;83(3):202-209. The chapter appendix was not included in the original article.

M. Caraël and J.R. Glynn (eds.), HIV, Resurgent Infections and Population Change in Africa, 11–25.
© Springer Science + Business Media B.V. 2008

Introduction

The international community is paying increasing attention to the formulation and use of indicators and targets against which human development can be measured. The Millennium Development Goals, for example, have been widely adopted and provide a focus for the diverse attempts being made to improve the health and welfare of the world's population (1). Mortality is included in these goals as well as being a component of the well established Human Development Indices used in the Human Development Report (2).

The 2003 Human Development Report focuses on the Millennium Development Goals and states: "The range of human development in the world is vast and uneven, with astounding progress in some areas amid stagnation and dismal decline in others. Balance and stability in the world will require the commitment of all nations, rich and poor, and a global development compact to extend the wealth of possibilities to all people." Thus there is a central vision of reducing global inequities, and this vision is shared by the Director-General of the World Health Organization (3, 4). With respect to income, there is an established tradition of using measures such as the Gini coefficient to estimate trends in global inequities (5). However, with respect to health, there are no quantitative indicators being used to summarize the extent to which the mortality experience of the world's population is converging over time. In this paper we present a novel measure, the Dispersion Measure of Mortality (DMM), that performs precisely this function. Before discussing this measure it is necessary to describe global trends in mortality.

Over the past 50 years major demographic changes have affected all regions and countries. As a result of changes in fertility and mortality the world's population has increased from 2.5 billion to 6 billion. Declines in mortality rates, especially during childhood, have been particularly remarkable (Fig. 1). For the world as a whole life expectancy at birth has increased from 46.5 years during the period 1950–55 to 65.0 years during the period 1995 to 2000 (Fig. 2). However, over the past decade the belief that we were on a path of inexorable improvement in mortality that would benefit people all over the world has been undermined. In the 1990s the impact of the HIV/AIDS epidemic, particularly in sub-Saharan Africa (6), and the serious health crisis in the former Soviet Union (7) have shown that mortality reversals can no longer be regarded as rare and exceptional phenomena. The situation we find ourselves in is new. Before the 1970s there were almost no examples of long-term reversals in mortality, with the obvious exceptions of those caused by war and famine. Reflecting this, many of the classic analyses of the 1970s that examined long-term demographic and epidemiological trends considered that further significant gains in longevity in countries with low mortality were unlikely but that death rates in countries with high mortality would fall, resulting in a worldwide convergence in mortality (8, 9).

The recent reversals of mortality highlight an important question: that is, to what extent have the improvements in mortality over the past 50 years been accompanied by convergence in the mortality experience of the world's population? Given the importance of this question it is striking that few researchers have attempted to explicitly address it. Mortality convergence is discussed by McMichael et al. who raise concerns about whether it can be sustained given recent setbacks (10). Similarly

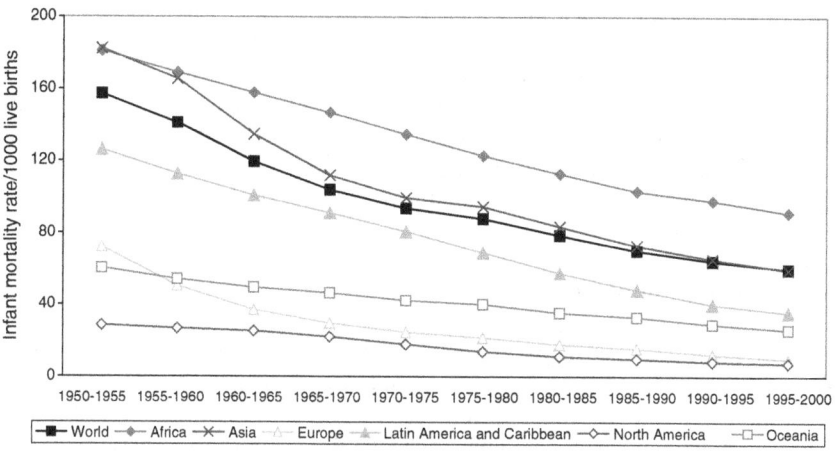

Fig. 1. Worldwide trends in infant mortality 1950–2000

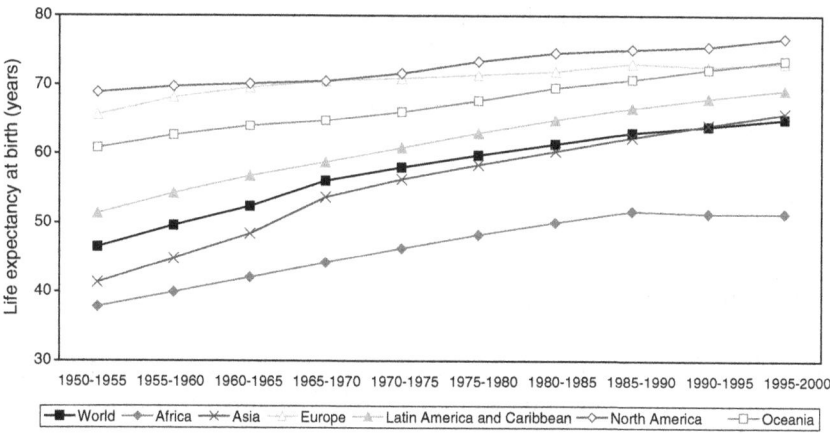

Fig. 2. Worldwide trends in life expectancy at birth 1950–2000

Wilson, in a systematic attempt to address the issue, concluded that there had indeed been convergence over the past 50 years (11). However, neither paper provided a quantitative summary measure of global mortality convergence.

Methods

We adopted a novel approach to measuring global mortality convergence, making use of a simple measure to provide a DMM calculated for consecutive 5-year periods from 1950 to 2000. Trends in the DMM indicate global convergence and divergence. Our analysis uses estimates of life expectancy at birth, infant mortality, and live births for 10 five-year periods (1950–55 to 1995–2000) and population estimates for mid-points of these periods (1952, 1957, 1962, etc.) taken from the United Nations 2000 revision of *World population prospects* (12). We also used data on mortality occurring among children less than 5 years old for 1990–95 and 1995–2000, the only two periods for which such data are available. Data from all 152 countries with populations of at least 1 million in 2000 were used. The excluded countries, mainly small island states, accounted for 0.27% of the world's population in 2000. Mortality trends in the only 10 excluded countries where the population exceeded 500,000 are similar to those of the countries included in the analysis.

Dispersion Measure of Mortality

The DMM measures the degree of dispersion that exists at any point in time in the mortality experience of the world's population. It is calculated as the average absolute inter-country mortality difference, weighted by population size, between each and every pair of countries. This approach draws on more generic mathematical work on measures of dispersion (13). Changes in the DMM over time indicate whether mortality is becoming more or less similar across the globe; decreases indicate convergence, while increases indicate divergence. The DMM for life expectancy at birth is measured in years of life, and the DMM for infant mortality is measured in infant deaths per thousand live births. So

$$\text{DMM} = \frac{1}{2(Wz)^2} \sum_i \sum_j \left(|M_i - M_j| * W_i * W_j \right)$$

where:

    i, j are countries, and $1 \leq i, j \leq 152$
    z is the world
    M is the mortality rate
    W is the weighting, and $\sum_i W_i = \sum_j W_j = W_z$

When applied to life expectancy at birth, M = life expectancy at birth, $Wz = 1$ and Wi represents relative population size of country i adjusted, however, in order to ensure that $\sum_i W_i * M_i = M_z$.

This adjustment is made because, generally speaking, the weighted average of country-specific life expectancies does not equal overall life expectancy (because life expectancies are based on life table stationary populations that differ from real populations). A simple transformation of population weights allows us to obtain weights so that the above equation is true while ensuring the minimum deviation from the original population weights (14). In the case of infant mortality, M = infant mortality rate and W = live births (as used for the denominator in calculating the infant mortality rate).

The routinely available mortality data used to construct the DMM are also used widely elsewhere (for example in the human development indices). However, the validity of all applications of global mortality data is subject to concerns about the quality of the data. For many countries the demographic data used to construct global indices are imprecise. In order to examine how far the trends in the DMM that we report could reflect these concerns, and in particular for recent changes, we undertook a series of sensitivity analyses.

The data are poorest for sub-Saharan Africa, the region where two-thirds of the countries experiencing recent mortality reversals are situated. Could data quality alone have accounted for our findings? If the reversals had been greater or had occurred in more countries than indicated by the data, or both, then our findings of divergence would stand. However, to test whether the findings would hold even if the documented reversals exaggerated the real situation we hypothesized that in the 24 countries with reversals occurring between 1980-85 and 1995-2000 that firstly, the decline in life expectancy at birth was actually only half that indicated by the data, and secondly that mortality had stagnated but not reversed. (These two scenarios were chosen in order to make generous allowances for data quality.) Mortality in the remaining countries was as indicated by their data. In both cases we recalculated the DMM using the hypothetical data.

India and China have played an important part in world demographic trends as a result of contributing 35–40% of the world's population. Consequently, these countries have a very large weighting in the calculation of the DMM. We tested whether replacing national data with subnational data for India (25 states) and China (28 provinces), thereby making the units of analysis nearer in size to other countries, had any bearing on our findings.

Findings

Between 1950 and the late 1980s the DMM for life expectancy at birth fell progressively after which time it started to increase (Fig. 3). Thus a long period of global convergence in life expectancy at birth has been replaced since the late 1980s by divergence. This occurred despite the fact that global life expectancy at birth improved throughout the period 1950–2000 (Fig. 2).

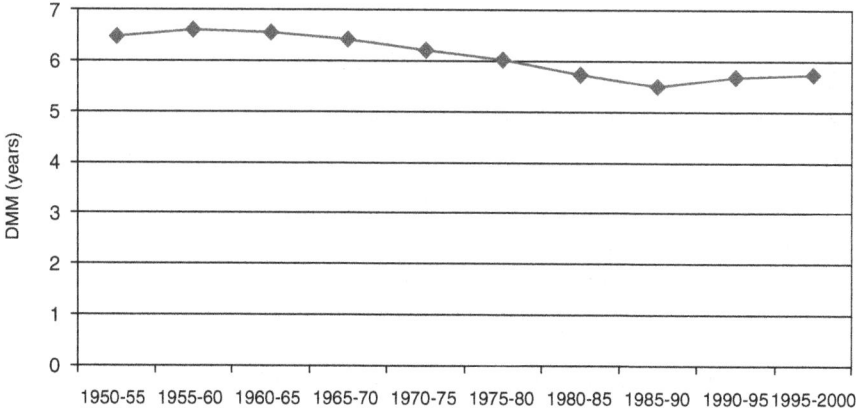

Fig. 3. Trend in the Dispersion Measure of Mortality (DMM) for life expectancy at birth: 1950–2000

In order to see what lies behind these summary trends we looked at net changes in life expectancy at birth for individual countries in three consecutive 15–20 year periods. Over the first period, 1950–55 to 1965–70, life expectancy at birth increased in all countries (Fig. 4A). Increases ranged from 1–12 years (with the exception of China where the increase was almost 19 years); the smallest increases occurred mostly in countries with low mortality. In most countries life expectancy at birth continued to improve over the period 1965–70 to 1980–85, although in parts of the

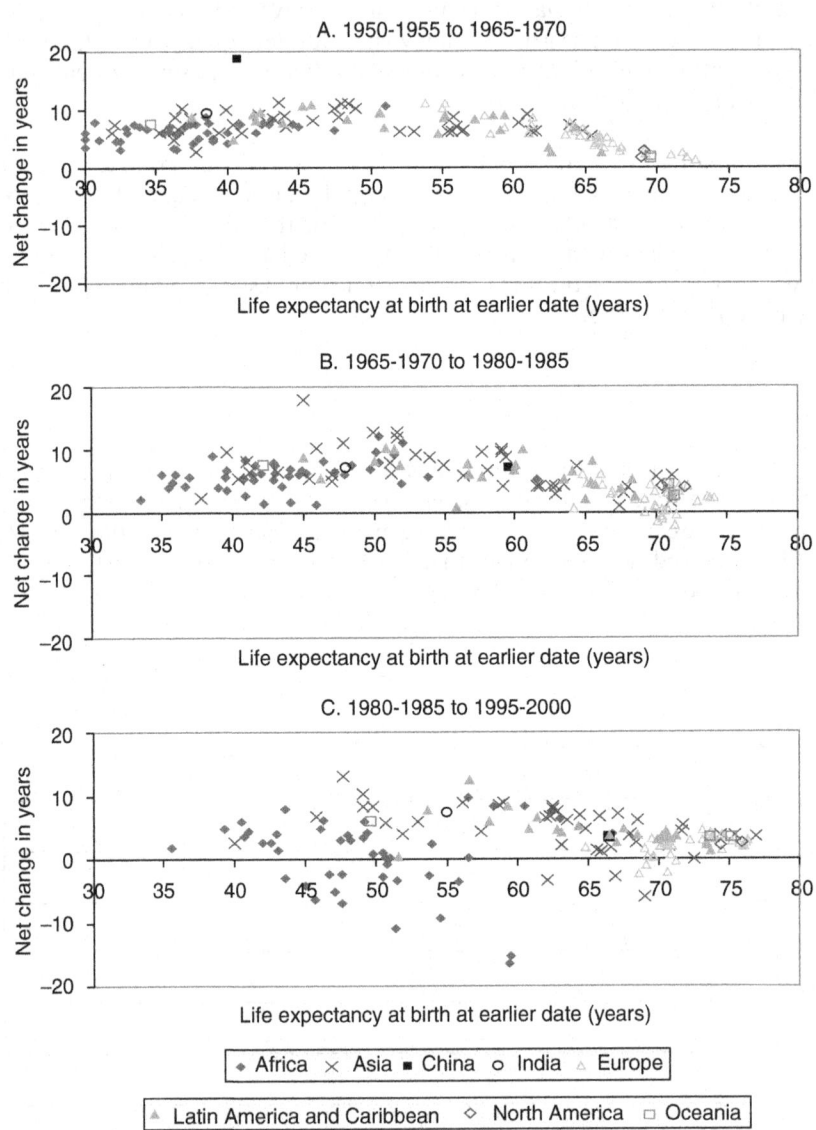

Fig. 4. Net change in life expectancy at birth for individual countries by time period
Note. Each point represents a single country

former Soviet Union, including the Russian Federation, life expectancy fell and in many countries in central and eastern Europe it stagnated (Fig. 4B). Most recently (1980–85 to 1995–2000) the pattern became much more diffuse, with 24 countries (accounting for 7.6% of the world's population in 1997) experiencing falls in life expectancy at birth (Fig. 4C). Situations in these countries spanned high mortality to low mortality and included 16 (out of 41) countries in sub-Saharan Africa, the remainder being in Asia and the former Soviet Union. In eight countries (in sub-Saharan Africa and the Democratic People's Republic of Korea) life expectancy fell by more than 5 years.

Given that infant mortality is an important component of life expectancy at birth it might be expected that trends in the DMM for this outcome would be the same as those for life expectancy at birth. However, in contrast to the trend for life expectancy at birth, the DMM for infant mortality decreased throughout the entire period 1950–2000, indicating persistent convergence over the past 50 years (Fig. 5). A more detailed analysis (not shown) concludes that during the first two 15–20 year periods all countries had a net decrease in infant mortality. However, between 1980–85 and 1995–2000 there was a net increase in infant mortality in 5 of the 152 countries, although these reversals were clearly not sufficient to reverse the overall trend of global convergence in infant mortality.

The DMM for mortality among children younger than 5 years (for the two data points available) decreased from 32.6 in 1990–95 to 31.2 in 1995–2000, indicating that convergence occurred during the 1990s.

Of the 24 countries experiencing net declines in life expectancy at birth between 1980–85 and 1995–2000, 19 (in sub-Saharan Africa and the former Soviet Union) showed simultaneous improvements in infant mortality (Fig. 6). The remaining five countries (Botswana, Burundi, Iraq, Kazakhstan, and the Democratic People's Republic of

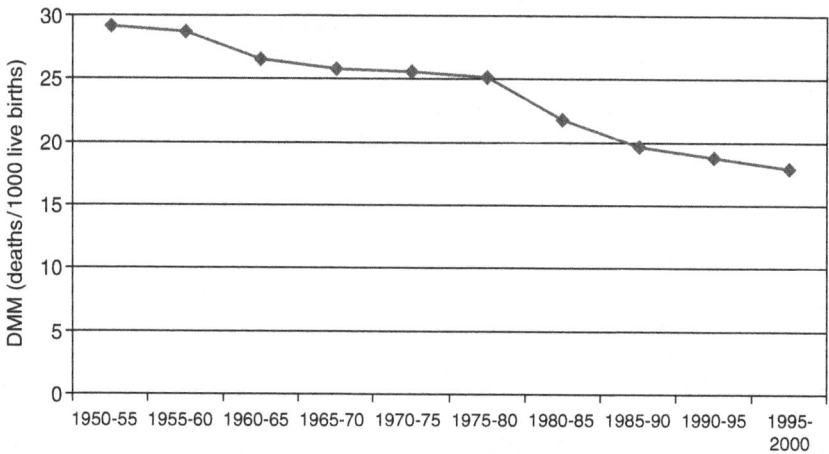

Fig. 5. Trend in the Dispersion Measure of Mortality (DMM) for infant mortality: 1950–2000

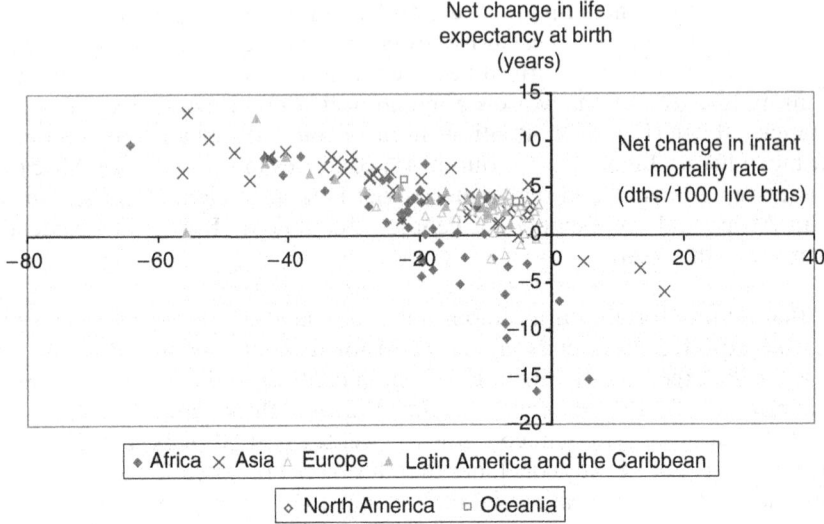

Fig. 6. Net change in life expectancy at birth and infant mortality rate: 1980–1985 to 1995–2000
Note. **Each point represents a single country**

Korea) experienced deteriorations in both infant mortality and life expectancy at birth. The causes behind these exceptional trends are likely to be diverse, although they will include the health effects of political and economic isolation, as in the cases of Iraq and the Democratic People's Republic of Korea.

When the mortality reversals between 1980–85 and 1995–2000 were assumed to be only half the size indicated by the data, the DMM trend for life expectancy at birth still showed a slight divergence in mortality in the 1990s preceded by a slight convergence between the late 1980s and early 1990s (Fig. 7A). When mortality was assumed to have stagnated but not reversed in these same 24 countries, the recalculated trends indicated continued convergence (Fig. 7B). Replacing national data with subnational data for India and China for the two time periods tested increased the DMM in 1950–55 from 6.5 to 6.8 years and decreased it in 1975–1980 from 6.0 to 5.9 years.

Discussion

This paper provides the first systematic quantification of global mortality convergence. It shows that the former trend of worldwide convergence towards low mortality has reversed. For life expectancy at birth, the switch in the late 1980s from convergence to divergence tells us that humanity has entered a phase during which progress in reducing mortality differences between many populations is now more than offset by the scale of the mortality reversals seen in others, notably in parts of sub-Saharan Africa and the former Soviet Union. Since the late 1980s the world has not only failed to become a more equal place in terms of mortality, but it has

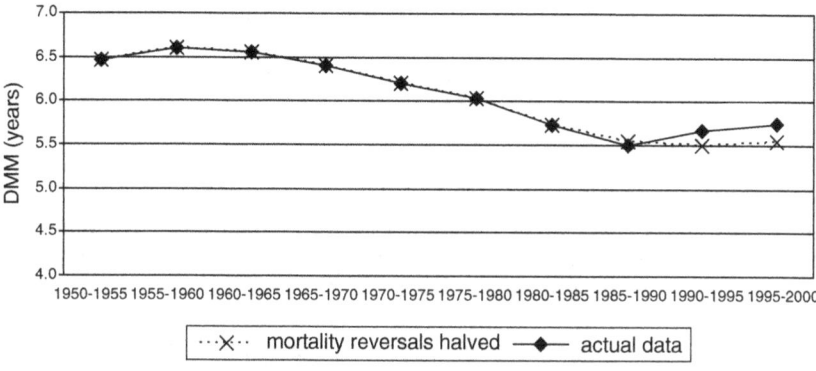

A. Scenario 1: mortality reversals halved

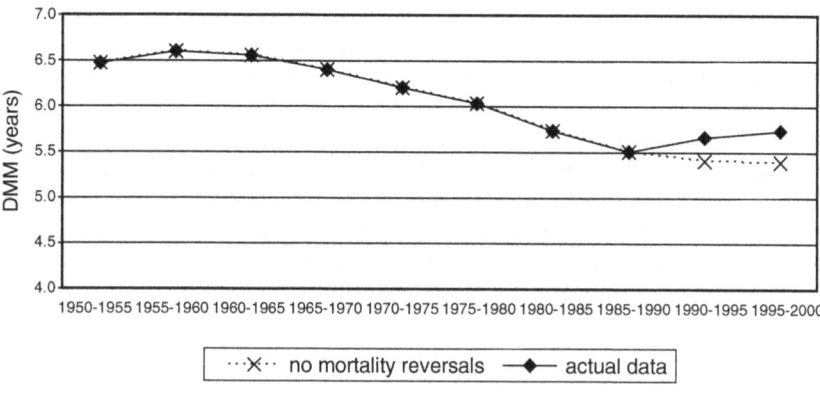

B. Scenario 2: no mortality reversals

Fig. 7. Hypothetical scenarios of trends in the Dispersion Measure of Mortality (DMM) for life expectancy at birth: 1950–2000

actually become less equal. This has occurred despite continued general improvements in mortality as reflected in the trends in global life expectancy at birth and infant mortality.

The fact that we observed recent global divergence in life expectancy at birth while infant mortality continues to converge indicates that it is mortality reversals occurring among those aged older than 1 year that are driving the divergence. The fact that in the 1990s we also saw convergence in mortality among children less than 5 years old indicates that the divergence during this decade is not the result of child mortality. We conclude, therefore, that the shift from global convergence to divergence is being driven by reversals in adult mortality. With respect to the former Soviet Union, including the Russian Federation, there is strong evidence that the reversals in life expectancy at birth are almost exclusively due to increases in adult mortality (7).

The DMM provides a novel approach to objectively measuring global mortality convergence; it goes beyond an enumeration of the countries showing improvements or reversals in mortality. The DMM quantifies the global dispersion of mortality at a point in time, and trends in the DMM indicate whether mortality of the world's population is, on aggregate, becoming more similar or less similar. In using information for all countries with a population of at least 1 million and weighting for the population size of each country (or live births in the case of infant mortality) the DMM has advantages over other commonly used summary measures of mortality contrast that only use information from the extremes of the mortality or socioeconomic distribution and do not weight for size of the unit. Being based on absolute differences in mortality, the DMM avoids a problem frequently encountered when using relative measures to examine time trends in inequality. Relative measures are strongly affected by the value of the reference mortality rate and consequently, in periods of falling mortality, tend to increase over time as the denominator decreases. The DMM provides different and complementary information to that given by the overall mortality level. Progress in one does not necessarily imply progress in the other. Global mortality rates may improve while the mortality distribution worldwide simultaneously diverges (in other words becomes less equitable).

Wilson, in his assessment of mortality convergence, failed to identify this transition from convergence to divergence in the late 1980s (11). This was primarily due to the fact that he contrasted three non-adjacent time periods (1950–55, 1975–1980, 2000) and hence failed to capture the period of reversal that occurred between the last two periods. In addition, he did not use a summary statistic and relied instead upon visual inspection of graphical data and on interquartile ranges that use only part of the available information.

Data source and quality

Before discussing these findings further it is important to mention the issue of data quality, although quality is an issue for any measures that use global mortality data to look at trends over time. The United Nations data used for this analysis are the best that are available for long-term trends. However it is well known that the source and quality of demographic data varies from place to place and over time. Most of Europe, north America (the USA and Canada) and Oceania had good registration systems and regular censuses covering the whole of the period studied. In contrast, many low- and middle-income countries, with the exception of some in Latin America and south-east Asia, have no (or incomplete) registers of births and deaths. In particular, it is worth noting that data are poorest in sub-Saharan Africa. Questions are asked in surveys and censuses in such countries on child survival, birth histories, orphanhood, sibling histories, and recent deaths in the household. Responses to these questions are often the main source of demographic information for such countries, from which indirect methods are used to estimate mortality and fertility (6, 15–17).

The quality of mortality data in itself is unlikely to affect trends in the DMM, although it may affect the absolute level of the DMM. The sensitivity analyses we undertook indicate that our findings remain the same even if we use some worst-case scenarios for data quality. Global divergence in life expectancy at birth would still be apparent in the 1990s even if the mortality reversals were only half the size indicated by the data. Moreover, no global divergence would be apparent in recent years if the countries whose data indicated reversals actually only had stagnating mortality. In other words, we conclude that the global divergence we observe results from mortality reversals in some countries alongside continued improvements in others.

Implications for policy

We suggest that global convergence in mortality needs to be adopted by the international community as one of the criteria for judging progress towards a more equitable world. The DMM has the potential to do this simply and transparently. It is a tool that can be used to monitor moves to reinstate and accelerate the trend towards global mortality convergence.

A prerequisite for effectively analysing and monitoring trends and formulating policy is the availability of reliable and comprehensive data. The crucial importance of improving data and developing better statistical measures has been highlighted (2, 18), and with the development of the Health Metrics Network (19) there are hopes that the need to strengthen health information systems will be seriously addressed.

The Millennium Development Goals have been internationally accepted as a framework for setting development objectives (1). With respect to mortality per se their main focus is on reducing mortality among children less than 5 years old. However, as this paper has shown, mortality among children is not the main factor behind the global divergence in life expectancy at birth. Our analysis suggests that adult mortality should be given greater emphasis as a global public health priority than is the case in the Millennium Development Goals (20).

Conclusion

Although in one sense the world has become a better place as mortality declines, in another way it has become worse as the distribution of life expectancy at birth worldwide has started to diverge; this indicates that global inequality in mortality is increasing. So far this divergence is relatively small and has been of limited duration compared with the earlier convergence. What is not clear is whether the divergence will continue or become larger or whether it will be reversed. Moreover, there are worrying signs that unless action is taken we may for the first time see global divergence in childhood mortality (2, 21). It is essential that policy-makers address these serious developments. The direction of future trends depends upon action today. Future global progress should be judged not only in terms of whether overall life expectancy continues to improve but also according to whether mortality convergence can be re-established and accelerated. The Dispersion Measure of Mortality offers a simple summary measure that can be used to monitor progress in this direction.

Acknowledgements

We are very grateful to Chris Wilson for providing us with estimates of life expectancy at birth for the states of India and provinces of China (see reference 11 for a full description of these data). The authors thank Andy Haines, Martin McKee, Liam Smeeth, Ian Timaeus and Gill Walt for their comments on an earlier draft. Kath Moser is supported by the Dreyfus Health Foundation.

Appendix

Adjustment of Population Weights for Estimation of Inter-Country Inequalities in Life Expectancy at Birth

Below we provide a brief description of a method for adjustment of population weights for linking life expectancies in sub-populations with life expectancy of the overall population. A more detailed description of this method is published elsewhere (14).

If a closed birth cohort consists of several sub-groups then the dynamics of its size is fully determined by mortality schedules in the sub-groups and their proportions in the overall birth cohort at the beginning of the follow up. Life expectancy for the whole birth cohort is the sum of the group-specific life expectancies weighted by population-weights of the sub-groups. However, a period life table is based on a hypothetical ("synthetic") cohort. This makes a link between the longevity of the overall population and group-specific lengths of life more complicated.

Let us consider the whole world population consisting of N country-populations with population weights $W_i, \sum_{i=1}^{N} W_i = 1$ and country-specific mortality measures equal to life expectancies at birth $M_i = e_0^i$. For the age-specific forces of mortality the following simple relationship is true:

$$\mu_x = \sum_{i=1}^{N} \mu_x^i W_x^i \quad \text{where } W_x^i \text{ denotes population weight of group } i \text{ in age group } x.$$

The survival function l_x is defined as $\exp(-\int_0^x \mu_t dt)$. Consequently, the exact link between life expectancy at age x for the whole population and specific mortality schedules can be expressed as:

$$e_0 = \int_0^\infty l_t dt = \int_0^\infty \left[\exp\left(-\int_0^t \sum_{i=1}^{N} \mu_x^i W_x^i dx \right) \right] dt$$

It is very difficult to develop an exact relationship between the latter expression of the global life expectancy and country-specific life expectancies

$$e_0^i = \int_0^{\infty} \left[\exp\left(-\int_0^t \mu_x^i dx \right) \right] dt.$$

Instead, one might think of an approximate linear decomposition for the global life expectancy. This could be achieved by a division of the global life table cohort at age 0 into country-specific fractions θ_i. Their sum should be equal to one, and the sum of person-years lived by all fractions should be equal to the total number of person-years lived by the global cohort (i.e. global life expectancy).

$$\sum_{i=1}^{N} \theta_i = 1$$

$$e_0 = \sum_{i=1}^{N} \theta_i e_0^i,$$

(1)

If $N=2$ then there is only one solution satisfying condition (1). If $N>2$, there are multiple solutions. This means, some additional constraint is needed. A reasonable approach would be to choose the weights θ_i characterized by a minimum Euclidian distance from population country-weights W_i

$$\sum_{i=1}^{N} (\theta_i - W_i)^2 \rightarrow \min.$$

(2)

It can be shown (14) that the problem of minimization with constraints can be solved by a system of linear equations:

$$\mathbf{A} \cdot \mathbf{z} = \mathbf{b}$$

(3)

In this expression matrix $\mathbf{A}$ has the dimension $(N+2) \bullet (N+2)$ and vector $\mathbf{b}$ has the dimension $(N+2)$:

$$\mathbf{A} = \begin{bmatrix} 2 & 0 & 0 & .. & .. & .. & 0 & 1 & e_0^1 \\ 0 & 2 & 0 & .. & .. & .. & 0 & 1 & e_0^2 \\ 0 & 0 & 2 & .. & .. & .. & 0 & 1 & e_0^3 \\ .. & .. & .. & .. & .. & .. & .. & & .. \\ .. & .. & .. & .. & .. & 2 & 0 & .. & .. \\ 0 & 0 & 0 & .. & .. & 0 & 2 & 1 & e_0^N \\ 1 & 1 & 1 & .. & .. & .. & 1 & 0 & 0 \\ e_0^1 & e_0^2 & e_0^3 & .. & .. & .. & e_0^N & 0 & 0 \end{bmatrix}, \quad \mathbf{b} = \begin{bmatrix} 2W_1 \\ 2W_2 \\ 2W_3 \\ .. \\ .. \\ 2W_N \\ 1 \\ e_0 \end{bmatrix},$$

(4)

Vector $\mathbf{z}$ of solutions of system (2) has dimension $(N+2)$ and its first N rows are the optimum weights θ_i. This vector can be calculated from:

$$\mathbf{z} = \mathbf{A}^{-1} \cdot \mathbf{b}$$

(5)

24 K. MOSER ET AL.

The adjusted population weights θ_i make it possible to present the global life expectancy as a weighted average of the country-specific life expectancies.

In the present study the absolute deviation (1) was used. In some cases, however, it is reasonable to use instead the relative deviation: $\sum_{i=1}^{N}\left[\left(\theta_i - W_i\right)/W_i\right]^2$ Correspondingly, the formula for matrix **A** is somewhat different:

$$\mathbf{A} = \begin{bmatrix} 2(W_1)^{-2} & 0 & 0 & \cdots & & & 0 & 1 & e_0^1 \\ 0 & 2(W_2)^{-2} & 0 & \cdots & & & 0 & 1 & e_0^2 \\ 0 & 0 & 2(W_3)^{-2} & \cdots & & & 0 & 1 & e_0^3 \\ \cdots & \cdots & \cdots & \cdots & \cdots & & \cdots & \cdots & \cdots \\ \cdots & \cdots & & \cdots & 2(W_{N-1})^{-2} & 0 & & \cdots & \cdots \\ 0 & 0 & 0 & \cdots & 0 & 2(W_N)^{-2} & 1 & e_0^N \\ 1 & 1 & 1 & \cdots & & 1 & 0 & 0 \\ e_0^1 & e_0^2 & e_0^3 & \cdots & & e_0^N & 0 & 0 \end{bmatrix}.$$

References

1. United Nations Millennium Project (2000). *Millennium development goals*, from http://www.unmillenniumproject.org/html/dev_goals.shtm

2. United Nations Development Programme (2003). *Human development report 2003.* (New York: Oxford University Press)

3. Lee, J. W. (2003). Global health improvement and WHO: Shaping the future. *The Lancet, 362,* 2083–2088

4. World Health Organization (2003). *The World Health Report 2003 – Shaping the future.* (Geneva: WHO)

5. Korzeniewicz, R. P. & Moran, T. P. (1997). World economic trends in the distribution of income, 1965–1992. *American Journal of Sociology, 102,* 1000–1039

6. Timaeus, I. (1998). Impact of the HIV epidemic on mortality in sub-Saharan Africa: Evidence from national surveys and censuses. *AIDS, 12* (Suppl 1), S15–S27

7. Shkolnikov, V., McKee, M. & Leon, D. (2001). Changes in life expectancy in Russia in the mid-1990s. *The Lancet, 357,* 917–921

8. Preston, S. H. (1976). *Mortality patterns in national populations.* (New York: Academic Press)

9. Omran, A. R. (1971). The epidemiological transition: A theory of the epidemiology of population change. *Milbank Memorial Fund Quarterly, 49,* 509–538

10. McMichael, A. J., McKee, M., Shkolnikov, V. & Valkonen, T. (2004). Mortality trends and setbacks: Global convergence or divergence? *The Lancet, 363,* 1155–1159

11. Wilson, C. (2001). On the scale of global demographic convergence 1950–2000. *Population and Development Review, 27,* 155–171

12. United Nations (2001). *World population prospects: The 2000 revision.* (New York: United Nations)

13. Kendall, M. & Stuart, A. (1977). *The advanced theory of statistics.* 4th edn., Vol. 1. (London: Charles Griffin)

14. Shkolnikov, V., Valkonen, T., Begun, A. & Andreev, E. (2001). Measuring inter-group inequalities in length of life. *Genus, LVII*(3–4), 33–62

15. Brass, W. (1996). Demographic data analysis in less developed countries: 1946–1996. *Population Studies, 50,* 451–467

16. Timaeus, I. (1999). Mortality in sub-Saharan Africa. (In J. Chamie & R. Cliquet (Eds.), *Health and mortality: Issues of global concern* pp. 108–131). New York: Population Division, United Nations and Population and Family Study Centre, Flemish Scientific Institute)

17. United Nations (2002). *World Population Prospects: The 2000 revision. Volume III: Analytical report.* (New York: United Nations)

18. Lee, J. W. (2003). *Speech to the fifty-sixth World Health Assembly, 2003.* Retrieved from http://www.who.int/dg/lee/speeches/2003/21_05/en/

19. Evans, T. & Stansfield, S. (2003). Health information in the new millennium: A gathering storm? *Bulletin of the World Health Organization, 81,* 856

20. Lock, L., Andreev, E., Shkolnikov, V. & McKee, M. (2002). What targets for international development policies are appropriate for improving health in Russia? *Health Policy and Planning, 17,* 257–263

21. Victora, C. G., Wagstaff, A., Schellenberg, J. A., Gwatkin, D., Claeson, M. & Habicht, J. P. (2003). Applying an equity lens to child health and mortality: More of the same is not enough. *The Lancet, 362,* 233–241

CHAPTER 2. THE IMPACT OF POPULATION GROWTH ON THE EPIDEMIOLOGY AND EVOLUTION OF INFECTIOUS DISEASES

GEOFFREY P. GARNETT
*Current address: London School Hygien and Tropical medicine
Department of Infectious Disease Epidemiology,
Imperial College London, London, UK*

JAMES J.C. LEWIS
*Department of Epidemiology and Population Health, London School
of Hygiene and Tropical Medicine, London, UK*

Abstract. It is generally expected that in developing countries the epidemiological transition, with improved health and lower mortality rates, will eventually lead to a demographic transition with lower fertility rates. The reductions in mortality characterising the epidemiological transition are often associated with controlling the infectious diseases within populations, which leaves the chronic diseases associated with old age, cancer and heart disease dominating the causes of death. However, if the demographic transition does not occur quickly, populations can grow rapidly, creating an increased potential for spread of infectious disease. These infectious diseases could, in turn, increase death rates amongst young people and reverse the epidemiological transition. The relationship between population growth, size and infection depends upon the changes in contact pattern associated with there being more people. If facilities can keep pace with growth, then the increase in contact rates can be kept to a minimum, and the potential reversal in the epidemic transition prevented. This makes development a crucial adjunct to population growth if the global community is not to be increasingly exposed to pandemics of infectious disease. Here we review the epidemiological and demographic theory which relates population growth and infectious disease.

Introduction

The biology of obligate infectious organisms is inextricably linked with the biology and behaviour of their host populations. Organisms that invade another species to gain the building blocks or energy for their survival and reproduction rely on transmission from host to host if they are to succeed. This transmission is a function of the natural history of the infection and the contact patterns of the host [1]. Clearly, the demography of the host population has an enormous role to play in determining both the supply of hosts and the contact patterns between them. Since the opportunities for parasitic organisms

27

M. Caraël and J.R. Glynn (eds.), HIV, Resurgent Infections and Population Change in Africa, 27–40.

are a function of host demography, changes in host population size, density and structure alter the environment within which pathogens are selected and play a role in their evolution. Concomitantly infectious diseases contribute to the demography of host populations influencing patterns of mortality and fertility. In this review we will describe the different ways in which demographic changes influence the epidemiology of infectious diseases and explore the patterns of population growth and movement that are likely to play an important role in the emergence and re-emergence of infectious diseases.

Parasites, in the current context, include all organisms that live within another organism, and do that organism harm, and include representatives of the prions, viruses, bacteria, fungi, protozoa, helminths and insects. These pathogenic organisms range widely in the frequency and severity of the disease symptoms they cause and the transmission routes through which they spread. The routes of transmission determine how the infections will be influenced by demography, as do the strategies used by the organisms to exploit their niche. Popular writings often depict the infection enjoying an easy life of rich pickings from an unwitting host [2]. In truth, the immune responses of the host and the hurdles to transmission, impose severe selective pressures on the parasites. Thus, there are always strategies employed by the parasite to avoid the immune system, either through racing the production of immune effectors or avoiding them through cryptic or changing surfaces. This tends to generate two types of life histories: either short-lived rapid-reproduction parasites such as the simple viruses and bacteria (e.g. measles, mumps, rubella, influenza and gonorrhoea), or long-lived slow-reproducing infections (e.g. herpes simplex, tuberculosis, syphilis and HIV). Since the resolution of infection within the host destroys that population of infectious organisms, infectious diseases are in part subject to group selection. However, it should be remembered that the individual organism is also competing intra-specifically within the host and that future generations of infection will represent the genotypes of organisms that manage to transmit. In any consideration of evolutionary strategies it is important to remember that evolution is blind. The flu virus does not consider the future problem of widespread immunity following an influenza pandemic and *Neisseria meningitides* does not consider its future success when it invades the host in a selective dead end, with catastrophic consequences for the host and itself. What we observe in nature are either transient epidemics of infectious disease, which spread with short term success, but which will die out, or infectious diseases that have found a strategy to allow them to persist.

In developing our understanding of the interaction between demography and infectious disease epidemiology, it is worth considering the type and quality of evidence available to us, and how we progress from anecdote to general rules and from speculation to theory. A detailed knowledge of the natural history and transmissibility of infections from observational studies, allows us to speculate about how changes in host population structure may have influenced their epidemiology. Historical and archaeological records of population size and organisation, along with evidence of patterns of disease and death, provide examples of coincident changes, including the invasion of new pathogens as civilizations were formed, through to the reductions in disease associated with improved hygiene and living conditions [3]. Other ecological comparisons between populations are instructive, allowing us to compare the success of different types of organism in different locations [4]. Theory has a role to play, since if we can predict patterns of disease based on our hypotheses, we can then test the hypotheses by comparison with experimental and observational data [5]. In understanding the contribution of infections to demography, records of mortality and its causes are vital. However, in the frequent absence of detailed records we have to rely on theoretical estimates based on what we know of the distribution and consequences of particular infections. This is particularly true of the influence of infectious diseases on fertility where limited numbers of detailed studies have to be related to the global distribution of infections. In studying both the impact of demography on infections and vice versa, general principles are derived from particular examples. However, the examples are never typical since it is specific pathogens such as bubonic plague, tuberculosis, malaria, influenza and HIV that dominate the relationship between infections and demography. Thus, throughout our discussion we have to relate to the particular characteristics of the key pathogens.

Three variables influence the potential for spread of an infection: the duration of infectiousness (D); the contact rate (c); and the likelihood of transmission if there is a contact (p): the duration of infectiousness determines how long an infection stays prevalent to expose others; the contact rate and transmission probability are variables in the transmission from infectious to susceptible individuals [1]. The product of these three variables is termed the basic reproductive number R_0, such that $R_0 = Dcp$ and represents the number of infections caused by one infectious individual in an entirely susceptible population. Thus, the basic reproductive number has to be above one for there to be a risk of an infection spreading. The influence of population size on the contact rate is central to the impact of population growth on infectious disease epidemiology. The incidence of infection is the product of the number of susceptibles (X) and the "force of infection" (λ); the per susceptible risk of acquiring infection, which is a function of the number of infectious individuals (Y) within the population, such that $\lambda = pc\ Y/N$, where N represents the population size.

The Impact of Population Size and Density on Contact Patterns

Whether the growth of a population influences the potential spread of an infectious disease depends upon how the number of individuals influences the patterns of contact and exposure. If population growth leads to greater crowding, more contaminated water supplies, or higher numbers of sexual contacts per person, then the contact rates allowing the transmission of many diseases will increase, making epidemics more likely. Alternatively, if expanding populations have additional geographic space, additional services and no change in sexual norms then the number of contacts can remain constant and no change in risk of epidemics occur. The two types of increase are illustrated in **Fig. 1**. Two extreme patterns have been identified [6]: first "density dependent transmission" in which the number of contacts increases as population size and hence density increase; in its extreme form there is a linear relationship ($c = c_D N$) and the transmission term takes the form

$$X\lambda \equiv Xpc\,Y\!\!\Big/_{\!N} \equiv Xpc_D N\,Y\!\!\Big/_{\!N} \equiv Xpc_D Y.$$

In this case $R_0 = Dc_D Np$, and hence there is a threshold population size, below which the basic reproductive number is less than one, above which it is more than one. With the transmission term above, the threshold population size for the inva-

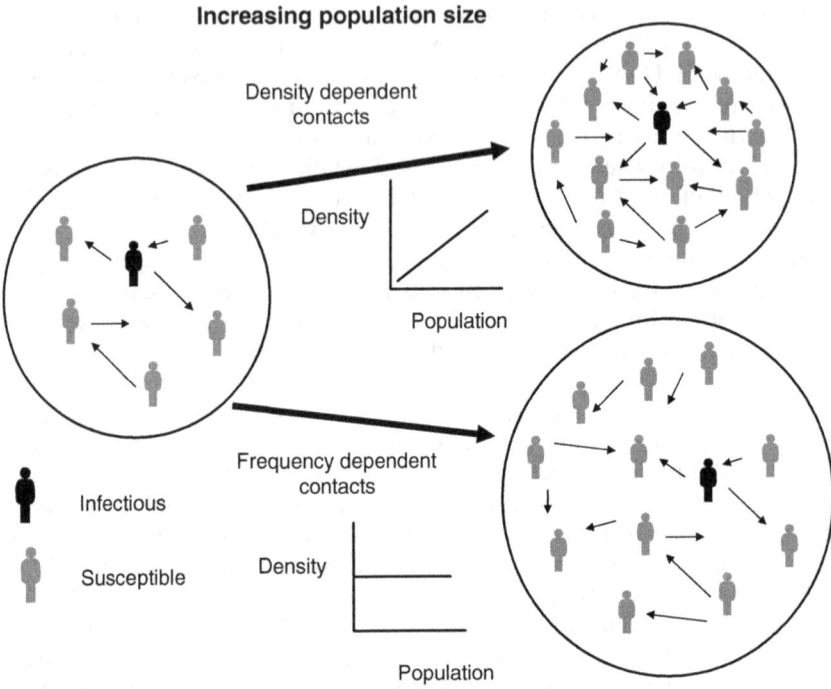

Fig. 1. Illustration of the two patterns of population growth: the first, in which density and contacts for infection increase; the second, where density remains constant and contacts remain constant

sion of an infection is given by the equation: $N_T = 1/(Dc_D p)$. Thus, the greater the transmission probability and duration of infection the smaller the population size in which an infection can invade. If population size does increase the contact rate, then growing populations will allow epidemics of organisms that have lower transmission probabilities and durations if they cross species barriers or evolve from other pathogenic or commensal organisms. The alternative type of transmission pattern is "frequency dependent transmission" where the rate of contact is independent of population size ($c = c_F$) and the transmission term takes the form $X\lambda = Xpc_F Y/N$. In this case there is no threshold population size for the invasion of the population since the basic reproductive number is independent of population size $R_0 = Dc_F p$. There has been much debate about which form is "correct", together with evidence from the field and from animal experiments [7, 8]. In reality it is likely that the relationship between population size and contacts will depend upon the local circumstances and the particular routes of transmission. So for example if safe water supplies are guaranteed as a population grows there will be no increased risk of water borne infections; if mosquito breeding sites are not allowed to proliferate than there should be no increase in mosquito vectored pathogens; if people maintain steady numbers of sexual relationships then sexually transmitted infections (STIs) will not increase; if hand washing and food hygiene is maintained then nosocomial infections and directly transmitted faecal orally transmitted infections should not increase; if rates of injecting drug use behaviour do not increase, sterile medical supplies are maintained and blood supplies are screened, then blood born pathogens should not increase; and, hardest to envisage, if crowding and density of population stay the same, then increased population size should not increase the rate of spread of infections borne in aerosols. However, growing populations place strains on the resources available; where these resources cannot keep pace, rates of contact and risks of epidemics will increase. If, with growing populations, individuals want to take the opportunity to mix in larger social groups or have more sexual partners then the infections which depend upon these forms of contact will thrive. It is likely therefore that growing populations do lead to a greater risk of infectious disease spread, but there are opportunities to combat this trend.

The Supply of Susceptibles Through Birth and Immigration

Analyses of the persistence of measles in cities and islands indicated that there was a threshold population size required for the persistence of the virus (i.e., the consistent presence of infection in the community) [9]. This was initially taken as evidence for a threshold population size for *invasion* and hence a density dependent transmission term. It also supported the belief that larger populations associated with the introduction of agriculture in early human history allowed for the invasion of directly transmitted simple viral infections such as measles and smallpox [10]. However, the ability of an infection to invade a population is not synonymous with the ability of an infection to persist [11]. Either through mortality decreasing population sizes or through inducing acquired immunity, infections are likely to reduce the numbers of susceptibles available to maintain chains of infection. New susceptibles are required to maintain an endemic infection and these susceptibles can be provided by loss of immunity, immigration or births. Thus, large populations and growing populations accrue susceptibles rapidly making it more likely that an infection will be able to persist [12]. A very rapid supply of susceptibles, as is the case for bacterial infections where recovery is back into a susceptible state or in the case of large growing populations, allows a continual high level of incidence. A slow supply of susceptibles is likely to lead to reductions in infection numbers or even stochastic fade out and elimination of the infection. Low numbers of infections will allow a build up of susceptible numbers in the population and new epidemics occur, leading to oscillation between epidemic and interepidemic periods. In a deterministic system we would expect to see damping of the oscillations over time, but epidemics continue because of seasonal variations in contact rates, as occurs with school attendance, and due to stochasticity [1]. The faster the rate of resupply of susceptibles as a function of population size and population growth, the more frequent epidemics will be and the more stable with a regular endemic level of infection the system will be [12].

The need to maintain susceptibles applies in the case of both density dependent and frequency dependent transmission. In the former it is both the number and proportion of the population susceptible that matters. The effective reproductive R_t number is the number of new infections caused by a single infection at any given time and equals 1 at the endemic steady state. The effective reproductive number in a homogeneous population is simply the basic reproductive number times the proportion of the population susceptible.

$$R_t = R_0 \frac{X}{N} = R_0 x.$$

Thus, at the endemic steady state the proportion of the population susceptible x is simply the inverse of the basic reproductive number. As the number of susceptibles increases, an epidemic becomes possible once the proportion susceptible exceeds this inverse of the basic reproductive number. If an infection causes mortality and drives down a population size, but does not induce acquired immunity, the recruitment of numbers to the population is what matters. In the case of frequency dependent transmission a fatal infection that can spread has the potential to drive a population extinct if death rates exceed birth rates, unless something else reduces the spread of infection, such as behaviour change.

The predicted changes of disease incidence have been observed in a detailed analysis of the spatial and temporal patterns of measles incidence within the UK [13]. Here, before the introduction of vaccination, epidemics of measles originated in the large cities of London and Manchester from which they spread as travelling waves. During the "baby boom" years of the 1960s in the UK there was an increased rate of supply of susceptibles, and an even more regular pattern of epidemics every two years was seen. Vaccination when it is introduced greatly increases the time taken for sufficient numbers of susceptibles to accrue and thereby increases the interepidemic period [13]. Within this analysis, Liverpool, prior to vaccination, is particularly interesting since it had higher than average birth rates associated with a large immigrant, Catholic population and consequently had yearly epidemics of measles [12], as had New York [14].

Thus, large and growing populations are more likely to maintain an infection and suffer repeated epidemics prior to vaccination. The mean age of infection also depends upon the frequency of epidemics and the birth rate. A higher rate of births should lead to a higher reproductive number and thereby a lower age of infection. This has been observed in Guinea-Bissau where infection with measles amongst urban children occurred at a lower age than in their rural counterparts [15]. Additionally, the high incidence of meningitis in West Africa reflects the high reproductive number of the bacterial infection in these communities [16]. In growing populations such as these the period between loss of maternally derived antibodies and infection is limited, leaving a limited period for vaccination as children age [17]. This led to efforts to develop a measles vaccine able to immunize children in the presence of maternally derived antibodies (which unfortunately had to be withdrawn following observations of increased non-specific death rates associated with vaccination) [18]. As vaccination becomes widespread, the mean age of infection increases, because susceptible individuals take longer to come into contact with infection, which should allow a greater window of opportunity to vaccinate. However, if there is poor vaccination coverage or efficacy, the growing population makes outbreaks more likely, since the speed of growth in susceptible numbers is greater and the critical number or proportion of the population susceptible is likely to be realised sooner.

The increase in the mean age of infection that follows vaccination programmes can be problematic since for many infections severity increases with age. Examples include polio infections, where paralysis rates were associated with an increased age of infection with improved hygiene [19]; chickenpox, where encephalitis and pneumonia are associated with infection in teenagers and young adults [20]; mumps, where orchitis is associated with post pubertal infection in males [21]; and rubella, where there is a risk of congenital rubella syndrome when pregnant women acquire infection. Indeed, in Greece—with vaccine coverage rates of less than 50%—there was an increase in the absolute rates of congenital rubella syndrome compared to the period before the vaccination programme was implemented [22].

The Impact of Epidemic and Endemic Disease on Mortality

There is no doubt that infectious diseases are a major cause of mortality in populations, which because of the young age of many of those infected and dying, can contribute to the loss of many life years. In healthy well nourished hosts the fatality rate (the proportion of infections leading to death rather than recovery) associated with the majority of infections is low. When health care provision and nourishment is adequate then mortality associated with infectious diseases is concentrated in those with underlying vulnerability, such as the elderly and immunocompromised, where rates of death from competing causes are high and the demographic impact of the infection is slight [23]. In resource-poor settings deaths from respiratory and diarrhoeal diseases are common in infants and young children. Here it is estimated that measles, malaria, tuberculosis, and pneumococcal infections cause 5 million deaths each year, which is nearly a tenth of global deaths [23]. It is relatively rare for infections to be associated with death in young adults; and it is perhaps particularly their fatality rate in young adults that makes the bubonic plague, syphilis, Spanish flu and AIDS notable historic events [3].

The demographic impact of an infectious disease depends upon the incidence of infection, the fatality rate, the age at which deaths occur and how long lasting the pandemics are. The importance of this last point was neatly captured by Thomas Short, following an analysis of bills of mortality, when he comments that "endemics may reign centuries but not epidemics" [24]. Over the long term a relatively small but continuous increase in mortality rates has a greater effect than acute large scale mortality. This is illustrated in **Fig. 2** where three acute mortality events in an exponentially growing population are compared with increases in the mortality rate over time. The time taken to recover from a given die off will depend upon the subsequent per capita population growth rate and is given by the equation

$$T = \ln (1 - \delta)/-r,$$

where δ is the fraction of the population dying and r is the per capita growth rate. Estimates of the initial mortality associated with the Black Death in Europe in 1347 and 1348 have altered from a high of 85% to a low of 5%, but are now believed to have been around 50% on the basis of records from institutions such as monasteries. However, it was the repeated epidemics, which followed the first and kept returning into the fifteenth century that reduced the populations [25].

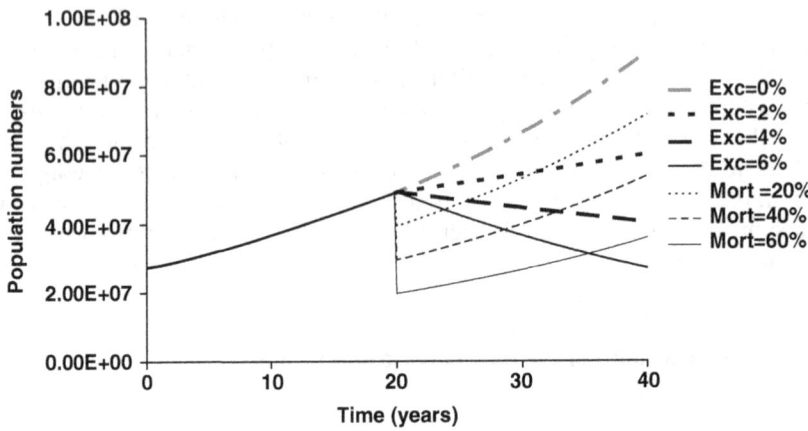

Fig. 2. The impact of infection associated mortality on a population growing at 3% per year. An acute mortality event killing off 20, 40 and 60% of the population (mort) is compared with a continuous 2, 4 and 6% increase in the mortality rate (Exc)

The demographic impact of AIDS is a source of debate. The virus is associated with an almost unprecedented high fatality rate, with seemingly all those infected dying eventually; and the infection is predominantly amongst young adults. This has to be balanced against the length of time it takes for HIV infection to progress to AIDS and death, and the low prevalence of the virus found in many populations. In the absence of treatment HIV takes an average of 10 years to cause death [26], this means that at an endemic state each 10% increase in HIV will increase the death rate by 1%. In addition vertical transmission of HIV to around 30% of children born to infected mothers [27] would lead to rapid childhood death in 3% of births with prevalence at 10% in women attending antenatal clinics. Thus, the prevalences of 30% seen in some locations in sub-Saharan Africa [28] might be expected to reduce a 3% population growth rate to zero. However, such prevalences are only generally observed in urban and semi-urban locations where fertility and birth rates are relatively high and growth rates in the absence of HIV would have exceeded 3% [29]. Thus, predicted negative population growths have not been observed in detailed studies. Furthermore, the observed prevalences are probably at the peak epidemic prevalence. As mortality due to AIDS increases then those initially most at risk of acquiring and transmitting infection are no longer present, and populations tend to reduce their risk behaviours [30, 31]. To maintain over time a given increase in death rates the prevalence of HIV would also have to be maintained. Thus, in a stable population a continued incidence of 3% across the population would be required to maintain a 3% increase in death rates. The AIDS epidemic is likely to reduce life expectancy and growth rates in many developing countries. However, if the death and disease associated with the virus undermines development and health it may delay or prevent the demographic transition and in the long run lead to larger rather than smaller populations.

The Impact of Infectious Diseases on Fertility

A number of infections have the potential to influence fertility as well as mortality. Gonorrhoea and chlamydia can cause pelvic inflammatory disease and lead to scarring of the fallopian tubes, causing sterility. Syphilis and HIV seem to reduce observed fertility in part due to early spontaneous abortions [32, 26]. The use of antenatal screening for syphilis and HIV allow for treatments to reduce neonatal syphilis and vertical transmission of HIV, but these are too late to prevent early foetal loss. The biological proximate determinants of fertility reduce population growth, as observed in Uganda and other African countries [33]. If they are removed, they are likely to be replaced by other proximate determinants limiting fertility, such as increased contraception and abortion [34]). As sexually transmitted infections (STI) are generally transmitted in a frequency dependent fashion (i.e., risk depends upon the distribution of numbers of sexual partners of individuals which are unlikely to be greatly influenced by overall population size [35]), then population growth should have little impact on the spread of these sexually transmitted diseases which reduce fertility. However, there is some evidence of increased risk behaviour in urban populations and among migrant labourers [36]. This, along with the lack of access to timely and appropriate health care and the exchange of sex for material goods and money, would increase rates of sexual partner change and the incidence of STI. Thus if population growth is associated with worsening socio-economic conditions then it could increase infertility along with death rates.

The impact of STIs on fertility depends upon the incidence of infection, the rate of complications and infertility and the age of infection amongst women in relation to their childbearing years. A recent survey of data from sub-Saharan Africa suggested a population attributable decline in total fertility of 0.37% (95% CI: 0.30%, 0.44%) with each percentage point of HIV prevalence [37, 38]. The high incidence of chlamydia in young women, which can lead to permanent primary or secondary sterility, means that it potentially has a major impact on birth rates. However, the actual rates of tubal occlusion are difficult to estimate since natural history studies are clearly unethical, and sterility can be difficult to detect especially if it follows earlier child birth. Assuming that 60% of chlamydial infections lead to salpingitis and that 20% of these develop bilateral tubal occlusion, then 12% of infections would lead to infertility. Then, as seems reasonable, assuming a six month duration of infection the incidence of infection would be twice its prevalence. Thus if women have a 5% prevalence of infection they should have a 10% incidence and a risk of sterility of 1.2% per year. The expected cumulative incidence of infertility as a function of years in the reproductive age classes associated with different incidences of an STI such as chlamydia or gonorrhoea is illustrated in **Fig. 3**. Assuming a constant net birth rate per woman over the 35 reproductive years the reduction in the total fertility rate associated with a particular prevalence of the bacterial STI can be calculated (**Fig. 4**). This relationship clearly depends upon the estimated rates of sterility associated with incident STI infection and the relationship between age specific rates of acquiring infection and births. Since high risk sexual behaviour and risk of STI infection is associated with sexual debut and pre-marital sex [39] our calculations, based on a constant age specific fertility, are likely to be conservative.

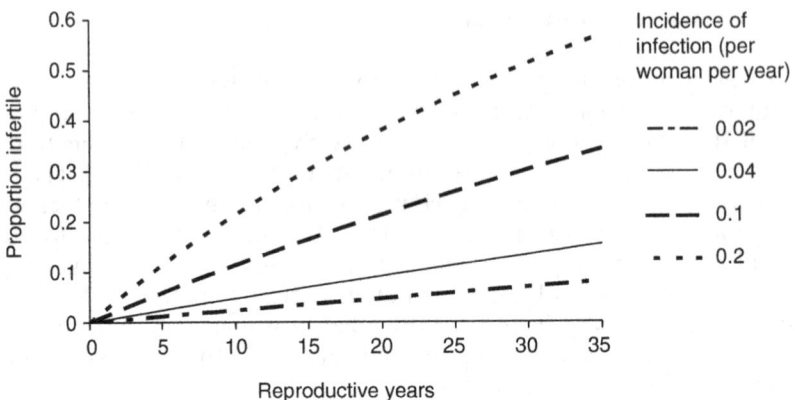

Fig. 3. The relationship between incidence per woman per year and the cumulative rate of infertility assuming that new infections are independent of past infection and a 12% risk of infertility for each infection

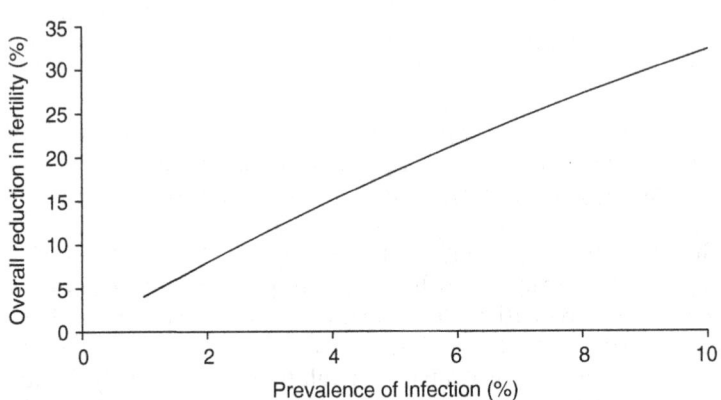

Fig. 4. The reduction in total fertility rate associated with different prevalences of a bacterial STI which causes sterility in 12% of infections and does not induce immunity. The results assume a constant age specific net fertility rate in the absence of sterility and a constant age specific incidence of infection

The Future: The Epidemiologic and Demographic Transition and the Re-Emergence of Infections

Population growth has three major consequences for infectious disease: (1) the sheer scale of cities provides more opportunities for a disease to persist with a rapid supply of susceptibles. (2) The conditions associated with a growing population and poverty generates increasing contact rates creating the conditions for epidemics. (3) The increases in travel and migration increase global contacts and turn epidemics into pandemics. Surveillance and health systems which are driven by the efficient management of current morbidity are ill equipped to deal with novel overwhelming spread of infections. Recent examples of emerging threats include severe acute respiratory syndrome (SARS) in East Asia [40], Ebola in Central Africa [41], avian flu in East Asia [42], and before that, Pulmonary Hantavirus Syndrome (PHS), which was associated with a 60% fatality rate leading to 51 deaths on its initial emergence [43]. Either these have failed to spread from person to person—or, if, like SARS, they have started inter-human transmission–they have had a low reproductive number and have been identifiable and preventable. (For SARS symptoms appear before infectiousness develops allowing for effective quarantine.) As we can learn from the great pandemics of history, the Black Death in Europe in 1347 and 1348 [3], syphilis in 1495 [44] and influenza in 1917–18 [45], such outbreaks can become devastating pandemics.

The impression is that the number of such events has been increasing, but improvements in modern communication and news network may have made apparent events of limited temporal and geographic scope, which would in the past have gone unnoticed. Such outbreaks are likely to be associated with increasing penetration of and contact with the environment [46], which has been on going for some time. However, the growth of populations may well have increased their frequency.

The possibilities of new pathogens jumping from animal to human increases as the absolute number of contacts with animals increases as human numbers increase and the evolution of novel infection types from non-pathogenic organisms also increases as the population size of the non-pathogenic organisms associated with humans expands. Once they do emerge their wide spread becomes increasingly likely. Large urban centres have grown rapidly in Asia and South America, and such expansion is expected to continue over the next few decades, with megacities, where the population is over 10 million appearing in India, China, Brazil and Indonesia (**Table 1**) [47]. These large populations provide places within which infections are likely to thrive. There is also the greatly increased connectivity of the world's population, with increasingly frequent and increasingly rapid travel. With air travel the majority of the world's population live within 36 hours journey time of each other [48].

Table 1. The number of cities with populations greater than 10 million [47].

	1950	1975	2000
Africa	0	0	0
Asia	0	1	8
Latin America	0	2	4
Europe	0	0	0
Japan	0	1	2
North America	1	1	2

Population growth along with the young, poorly resourced communities it creates is a major concern for both the local health and wellbeing of the populations, but also for global health. To tackle the symptoms, improved surveillance, quarantine and containment facilities in health care, along with the capacity for rapid aetiological research and the development of diagnostics and treatments are required to combat infectious disease. However, to tackle the cause, population growth needs to be accompanied by the provision of housing and services to reduce contact patterns, and by good vaccination coverage and health care; and the demographic transition needs to slow the growth of populations.

References

1. Anderson, R. M. & May, R. M. (1991). *Infectious diseases of humans: Dynamics and control.* (Oxford: Oxford University Press)

2. Nikiforuk, A. (1993). *The fourth horseman: A short history of epidemics, plagues and other scourges.* (London: Phoenix)

3. McNeill, W. H. (1976). *Plagues and peoples.* (New York: Penguin Books)

4. Ewald, P. W. (2002). *Plague time: The new germ theory of disease.* (New York: Anchor Books)

5. Little, T. J. & Ebert, D. (2001). Temporal patterns of genetic variation for resistance and infectivity in a Daphnia-microparasite system. *Evolution; International Journal of Organic Evolution, 55*(6), 1146–1152

6. McCallum, H., Barlow, N. & Hone, J. (2001). How should pathogen transmission be modelled? *Trends in Ecology and Evolution, 16*(6), 295–300

7. de Jong, M. C. M., Diekmann, O. & Heesterbeek, H. (1995). How does transmission of infection depend on population size? (In D. Mollison (Ed.), *Epidemic models: Their structure and relation to data* (pp. 84–94). Cambridge: Cambridge University Press)

8. Begon, M., Bennett, M., Bowers, R. G., French, N. P., Hazel, S. M. & Turner, J. (2002). A clarification of transmission terms in host-microparasite models: Numbers, densities and areas. *Epidemiology and Infection, 129*(1), 147–153

9. Black, F. L. (1996). Measles endemicity in insular populations: Critical community size and its evolutionary implication. *Journal of Theoretical Biology, 11*, 207–211

10. Bartlett, M. S. (1960). The critical community size for measles in the United States. *Journal of the Royal Statistical Society, 123*, 37–44

11. Anderson, R. M. & May, R. M. (1986). The invasion, persistence and spread of infectious diseases within animal and plant communities. *Philosophical Transactions of the Royal Society of London. Series B, Biological Sciences, 314*(1167), 533–570

12. Finkenstadt, B. & Grenfell, B. (1998). Empirical determinants of measles metapopulation dynamics in England and Wales. *Proceedings of the Royal Society of London. Series B, Biological Sciences, 265*(1392), 211–220

13. Grenfell, B. T., Bjornstad, O. N. & Kappey, J. (2001). Travelling waves and spatial hierarchies in measles epidemics. *Nature, 414*(6865), 716–723

14. London, W. P. & Yorke, J. A. (1973). Recurrent outbreaks of measles, chickenpox and mumps. I. Seasonal variation in contact rates. *American Journal of Epidemiology, 98*(6), 453–468

15. Aaby, P., Bukh, J., Lisse, I. M. & da Silva, M. C. (1988). Decline in measles mortality: Nutrition, age at infection, or exposure? *British Medical Journal (Clinical Research Ed)*, *296*(6631), 1225–1228

16. Sultan, B., Labadi, K., Guegan, J. F. & Janicot, S. (2005). Climate drives the meningitis epidemics onset in West Africa. *PLoS Medicine*, *2*(1), e6

17. McLean, A. R. & Anderson, R. M. (1988). Measles in developing countries. Part I. Epidemiological parameters and patterns. *Epidemiology and Infection*, *100*(1), 111–133

18. Aaby, P., Samb, B., Simondon, F., et al. (1996). Five year follow-up of morbidity and mortality among recipients of high-titre measles vaccines in Senegal. *Vaccine*, *14*(3), 226–229

19. Evans, A. S. & Kaslow, R. A. (1997). *Viral infections of humans: Epidemiology and control*. 4th edn. (New York: Plenum Publishing)

20. Garnett, G. P. & Grenfell, B. T. (1992). The epidemiology of varicella-zoster virus infections: A mathematical model. *Epidemiology and Infection*, *108*(3), 495–511

21. Siemer, S. W., Uder, M., Scholz, M., Steffens, J., Jeanelle, J. P. & Humke, U. (1997). Are low vaccination rates responsible for increased incidence of mumps orchitis in adolescents and adults? *Der urologe. Ausg A*, *36*(5), 456–459

22. Panagiotopoulos, T., Antoniadou, I. and Valassi-Adam, E. (1999). Increase in congenital rubella occurrence after immunisation in Greece: Rretrospective survey and systematic review. *BMJ (Clinical Research ed.)*, *319*(7223), 1462–1467

23. The World Bank (1993). World Development Report. Washington

24. Short, T. (1750). *New observations, natural, moral, civil, political and medical, on city, town and country bills of mortality*. (London: Longman & Millar)

25. Platt, C. (1996). *King death: The black death and its aftermath in late medieval England*. (London: UCL Press)

26. UNAIDS Epidemiology Reference Group (2002). Improved methods and assumptions for estimation of the HIV/AIDS epidemic and its impact: Recommendations of the UNAIDS Reference Group on estimates, modelling and projections. *AIDS*, *16*(9), W1–14

27. Dabis, F., Elenga, N., Meda, N., et al. (2001). 18-Month mortality and perinatal exposure to zidovudine in West Africa. *AIDS*, *15*(6), 771–779

28. UNAIDS. AIDS epidemic update (2003). Retrieved from http://www.unaids.org/en/Resources/Publications/Corporate+publications/AIDS+epidemic+update+-+December+2003.asp

29. Sewankambo, N. K., Wawer, M. J., Gray, R. H., et al. (1994). Demographic Impact of HIV-infection in Rural Rakai District, Uganda - Results of a population-based cohort study. *AIDS*, *8*(12), 1707–1713

30. Kamali, A., Quigley, M., Nakiyingi, J., et al. (2003). Syndromic management of sexually-transmitted infections and behaviour change interventions on transmission of HIV-1 in rural Uganda: A community randomised trial. *The Lancet*, *361*(9358), 645–652

31. Kilian, A. H., Gregson, S., Ndyanabangi, B., et al. (1999). Reductions in risk behaviour provide the most consistent explanation for declining HIV-1 prevalence in Uganda. *AIDS*, *13*(3), 391–398

32. Gray, R. H., Wawer, M. J., Serwadda, D., et al. (1998). Population-based study of fertility in women with HIV-1 infection in Uganda. *The Lancet*, *351*(9096), 98–103

33. Garnett, G. P., Swinton, J., Brunham, R. C. & Anderson, R. M. (1992). Gonococcal infection, infertility, and population growth: II. The influence of heterogeneity in sexual behaviour. *IMA Journal of Mathematics Applied in Medicine and Biology*, *9*(2), 127–144

34. Zaba, B. & Campbell, O. M. (1994). The impact of eliminating sterility on population growth. *Sexually Transmitted Diseases, 21*(5), 289–291

35. Garnett, G. P. & Anderson, R. M. (1996). Sexually transmitted diseases and sexual behavior: Insights from mathematical models. *Journal of Infectious Diseases. 174*(Suppl 2), S150–161

36. Brunham, R. C. (1997). Core group theory: A central concept in STD epidemiology. *Venereology, 10*(1), 34–39

37. Lewis, J. J. C., Ronsmans, C., Ezeh, A. & Gregson, S. (2004). The population impact of HIV on fertility in sub-Saharan Africa. *AIDS, 18*(Suppl 2), S35–S43

38. Brunham, R. C., Garnett, G. P., Swinton, J. and Anderson, R. M. (1991). Gonococcal infection and human fertility in sub-Saharan Africa. *Proceedings of the Royal Society of London. Series B, Biological Sciences, 246*(1316), 173–177

39. Gregson, S., Nyamukapa, C. A., Garnett, G. P., et al. (2002). Sexual mixing patterns and sex-differentials in teenage exposure to HIV infection in rural Zimbabwe. *The Lancet, 359*(9321), 1896–1903

40. Riley, S., Fraser, C., Donnelly, C. A., et al. (2003). Transmission dynamics of the etiological agent of SARS in Hong Kong: Impact of public health interventions. *Science, 300*(5627), 1961–1966

41. Leroy, E. M., Rouquet, P., Formenty, P., et al. (2004). Multiple Ebola virus transmission events and rapid decline of central African wildlife. *Science, 303*(5656), 387–390

42. Normile, D. (2004). Infectious diseases. Stopping Asia's avian flu: A worrisome third outbreak. *Science, 303*(5657), 447

43. Khan, A. S. & Young, J. C. (2001). Hantavirus pulmonary syndrome: At the crossroads. *Current Opinion in Infectious Diseases, 14*(2), 205–209

44. Quetel, C. (1990). *History of syphilis.* (Cambridge: Polity Press)

45. Cliff, A., Haggett, P. & Smallman-Raynor, M. (1998). *Deciphering global epidemics.* (Cambridge: Cambridge University Press)

46. Morse, S. S. (1994). The viruses of the future? Emerging viruses and evolution. (In S. S. Morse (Ed.), *The evolutionary biology of viruses.* (pp. 325–335). New York: Raven Press)

47. UN Population Division (2001). *World urbanization prospects: The 2001 revision.* (New York: UN)

48. Habib, N. & Behrens, R. (2000). *Travel health and infectious disease.* (London: Nuffield Trust)

CHAPTER 3. WHY CHILD MORTALITY IN SUB-SAHARAN AFRICA HAS CEASED DECLINING SINCE THE EARLY 1990S. THE EXAMPLE OF SENEGAL, A COUNTRY WHERE THE HIV EPIDEMIC HAS REMAINED AT A LOW LEVEL

GILLES PISON

Institut National d'Etudes Démographiques (INED), Paris, France

Abstract. The decline in child mortality in Sub-Saharan Africa that had been observed since the 1950s slowed down over the last fifteen years, and there has even been an increase in certain countries. This was not solely attributable to AIDS. In this paper the trends in Senegal have been examined in detail, as an example of a country little affected by AIDS but where trends in child mortality have closely resembled those of the whole region. In three Senegalese rural population observatories the decline in child mortality in the 1970s and 1980s was attributable to the reduction in deaths from infectious diseases, thanks largely to vaccinations. The situation reversed due to a combination of several factors: the development of chloroquine resistance leading to many malaria deaths; inefficiencies in the health services leading to failures in basic services, including vaccination; and a poor economic climate. These factors are common to many countries in Sub-Saharan Africa and explain why many of them have experienced this health crisis, irrespective of whether or not they are stricken by the AIDS epidemic.

Introduction

Life expectancy at birth worldwide has increased considerably over the last century, due mainly to a marked reduction in child mortality. To what extent has this been the case in Sub-Saharan Africa, and has the recent appearance of AIDS and reappearance of other diseases limited this progress and provoked a renewed rise?

We shall first examine these questions by starting with a general picture of the trends in child mortality in Sub-Saharan Africa over the last fifty years. Then, in the second part of this chapter, we shall study the situation in Senegal, where the trend in child mortality—particularly during the recent period—closely resembles that for the whole of Africa, but where the HIV epidemic has, up to the present, remained at a low level. In the third section we shall employ the data collected in three rural areas of Senegal where the population has been monitored for more than twenty years, in order to study

41

M. Caraël and J.R. Glynn (eds.), HIV, Resurgent Infections and Population Change in Africa, 41–65.
© Springer Science + Business Media B.V. 2008

the changes in child mortality and its causes in greater detail, and examine the reasons explaining the successes and failures of the battle against child death.

Child Mortality Trends in Sub-Saharan Africa

General Trends

Fig. 1 shows the evolution of infant mortality (the probability for a new born child of dying before his first birthday ($1q0$)) in Sub-Saharan Africa as a whole during the period 1950–2000, as indicated by the United Nations Population Division [1]. In order to permit comparisons, the diagram also shows the evolution throughout Asia, and in particular India.

Over the last 50 years, infant mortality ($1q0$) has declined in Sub-Saharan Africa, falling from a level of roughly 180 per 1000 in 1950–54 to 103 per 1000 in

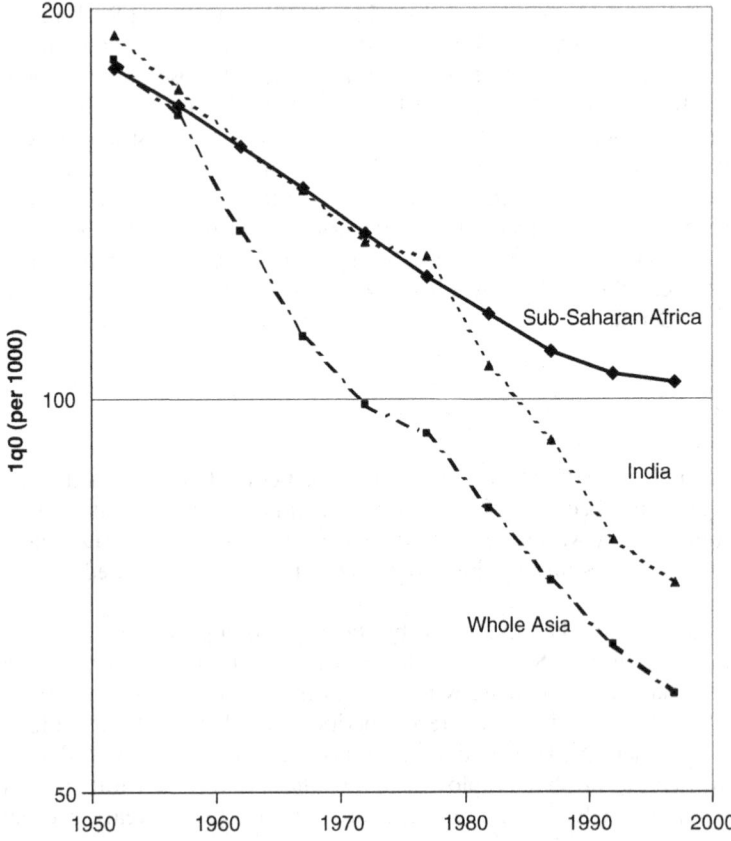

Fig. 1. Infant mortality trends ($1q0$) in Sub-Saharan Africa between 1950 and 2000
Source: **United Nations, Population Division, 2005 [1]**

1995–1999. The decline appears to have occurred at a steady rate until the late 1980s, and to have then slowed down during the last decade and even stagnated. The United Nations anticipate in their projections a further fall to 95 per 1000 in 2000–2004.

Although the decline in Sub-Saharan Africa over these 50 years seems high in absolute figures, it was considerably lower than that in Asia. Infant mortality in 1950–54 was at the same level in Asia as in Sub-Saharan Africa (around 180 per 1000 according to UN data), but between 1995–1999 it was no more than 59 per 1000 there as against 103 per 1000 in Africa. The rate of fall was slower in Africa than in Asia during this whole period (**Fig. 1**). In India, however, at least up to the late 1970s, the trend was quite close to that of Sub-Saharan Africa. Infant mortality was slightly higher there than in Africa in 1950–54 (190 and 180 per 1000 respectively), and declined at approximately the same rate in the two continents during the following 25 years—129 per 1000 in 1975–79 in India compared to 124 per 1000 in Africa. From 1980 onwards, the rate of decline increased in India, whereas in Africa it remained stationary and the levels diverged rapidly. In 1995–1999, infant mortality reached 72 per 1000 in India compared to 103 per 1000 in Africa.

The rapid fall in Africa from 1950 to 1980 can doubtlessly be attributed to the same causes as in other parts of the world where mortality was very high. Progress in infrastructure and in health programmes led to the spread of vaccination and effective treatments and to the consequent reduction in the infectious diseases that were chiefly responsible for child deaths. Socio-economic progress, especially in education, played an important part here in enabling all population classes to benefit from progress in health.

It could be thought that the halt in the lessening of mortality over the last 15 years seen in Sub-Saharan Africa but not in Asia, was due to a phenomenon unique to Africa: the AIDS epidemic being the first to come to mind. It is certainly very extensive in Sub-Saharan Africa, with important effects on mortality, and although these consequences have not yet been well assessed, they must have started appearing in the late 1980s. Some of those infected by HIV were children infected by their mother. UNAIDS [2] has estimated that, while in Sub-Saharan Africa there were slightly more than 25 million births annually, almost 600,000 children in the early 2000s were newly infected each year. Most of these were infected during pregnancy, delivery or via the mother's milk. The question remains as to whether the principal factor accounting for the halt in the reduction of child mortality lay with the AIDS epidemic, or whether other diseases or factors were also involved.

Comparison Between African Countries More Affected by AIDS and Those that Are Less Affected

The AIDS epidemic has affected the various Sub-Saharan African countries very differently. If we assume that AIDS is the main factor in the halt in the decline in mortality throughout the whole region, one would have expected that the mortality over the past fifteen years would have continued to fall in the countries little affected by the epidemic, whereas it would have stopped falling or even risen again in those greatly affected.

Let us first examine the evolution of child mortality according to the African country, this time using as indicator of child mortality the probability that a newborn will die before the age of 5 years (5q0). This indicator has the advantage of being less susceptible to estimation errors than the probability of death before 1 year, 1q0. In addition, it takes greater account of the risks of death in childhood where children, even if they have reached their first birthday, will still be exposed for many years to high mortality risks.

Fig. 2 shows the trends of child mortality (5q0) between 1960 and 1995 in various Sub-Saharan African countries according to Hill and Amouzou [3, 4]. All countries are represented, except those that have been excluded because they were considered unrepresentative of the region, or because no suitable data existed for them (Djibouti, Equatorial Guinea, Cape Verde, Mauritius, Reunion, Seychelles). Fig. 2 includes a total of 42 countries, and Hill et al. have assessed the 5q0 level and trends in each of them by employing the various sources of information on child mortality on a national scale: censuses, multi-round surveys, retrospective fertility surveys—such as the world fertility survey and demographic and health surveys—and the UNICEF surveys on multiple indicators carried out in 2000. The 5q0 estimates taken from these various sources when placed end to end do not generally constitute a coherent whole for a country. The quality of the data varies greatly from one source to another and the assessments may be marred by distortions according to the type of data and the methods applied to them. To extract a plausible estimate of the 5q0 trend from these different points, Hill et al. applied the same regression method for the various countries.

The trend shown in Fig. 2 is similar to that of Fig. 1: child mortality declined in most countries between 1960 and 1990, followed by a pause from 1990 to 1995.[1] In detail, certain countries display a downward trend, whereas in others, less numerous, it is upward. If the AIDS epidemic were the main reason for this difference, it would be anticipated that the countries most affected by AIDS would be in the second category and the less affected in the first. In Fig. 2, countries have been classified into three groups according to the proportion of persons infected by HIV in 1990 among those between the ages of 15 and 49 years, as estimated by UNAIDS: a first group of low HIV prevalence countries (less than 1%) (full line), a second one with intermediate level (between 1% and 5%) (dash line) and a third one with high prevalence (>=5%). Fig. 2 does not show a clear connection between the child mortality trend and the prevalence of HIV in a country. In order to verify whether there is indeed a connection between the importance of the HIV epidemic and the recent trend in child mortality, we present Fig. 3. Each point corresponds to one of the 42 countries in Fig. 2, and its position is a function of the proportion of persons infected by HIV in 1990 among those between the ages of 15 and 49 years, as estimated by UNAIDS (on the x axis), and the ratio between 5q0 in 1995 and 5q0 in 1985 (on the y axis). Countries for which this ratio was greater than 1 experienced a rise in child mortality between these two dates, while those where it was less, experienced a fall.

---

[1] Hill et al. estimated the mortality trend up to 2000, but the most recent data analysed in their study were collected in 2000. They are of a retrospective nature and therefore only provide an assessment for periods frequently originating from several years prior to 2000. The estimate they provide for the year 2000 is the result of a projection obtained by prolonging the trends from previous years. We prefer not to take account of them here, and to take into consideration solely the estimates up to 1995.

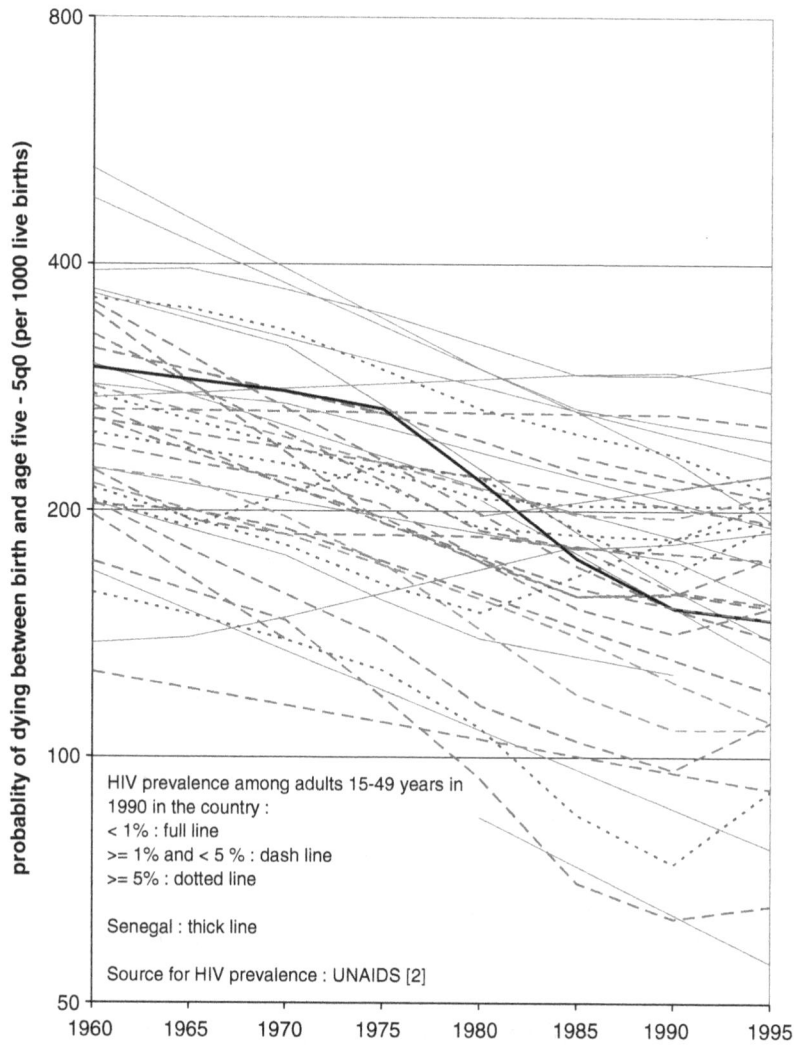

Fig. 2. Child mortality (5q0) trends between 1960 and 1995 in 42 countries of Sub-Saharan Africa (each curve corresponds to one country)
Source: **Hill and Amouzou [4]**

Fig. 3 does not show a clear connection between the child mortality trend between 1985 and 1995 and the prevalence of HIV in a country, even though the decline of child mortality seems more frequent in countries with a low prevalence. The AIDS epidemic does not appear to be the sole factor accounting for the slowing down of the decline in child mortality in Sub-Saharan Africa. Other factors must also have played a part.

Our comparison between countries by level of HIV infection is not perfect, however, since 5q0 has probably been under-estimated with a larger bias during the recent

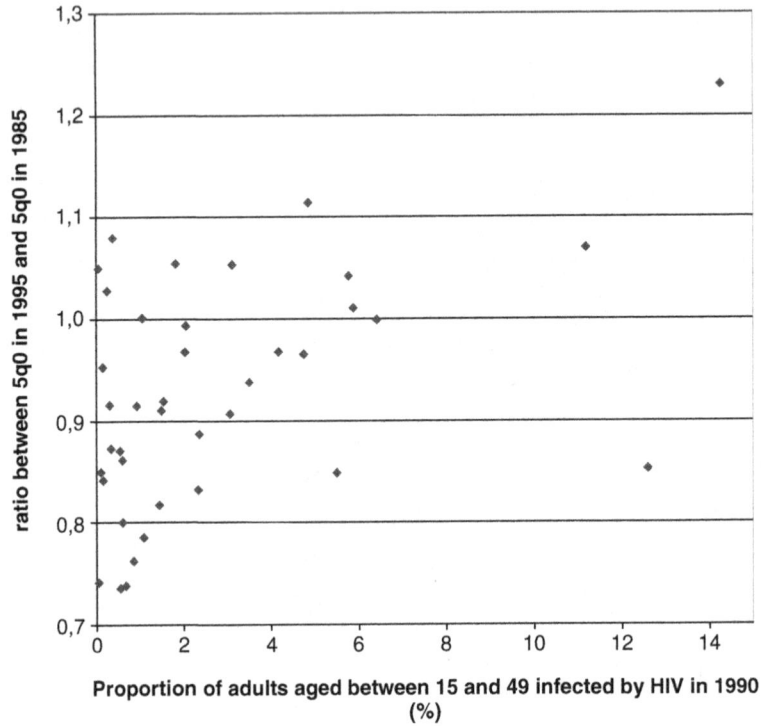

Fig. 3. Child mortality (5q0) changes between 1985 and 1995 and HIV prevalence in Sub-Saharan Africa—one dot corresponds to one country

period than during the earlier ones.[2] Nevertheless, the fact that even in the countries little affected by the HIV epidemic the fall in child mortality in Sub-Saharan Africa has been interrupted or greatly reduced, is an indication that factors other than AIDS have played a part.

To improve understanding of the reasons for the rapid fall in child mortality from the 1950s to 1980s and the subsequent halt in progress for fifteen years, we shall examine in detail the case of Senegal. This country offers the following four advantages:

---

[2] In all the countries, the information employed arose from the declarations of a sample of women between the ages of 15 and 49 years concerning the children that they had had and the state of each of them, whether living or dead. Deceased women were obviously unable to provide information on their own children, but these children had doubtlessly been subject to a higher mortality than the children whose mothers were still alive. First, they had shared the same socio-economic environment as their mothers, and if it had been unfavourable for the latter (which would partly explain why they were dead) it would also have been the same for their children. Second, the children of women who died young, before 50 years of age, became orphans early and were subject, after the death of their mother, to greater risks than the children whose mother was still alive. Because of this correlation between the mortality of mothers and their children, retrospective surveys investigating the mothers generally lead to an underestimation of child mortality. In populations highly affected by AIDS, the correlations are particularly marked: children whose mother is infected may themselves be infected by her at birth. In the absence of effective treatments, both mother and child therefore incur a high risk of dying rapidly. But the death of the child will not be reported if the mother is already dead at the time of the survey.

- child mortality has evolved here in a way that is typical of the whole region, and especially includes a rapid fall followed by a fifteen-year pause;
- up to the present, the country has been little affected by AIDS: the proportion of those between the ages of 15 and 49 infected by HIV at the end of 2001 is estimated at 0.5% [2];
- sources of information there are relatively numerous and enable the evolution of child mortality on a national scale to be retraced quite well;
- the country also possesses three population observatories in rural areas that have been able to monitor child mortality and its causes in detail over a long period.

Child Mortality Decline and Evolution of Health Conditions in Senegal

Child Mortality Declining in Senegal Since 1945

Eight surveys supply data that permit the national level of child mortality in Senegal to be estimated. The type and quality of data gathered varies among the surveys, as do the methodologies employed. Accordingly, it is preferable to focus on a simple, robust indicator of child mortality: the probability that a newborn will die before the age of 5 ($5q0$). **Fig. 4** shows $5q0$ estimates for Senegal since 1946. Although these

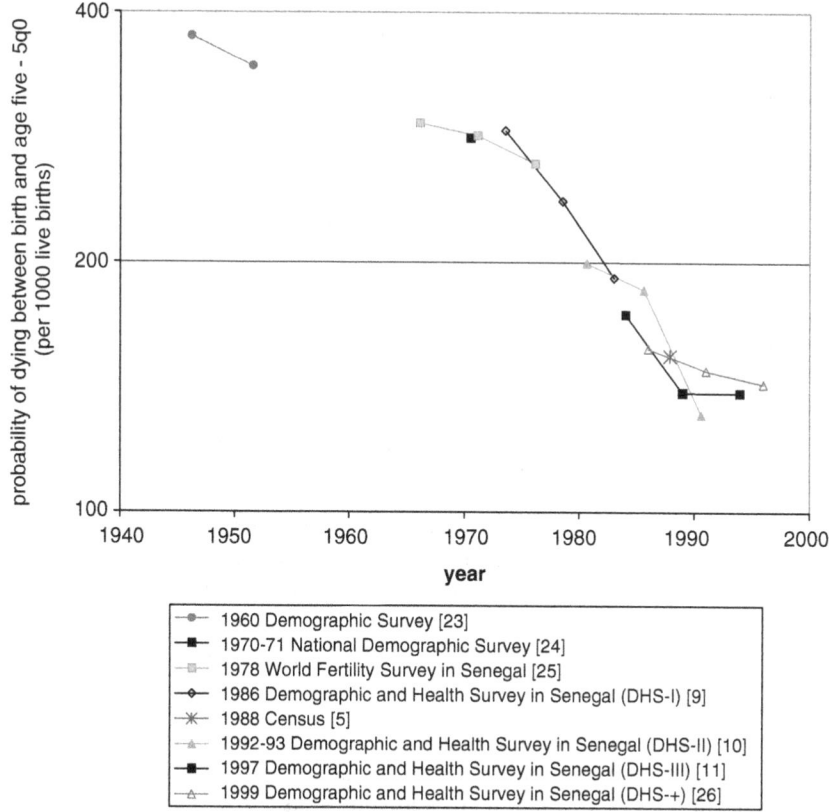

Fig. 4. **Child mortality trends in Senegal between 1945 and 1996**

measurements result from different surveys and estimation techniques, they are fairly consistent. In the 45 years following the end of the Second World War, child mortality (5q0) declined by two-thirds, falling from a level of roughly 400 per 1000 to 140 per 1000 in the late 1980s. The decline appears to have halted thereafter, and mortality to have stagnated at this level or decreased very slowly. Going back to the beginning of the period, the decline appears to have occurred rather slowly until the early 1970s, with a 25% drop in 25 years (from 373 per 1000 in 1946 to 280 per 1000 in 1970), and to have accelerated thereafter, with 5q0 falling by more than 50% in the next 20 years (to a level of 140 per 1000 around 1990), before the more recent halt in the decline.

Changes in Health Infrastructure and Health Programmes in Senegal Since 1945

Review

Until 1978, Senegal's health infrastructure (hospitals, maternity clinics) was focused on the cities. Public health programmes to improve sanitary conditions and control diseases were developed primarily in the towns, building on these infrastructures. The poorly served rural areas benefited only from periodic visits of mobile teams from the Major Endemic Diseases Department (Service des Grandes Endémies), whose activities began to deteriorate following independence in 1960. In 1978, following the recommendations made at the World Health Conference in Alma Ata in 1977, Senegal introduced primary health care. Paralleling the effort towards decentralization of the major health facilities (hospitals and dispensaries), this policy led to the training of community health workers and the establishment of village health centres and maternity clinics. Using these new village-based infrastructures, several mother and child health care (MCH) programmes were initiated: vaccinations, malaria prevention, rehydration of children suffering from diarrhoea, pregnancy monitoring and assistance in delivery, and food supplements for young children.

Health Infrastructures

The number of hospitals increased threefold between 1960 and 1988, reflecting the policy to equip each region with a hospital and to divide some hospitals in the cities into two [5]. The number of hospital beds has not grown proportionately however, and has not even kept pace with population growth. Thus, despite the proliferation of hospitals, the supply of beds per inhabitant has fallen slightly.

The number of health centres has changed very little, continuing to be one per departmental capital. These are normally run by a physician and are equipped with hospital beds. The number of dispensaries, on the other hand, has increased sharply: it more than tripled between 1960 and 1988. Operated by nurses, these dispensaries are found throughout the country. They are generally located in the district (arrondissement) capitals or rural communities.

Maternity clinics were rare and, until 1977, concentrated in the towns. Beginning in 1978, the primary health care policy led to the construction of a large number of such clinics in rural areas. In 1988, there were almost as many rural maternity clinics as there were dispensaries.

In 1960, the Dakar region, which accounted for 14% of the population, had three out of the five hospitals in the country and the vast majority of hospital beds. In 1988, it had 22% of the population, but only six out of 16 hospitals and half of the hospital beds. The distribution of facilities between Dakar and the rest of the country, while remaining unequal, appears to have improved considerably. Nevertheless, health personnel remain very concentrated in Dakar, where two-thirds of the countrys physicians, pharmacists and dentists and half of its nurses and midwives are to be found.

Health Programmes

Numerous programmes were implemented before 1978, each one having a specific scope of action. They were carried out either by MCH centres in urban settings, or by mobile teams (smallpox eradication and control of leprosy). After 1978, these programmes were integrated into the general primary health care programme carried out by the dispensaries and mobile teams for vaccination. Two of these specific programmes, the antimalaria campaign and vaccinations, are discussed in greater detail below.

Antimalaria Campaign. Malaria, which is endemic in Senegal and one of the major causes of child mortality, was the focus of specific eradication programmes beginning in 1953 [6]. Between 1953 and 1961, an eradication trial was conducted in the region of Thiès and the western part of the region of Fatick, in which homes were sprayed with DDT combined, after 1957, with chemoprophylaxis. This programme was a failure. In 1963, another antimalaria programme, using chloroquine-based chemoprophylaxis (called "chloroquinization") was launched throughout Senegal. Its impact appears to have been very unequal, throughout time and from one region to another, although there was little follow-up or evaluation. On the whole, its effects on malaria mortality and morbidity appear to have been limited [7]. This programme was discontinued in 1979 and malaria prevention was thereafter incorporated into primary health care.

Vaccinations. Initiated in Senegal in 1981, the Expanded Programme for Immunization (EPI) was designed to extend vaccination coverage to rural areas, which were at that time not well served, and to improve coverage in urban areas. Its objective was to protect children against seven diseases: tuberculosis, diphtheria, tetanus, pertussis, polio, measles and yellow fever. Its strategy was based on fixed vaccination centres and mobile teams:
– permanent centres: in urban areas, the MCH centres continued to operate as they had done previously; health centres in rural areas began systematic vaccination at dispensaries. They also provided coverage for people living within a 15 km radius by means of travelling vaccination teams;
– mobile teams: in rural areas, mobile teams were established to administer vaccinations beyond the 15 km radius covered by the dispensaries.

The programme targeted young children and also pregnant women, who were given tetanus vaccinations to protect their newborns against neonatal tetanus.

Since its beginning, the EPI (Expanded Programme for Immunization) has undergone three major acceleration efforts, one in the first quarter of 1987, the second in the first quarter of 1990 and the third in 1995. These led to the training and mobilization of administrative and health personnel, media information campaigns (especially by radio), and the provision of new equipment for dispensaries, especially in 1987.

The percentage of children aged 12–23 months who were fully vaccinated[3] increased considerably in the 1980s (**Table 1** and **Fig. 5**). Based on data from vaccination coverage surveys using the standard World Health Organization method, it progressed from 18% in July 1984 to 35% in July 1987, and to 55% in June 1990. The 1987 and 1990 percentages probably represent the maxima for the period 1987–90, since, in both years, the surveys were carried out just after an acceleration phase. The average for the period is possibly somewhat lower. Detailed analysis of vaccination dates confirms that the increased coverage rate coincides with the two acceleration campaigns that took place in early 1987 and early 1990 [5].

Complete vaccination coverage increased 1.2-fold in the Region of Dakar between 1984 and 1987, and 1.5-fold in the other urban areas [5]. The impact of the acceleration of the EPI in early 1987 was therefore relatively slight in the towns. In rural areas, on the other hand, where coverage was particularly low in 1984, there was a threefold increase in 1987, so that the gap in coverage levels compared to the towns was almost closed in one go.

The demographic and health surveys of 1986 and 1992 and the Senegalese survey of health indicators in 1999 collected information about the vaccinations received by children, but employed a different method from that recommended by the WHO.

Table 1. Vaccination coverage of children aged 12–23 months (%), by date and vaccine (1). All of Senegal.

Vaccine	Vaccination coverage surveys, standard World Health Organization method			Demographic and health surveys (DHS)		
	1984	July 1987	June 1990	1986	1992	1999
BCG		92	94	26	63	59
DTPP-1 (2)		81	91	27	61	55
DTPP-2		69	83	18	56	50
DTPP-3		47	63	9	49	42
Measles		63	76	20	45	41
Yellow fever		72	75	19	44	–
Fully vaccinated children (3)	18	35	55	7	41	36

Sources: 1984 : Claquin et al., 1987 [27]; July 1987 : Claquin et al., 1987 [27]; June 1990 : Evaluation du PEV au Sénégal, 1990 [28]; 1986 : Ndiaye et al., 1988 [9]; 1992 : Ndiaye et al., 1994 [10]; 1999 : Sow et al., 2000 [26].
Notes : (1) Measure based only on the information contained in health cards or vaccination cards. When these documents were lost, the child was not counted as being vaccinated. These are therefore minimum estimates. (2) The proportion of children vaccinated with polio vaccine, given independently from DTP vaccine from 1986, are not indicated here. (3) Vaccinated against seven diseases : tuberculosis, diphtheria, tetanus, pertussis, polio, measles and yellow fever.

---

[3] That is, vaccinated against seven diseases: tuberculosis, diphtheria, tetanus, pertussis, polio, measles and yellow fever.

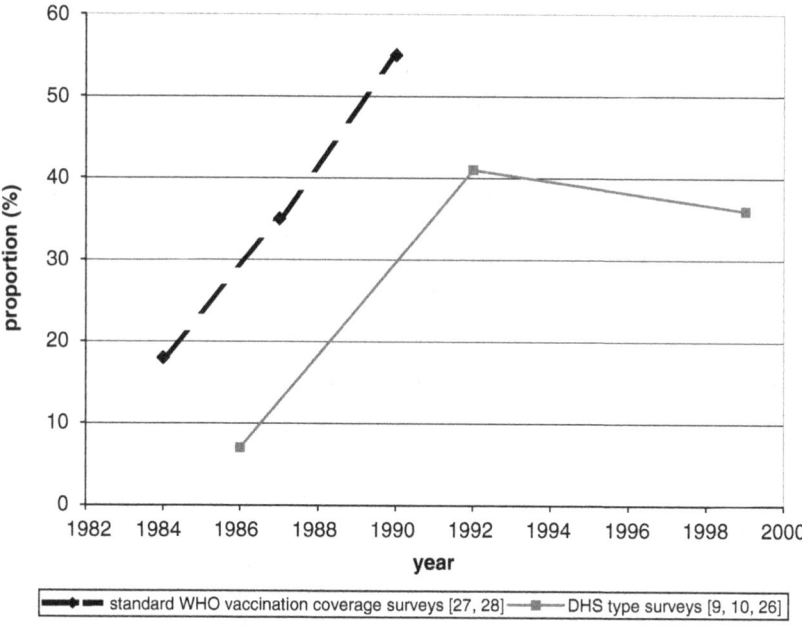

Fig. 5. Change in the proportion of children aged 12-23 months fully vaccinated in Senegal

In consequence, the levels of vaccination cover according to these surveys cannot be compared directly with those provided by the WHO-type surveys. They are, however, comparable between themselves, from one survey to another. The image that these surveys give of the evolution of vaccination coverage in the 1980s is similar to those of the WHO type: that of a considerable increase (**Table 1** and **Fig. 5**). These investigations have the advantage of providing information on the trend in vaccination coverage during the following decade. 1992 and 1999 are the only two observation points, but they indicate that vaccination coverage has diminished rather than continuing to increase. The proportion of children between the ages of 12 and 23 months who were fully vaccinated decreased from 41% in 1992 to 36% in 1999. The change was not regular. Subsequent to the restarting of the EPI in 1995, vaccination cover rose rapidly that year, but then started to decline rapidly, reaching very low levels in 2000 and 2001 [8].

Anti-tetanus vaccination of pregnant women greatly increased in the 1980s and 1990s, with the proportion of those having received at least one anti-tetanus injection during their pregnancy increasing from 31% for those giving birth during the period 1981–86, and then to 71% and 84% respectively for those who delivered in 1987–1992 and 1992–1997 [9, 10, 11]. The vaccines received during a pregnancy ensure protection over several years, and the children arising from later pregnancies are also protected, even if the mother has not been revaccinated. Consequently, the immunity to neo-natal tetanus resulting from the anti-tetanus vaccinations of pregnant women progressed even more than the figures indicate.

Spread of Vaccination, One Major Cause of the Decline in Child Mortality

Child mortality, as we have seen above, declined continuously in Senegal between World War II and the late 1980s. In 45 years, from 1945 to 1990, the probability of dying before the age of five was reduced by two thirds, from approximately 400 per 1000 to 140 per 1000. The decline accelerated in the late 1970s and early 1980s, when a new health policy oriented towards primary health care was initiated. The proliferation of health infrastructures in the various regions that resulted from this, and the implementation of the Expanded Programme for Immunization (EPI) probably contributed significantly to the accelerated decline.

The cessation of the fall in child mortality at the watershed between 1980 and 1990 coincided with a pause in improvements to the health infrastructures and programmes. In particular, the EPI, which had greatly advanced during the 1980s, then marked time with a decrease in vaccination coverage during the 1990s, despite the revival in 1995.

These observations suggest that the development of health infrastructures and programmes have been essential for the reduction in child mortality, especially in the countryside. The timing of this reduction also suggests that the immunization programme played a leading role in the acceleration of the decline in the 1970s and 1980s [12]. And the decrease of vaccination coverage is probably one factor explaining why the decline in child mortality ceased thereafter.

For a better understanding of the mortality trends of children in Senegal, we shall now examine the changes that have occurred in the causes of death. Unfortunately, reliable information is not available for causes of death on a national scale, but the observations made in the three rural population observatories existing in Senegal will give an idea of the changes that have taken place in this country.

Changes in Child Mortality and Cause of Death Recorded in the Three Rural Population Observatories of Senegal

The populations of three Senegalese rural areas—Bandafassi, Mlomp and Niakhar—have been monitored for more than twenty years [13, 14, 15, 16] (**Fig. 6**). Changes in child mortality and causes of child death have been documented precisely in these populations. As these population observatories are located in areas of the country that are very diverse, the mortality differences between them give an idea of the total geographic variations within the country.

The Bandafassi, Mlomp and Niakhar Population Observatories

Locations and Characteristics
The Bandafassi population observatory is situated in Southeast Senegal, and at 750 km is the farthest site from Dakar, the capital city (**Fig. 6**). The Niakhar observatory, situated in the West and most populated area of the country, is the closest (150 km from Dakar). Mlomp, located in the Southwest, like Bandafassi, is relatively distant (500 km) from Dakar.

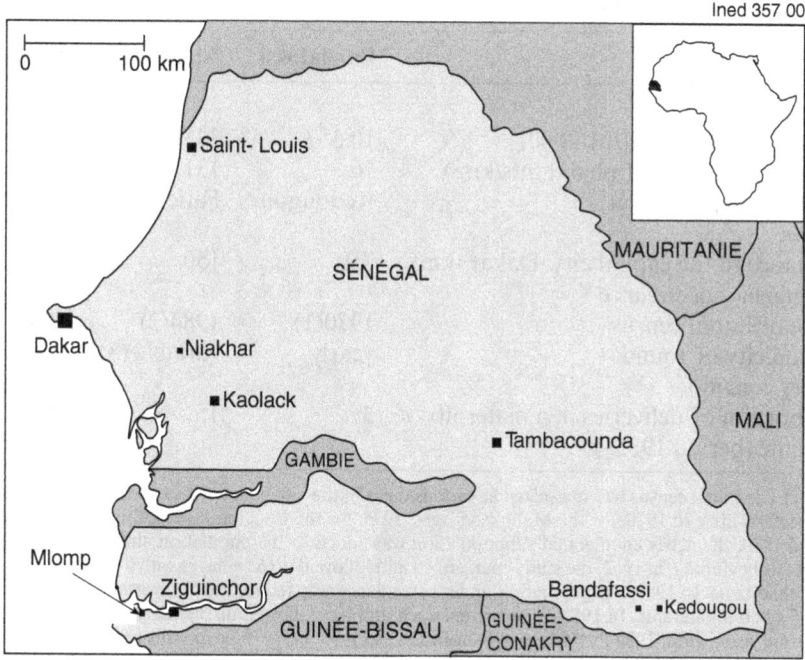

Fig. 6. Location of Bandafassi, Mlomp and Niakhar in Senegal

In 2000, the three sites had populations of about 10,000 inhabitants (Bandafassi), 30,000 (Niakhar), and 8,000 (Mlomp) (**Table 2**). Population density differed greatly from one site to the other, being highest in Niakhar (131 inhabitants per square km), lowest in Bandafassi (16) and intermediate in Mlomp (63). The ethnic composition also varies. In Niakhar, it is homogenous, with 95% of the population belonging to the Serer ethnic group, and in Mlomp also, one ethnic group, the Diolas, is dominant. The population of Bandafassi, however, is more diverse and divided into three ethnic groups: the Fula (57% of the population), the Bedik (28%) and the Malinke (16%).

The population of the three sites have access to health centres operated by nurses: one in Bandafassi, one in Mlomp, and three in Niakhar. Their level of activity varies. The Mlomp dispensary, operated by a nurse who is also a Catholic nun, is the busiest. In addition to an outpatient clinic it has 12 hospital beds and a small laboratory. All pregnant women of Mlomp attend prenatal visits and deliver in a maternity clinic, most frequently that in the area close to the health centre, which has 10 beds. Pregnant women at risk are systematically taken to Ziguinchor hospital (at a distance of 50 km) some time before delivery. Deliveries occurring in the Mlomp maternity clinic are assisted by two matrons supervised by the nurse from the health centre.

The health centres of the other two sites are less active, and the proportion of women delivering in a maternity clinic is low: 15% in Niakhar during the 1988–1997 period, and 3% in Bandafassi (Table 2). Throughout the whole of Senegal, about one woman in two delivered in a maternity clinic during the 1988–1997 period, with a higher proportion in towns (about 80%) than in rural areas (about 30%) [10, 11]. The proportions observed

Table 2. The rural population observatories of Senegal.

	Bandafassi	Niakhar	Mlomp
Population			
Total population (01/01/2000)	10 357	30 023	7 591
Population density (inhabitants/km^2)	16	131	63
District (département)	Kedougou	Fatick	Oussouye
Distance			
Distance to the capital city, Dakar (km)	750	150	500
Demographic surveillance			
Date of initial census	1970(1)	1984(2)	1985
Periodicity of rounds	yearly	variable (3)	yearly
Delivery conditions			
Proportion of deliveries in a maternity clinic (period 1985–1997)	3%	15%	99%

Notes: (1) The initial census was organized at various dates in the villages of the various subpopulations of the Bandafassi area: in 1970, for the Malinke villages; 1975, for the Fula ones; 1980, for the Bedik ones. In 1975 and 1980, the newly enumerated subpopulation was added to the population already being followed up. (2) At its beginning, in 1962, the study enumerated and followed up 65 villages with a total population of 35,000 inhabitants. In 1969, the population under surveillance was reduced to 8 villages with a total population of 4,000 inhabitants. In 1983, it was re-enlarged and has followed up 30 villages until now. (3) The rounds were yearly from 1984 to 1987, weekly from 1987 to 1997, every three months from 1997.

in Niakhar and Bandafassi are therefore well below the average for rural areas of the country. The exceptional situation in Mlomp, where the level is very high and well above the urban average, results from the efforts of health personnel in the area, and the delivery traditions of the Diola ethnic group, who do not favour delivery at home [17].

Mlomp also preceded the other sites with vaccinations. When it started, in 1971, the vaccination programme at first only involved a few of the children, but by the late 1970s it had gradually increased in influence until practically all children were fully vaccinated. The vaccination cover has subsequently been maintained at this very high level up to the present day. In Bandafassi, apart from vaccinations received during national campaigns, practically no child was vaccinated until 1987. It was only then, following the acceleration of the EPI organised at the beginning of that year, that children there began to be vaccinated on a regular basis, and led that year to a sudden increase in vaccination coverage. From a level approaching 0% it rose to 48% of the 12 to 35-months-old children in February 1987 [12]. Over the following years, due to the relaxation of effort, vaccination coverage tended to decrease, but the revival of the EPI in 1995 brought it once more to a peak, this time even higher than in 1987, with 80% of the children fully vaccinated. The effort was unfortunately once more relaxed throughout the subsequent years and coverage rapidly diminished to below 50% in 1999 [18].

Fertility is high in all three sites, but with appreciable differences between them. In 1990, it was highest in Niakhar, where the total fertility rate was, on average, 7.7 children per woman, lowest in Mlomp (5.0) and intermediate in Bandafassi (6.3).

Population Surveillance

The populations of each site have been monitored for several years by means of multi-round survey techniques [13, 14, 15, 16]. Following an initial census, villages have been repeatedly visited on a regular basis. The list of those present on the previous occasion is checked during every visit, and information is collected concerning the births, marriages, migrations and deaths (including cause of death) that have taken place in the meantime. Surveillance did not start the same year in the various sites, and the frequency of visits is different (**Table 2**). In Bandafassi and Mlomp, where surveillance started in 1970 and 1985 respectively, visits are carried out on an annual basis, whereas in Niakhar, where surveillance started in 1984, the frequency of visits has changed. It was annual from 1984 to 1986, weekly from 1987 to 1997, and subsequently three-monthly.

As in many rural African areas, most deaths occur without the presence of a doctor to certify the event or diagnose the cause. This is then determined by employing the "verbal autopsy" method, which involves collecting information on the circumstances of the death and the symptoms of the disease that preceded it from the family of the deceased person. The same questionnaire is employed for such interviews at the three sites [19, 20].

Information collected directly from the family is collated with clinical information from the health centre or hospital registers for those patients who died or had a clinical examination there before their death. In the case of Mlomp, most people who died had visited the health centre during their final illness, and information is consequently available from the register kept by the nurses since the beginning of the survey. Once it has been completed, the verbal autopsy questionnaire is submitted to two doctors for each of them to make an independent diagnosis. If they disagree, a third doctor rereads it and acts as an arbiter.

The diagnoses made through this method are more or less precise and reliable, depending on the causes of death. Neonatal tetanus, for example, is quite easily identified by this means, as is measles. There is a specific word for measles in every language, and everyone can identify it when an epidemic breaks out. When a mother who has lost her child is asked whether the cause of death was "measles" (using the name employed in her own language), she is seldom mistaken, and her personal diagnosis can generally be considered reliable. Due to the spread of immunization since the 1980s and the resulting decline in epidemics however, self-diagnosis of measles is not as reliable as it was previously. For many other diseases diagnosis made through the verbal autopsy method is not very reliable. Malaria, for example, is easily mistaken for other diseases that also involve fever (see below).

Information gathered by the population surveillance systems in force at the three sites is of high quality for African rural populations. In particular, the covering of events is almost complete and their dating precise. This ensures good reliability of the resulting demographic measures, in particular those relating to the mortality level and trends.

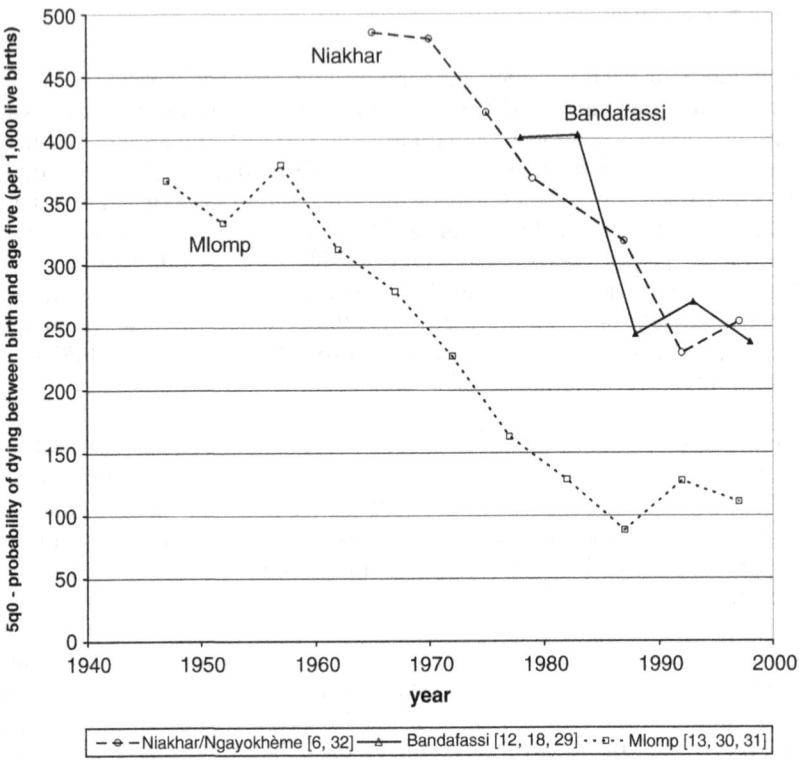

Fig. 7. Trends in child mortality (5q0) in the three rural areas under demographic surveillance in Senegal

Evolution of Child Mortality in the Three Population Observatories of Senegal

The mortality trends of children under five (5q0) in the three population observatories of Senegal are shown in **Fig. 7**. Similar patterns are found in the three areas studied: a first period with a plateau; a second period with a rapid fall; and then a third with a pause or increase. The differences lie in the timetable and levels. In Bandafassi, the farthest zone from Dakar, child mortality commenced its rapid decline the latest (after 1986), and this decline correlates with the acceleration of the Expanded Programme of Vaccination of 1987 [12]. In Niakhar, 150 km from Dakar, the fall began earlier, from the early 1970s. This was mainly attributed to a diminution in rainfall causing a reduction in malaria [6], but the fall continued at the same rate after the dry years had passed. The Mlomp zone was clearly different from the other two in that the fall started earlier (from the mid-1960s), and reached a much lower level—the risk of death before 5 years declined fourfold in 20 years. This rural zone, very distant from Dakar, has benefited since 1961, as mentioned above, from a dispensary and a private maternity clinic that quickly ensured that a large majority of the population in the area would have some quality health services [13].

There is a correlation between mortality decline and the availability of health services in these three rural zones. The educational level of women and household incomes at the time were low in all these areas. The rapid fall in child mortality in rural areas of Senegal during the late 1970s could therefore to a large extent have been connected to the decentralization of infrastructures, and to the new public health policy, which enabled the majority of them to have access to the health services that had previously been denied them.

The fall in child mortality recorded in the three observatories was interrupted in a similar fashion in the late 1980s, and then remained at about the same level (250 per 1000) at Bandafassi and Niakhar during the 1990s, and even rose slightly in Mlomp, from 88 per 1000 in 1985–89 to 111 per 1000 in 1995–99 (**Fig. 7**). The pause phenomenon is therefore to be found in the three observatories as in the whole country.

3. Distribution of the Causes of Death

Fig. 8 compares child mortality and its causes in Bandafassi, Mlomp and Niakhar during the second half of the 1980s (1984–1989 period in Bandafassi and Niakhar, and 1985–1989 in Mlomp), distinguishing neonatal mortality (**Fig. 8a**) from that between one month and five years (**Fig. 8b**).

Neonatal mortality was lowest in Mlomp (36 per 1000) and highest, more than double, in Bandafassi (87 per 1000), with an intermediate level of 55 per 1000 in Niakhar. The overall difference was due to differences in mortality for all the major causes of death. Neonatal tetanus, responsible at that time for one third of the neonatal deaths in Niakhar and one quarter in Bandafassi, and accounting in the two sites for the demise of about twenty newborns per thousand, was only 1 per 1000 in Mlomp. There were almost the same contrasts for deaths due to premature delivery and low birth weight (2 per 1000 in Mlomp as against 15 and 21 per 1000 in Niakhar and Bandafassi respectively). Beyond the neonatal period and up to

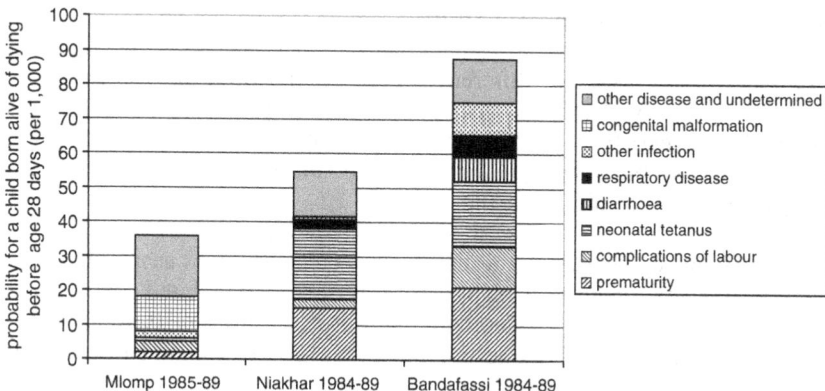

Fig. 8a. Neonatal mortality by cause of death in the three population observatories of Senegal (period 1984–1989)

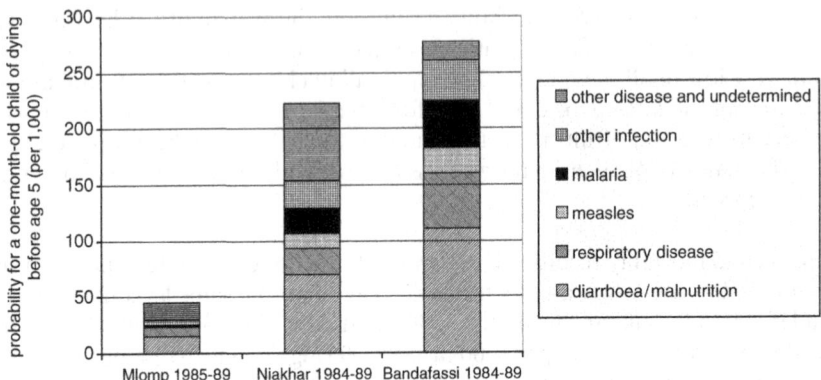

Fig. 8b. Mortality of children from age 28 days to age 5 years by cause of death in the three population observatories of Senegal (period 1984–1989)

five years (**Fig. 8b**), the overall difference in mortality level was even greater (45, 223 and 277 per 1000 in Mlomp, Niakhar and Bandafassi respectively), and it was linked once more to the differences in mortality for each of the major causes of death—diarrhoea and malnutrition, pneumonia, malaria etc. Measles, an important cause of death in Bandafassi and Niakhar at that time, was absent in Mlomp.

Unfortunately, we have no information on the causes of child mortality in Mlomp before the 1970s when it was still high there, but it is probable that the same causes as those present in Bandafassi and Niakhar in the recent period were dominant at the time. If we assume that the causes of death in Bandafassi and Niakhar in the second half of the 1980s reflected those prevalent in Mlomp, twenty years previously—at a time when death from all causes reached the same levels there—it is likely that there was a fall in each of the major causes of death.

Measles, a Fast Regressing Cause of Death

As just noted, there are great differences between the three sites in deaths from measles. This cause of death has nearly disappeared in Mlomp (only two deaths during the fifteen years from 1985 to 1999 among a total of some 300 deaths of children under 5 years), but it was still an important cause of death in Bandafassi and Niakhar during the second half of the 1980s.

As mentioned above, measles was a disease that villagers could easily identify, and information was consequently available on cases of measles-related deaths that had occurred since the inception of demographic observation in 1970, well before the introduction of verbal autopsy questionnaires in 1984. This enabled the evolution of measles-related mortality since 1970 to be traced, and **Table 3** indicates the variations in measles-related mortality rates according to four periods, two of which—1970–1979 and 1980–1986—occurred before the introduction of the immunization campaign in 1987 and the other two—1987–1989 and 1990–1993—subsequently.

Table 3 first shows the drastic change that occurred in 1987. Before then, measles was responsible for a high proportion of deaths. Among children from 1 to 20-months-old it accounted for about one out of every seven deaths (14% in 1970–1979 and 15% in 1980–1986), and of one out of every three (35% and 30% respectively) among children aged 21 to 59 months, thus making it the primary cause of death. From 1987, however, measles was responsible for only 3% and 5% of deaths at these ages.

Fig. 9a retraces the annual variations of the measles mortality rates in Bandafassi among all children under five-years-old over the whole period, from 1970 to 2001. The annual variations in Niakhar are also shown from 1984. The figure shows that measles

Table 3. Measles mortality rate by age-group and period: Bandafassi, 1970–1993.

	Age group			
	1–20 months		21 months–59 months	
Period	Measles annual mortality rate (per thousand)	Proportion of total deaths caused by measles (percent)	Measles annual mortality rate (per thousand)	Proportion of total deaths caused by measles (percent)
1970–1979	21.0	15	25.3	35
1980–1986	14.6	14	14.9	30
1987–1989	0.0	0	0.0	0
1990–1993	2.9	4	2.6	8

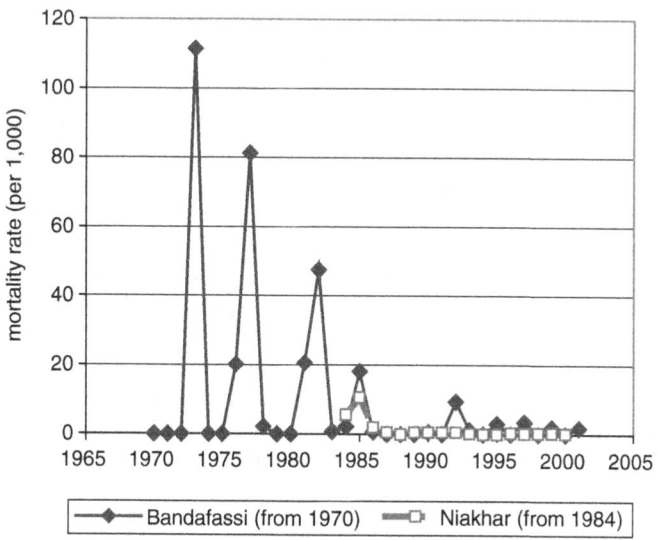

Fig. 9a. Annual fluctuations of measles mortality among children under five years old at Bandafassi and Niakhar

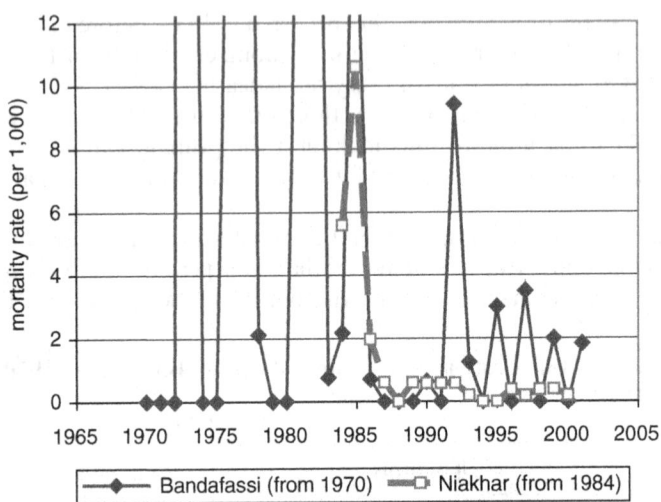

Fig. 9b. Annual fluctuations of measles mortality among children under five years old at Bandafassi and Niakhar (Y-axis with scale enlarged by a factor of 10)

occurred in the Bandafassi area only in epidemics with comparatively long intervals between them. In the period 1970–1995 there were four epidemics: in 1973, 1976–77, 1981–82 and 1985. A fifth epidemic occurred in 1992, with a lower mortality. Each of the epidemics affected only some villages [5, 12]. Before 1987 more than a decade often elapsed between two successive epidemics in the same village. Because of the long intervals, whenever a village was affected by an epidemic, it was massively hit—within only a few weeks, many children fell ill (practically all those who were born since the previous epidemic), with very high mortality rates. At least 15% of all children less than five-years-old died in the 1976–77 and the 1981–1982 epidemics [21].

The epidemiology of measles in Bandafassi changed after 1985. Almost seven years elapsed before a new epidemic occurred in 1992, and this led to relatively fewer deaths than previously. As the mortality rates were much lower after 1985 than previously, **Fig. 9b** shows the data using a larger scale on the y axis. After 1992, deaths from measles were observed more frequently (every two years) but the numbers in each epidemic were ten to fifty times lower than in the 1970s and the first half of the 1980s. Measles became increasingly endemic, and very much less lethal.

The observation was similar in Niakhar, but preventive measures did not commence until 1984; and the last big measles epidemic, which was national and also affected Bandafassi, was in 1985. Since then, measles has become a much less frequent cause of death in Niakhar, with a mortality that remained at more or less the same level until 2000, without diminishing.

Deaths from measles in both Bandafassi and Niakhar declined greatly in the 1980s; and this marked regression of one of the main causes of child mortality was the most spectacular consequence of introducing vaccinations in these two populations. The

lessening of vaccination coverage in the 1990s led to a slight rise in deaths from measles in Bandafassi, but this was far from the extremely high pre-vaccination levels. In
Niakhar, it remained at the same level in the 1990s without further decreasing.

Recent Considerable Rise in Deaths from Malaria

Deaths from malaria are more difficult to diagnose than those from measles. This disease, as mentioned above, cannot be identified with any certainty through the verbal
autopsy method, because of the difficulty in distinguishing it from other diseases that
also cause fever. So here, "malaria" is a broad category that includes "true malaria"
but also "unspecified fever". In Mlomp, however, malaria-related mortality could be
retraced with some accuracy, because many of the children who died following bouts
of fever had sought advice from the local health centre, where biological tests (using
thick blood films) were made in order to ascertain whether the malaria diagnosis
should be confirmed.

Fig. 10 shows the evolution of malaria-related mortality in the three areas since 1985.
In Mlomp, it was relatively low until 1991 (five times less than Bandafassi and eight

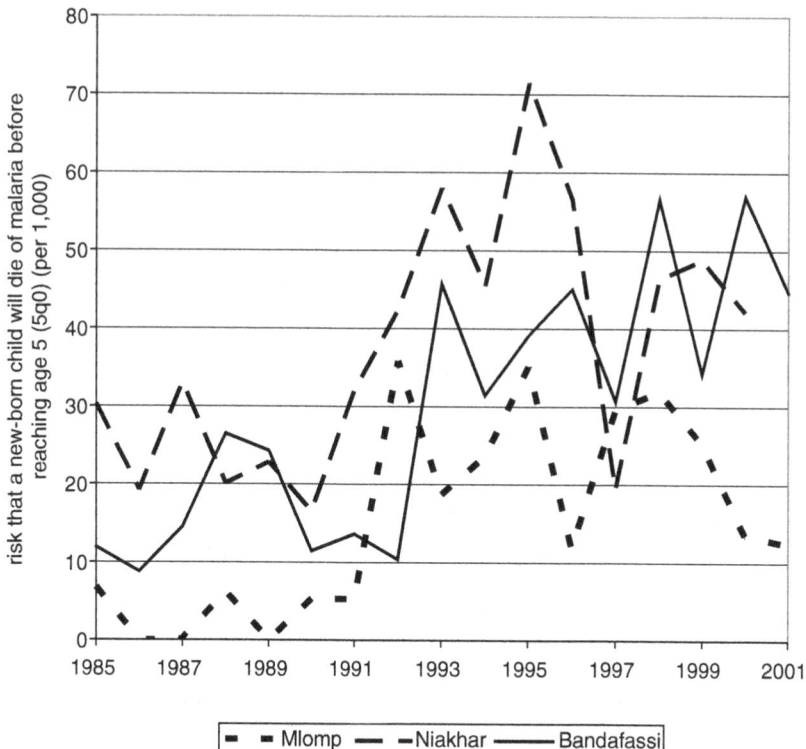

**Fig. 10. Evolution of malaria-related child mortality at Bandafassi, Mlomp and Niakhar
from 1985 to 2001**

times less than Niakhar); a sign that the fight against malaria organized by the health centre in the 1970s and 1980s was successful. Malaria-related mortality rose sharply between 1991 and 1993, and has subsequently remained at higher levels. During the periods 1985–1991 and 1993–2000, malaria increased 7-fold in Mlomp, 2.5-fold in Bandafassi and 2-fold in Niakhar. This rise was largely attributable to the appearance and spread of malaria strains in the late 1980s and early 1990s that were resistant to chloroquine, the anti-malarial widely used in Senegal both preventively and curatively up to the present day [22], and which had enabled malaria-related mortality to be drastically reduced in Mlomp from 1975 onwards. This unfavourable evolution in deaths from malaria is one of the reasons why overall child mortality stagnated in Bandafassi and Niakhar in the 1990s and rose again in Mlomp.

Conclusion

The slowing down of the decline in child mortality in Sub-Saharan Africa over the last fifteen years, and even its increase in certain countries, was not solely attributable to AIDS. In order to determine any other diseases or factors that also played a part, Senegal was chosen for study—a country very little affected by AIDS but where trends in child mortality have closely resembled those of the whole region and have remained stagnant throughout the last fifteen years. In addition, Senegal has the advantage of possessing relatively numerous information sources available for tracing the evolution of child mortality on a national scale, as well as three population observatories in a rural area where child mortality could be followed and the causes of deaths studied in detail over almost 20 years.

It is evident that Senegal experienced an appreciable and steady fall in child mortality from the end of World War II until the late 1980s. In 45 years, from 1945 to 1990, the risk of a newborn child dying before the age of five years was divided by three, dropping from about 400 per 1000 to 140 per 1000. The fall accelerated towards the end of the 1970s and early 1980s, at a time when a new public health policy oriented towards primary health care was introduced. This led in particular to the increase of primary health care infrastructures in the regions (they had previously been highly concentrated in Dakar), and to the introduction of the Expanded Programme for Immunization (EPI).

The three Senegalese rural population observatories showed that the decline in child mortality in the 1970s and 1980s was allied to the reduction in deaths from infectious diseases, thanks largely to vaccinations. Death from measles, previously one of the primary causes of child mortality, regressed drastically after the introduction of vaccinations. But in the 1990s, just as in the whole country, vaccination ceased to increase in Bandafassi and Niakhar (and even diminished in the former), and deaths from measles, while not returning to the previously very high levels, no longer fell. Deaths from malaria, on the other hand, greatly increased following the spread of chloroquine resistance within the country. Stagnation of the vaccination effort and revival of malaria mortality allied to chloroquine resistance explain the halt in the decline of infant mortality in Bandafassi and Niakhar. In Mlomp, where nearly all the children had been vaccinated for at least

20 years, it was the rise in malaria mortality that explained the resurgence of child mortality in the 1990s.

These observations are probably valid for the whole country, and deaths from malaria must have appreciably increased. The pause in the vaccination drive must also have impeded the struggle against death by infection. These two phenomena were the main reasons for the fifteen year cessation of the decline in under-five mortality in Senegal, an example of a country that, despite having so far escaped a severe AIDS epidemic and its consequences on mortality, has still experienced a health crisis leading to a halt in the decline of child mortality. This crisis was due to the conjunction of several factors, in particular: a new epidemiological situation created by resistance to chloroquine; a health service lacking in efficiency; inability to ensure basic health services (such as vaccinations); and an unfavourable economic situation. These factors are common to numerous countries in Sub-Saharan Africa and explain why many of them have experienced this health crisis, irrespective of whether or not they are stricken by the AIDS epidemic.

References

1. United Nations, Population division (2003). *World population prospects: The 2002 revision.* (New York: UN)

2. UNAIDS (2004). *Report on the global AIDS epidemic.* (Geneva, Switzerland: UNAIDS)

3. Hill, K., Pande, R., Mahy, M. & Jones, G. (1999). *Trends in child mortality in the developing world: 1960–1996.* (New York: UNICEF)

4. Hill, K. & Amouzou, A. (2006). Trends in Child Mortality, 1960 to 2000. (Chapter 3 in Jamison, D. et al. (Eds.), *Disease and Mortality in Sub-Saharan Africa.* Washington, DC: The World Bank)

5. Pison, G., Hill, K., Cohen, B. & Foote, K. (1995). *Population dynamics of Senegal.* (Washington: National Academy Press)

6. Cantrelle, P. et al. (1986). The profile of mortality and its determinants in Senegal, 1960–80. (In *Determinants of Mortality Change and Differentials in Developing Countries: The Five-Country Case Study Project* (pp. 86–116). New York: Population Studies n 94)

7. Garenne, M., Cantrelle, P. & Diop, I. L. (1985). Le cas du Sénégal. (In J. VALLIN et al. (Eds.), *La lutte contre la mort* (pp. 307–330). PUF, Paris: Cahier de l'ined)

8. WHO (2004). *Reported estimates of vaccine coverage.* Retrieved from http://www.who.int/vaccines/globalsummary/timeseries

9. Ndiaye, S., Sarr, I. & Ayad, M. (1988). *Enquête démographique et de santé au Sénégal 1986. Direction de la Statistique.* Demographic and Health Survey. (Columbia: Dakar and Westinghouse Institute for Resource Development)

10. Ndiaye, S., Diouf, P. D. & Ayad, M. (1994). *Enquête démographique et de santé au Sénégal (EDS-II) 1992–1993.* Direction de la Statistique. Demographic and Health Survey, (Calverton, Maryland: Dakar et Macro International)

11. Ndiaye, S., Ayad, M. & Gaye, A. (1997). Enquête démographique et de santé au Sénégal (EDS-III) 1997. Direction de la Statistique, Dakar et Macro International, Demographic and Health Survey, 238 p.

12. Desgrees du Lou, A. & Pison, G. (1996). The role of vaccination in the reduction of childhood mortality in Senegal. *Population An English Selection, 8,* 95–121

13. Pison, G., Trape, J. -F., Lefebvre, M. & Enel, C., (1993). Rapid decline in child mortality in a rural area of Senegal. *International Journal of Epidemiology*, *22*(1), 72–80

14. Pison, G., Desgrees du Lou, A., Langaney, A. (1997). Bandafassi: A 25 years prospective community study in rural Senegal (1970–1995). (In Das M. Gupta, et al. (Eds.). *Prospective community studies in developing countries* (pp. 253–275), Oxford: Clarendon Press)

15. Delaunay, V., Etard, J. F., Preziosi, M. P., Marra, A. & Simondon, F. (1992), (2001). Decline in infant and child mortality rates in rural Senegal over a 37-year period (1963–1999). *International Journal of Epidemiology*, 30, 1286–1293

16. Pison, G. (2005). Population observatories as sources of information on mortality in developing countries. *Demographic Research*, *13*(13), 301–334. Retrieved from http://www.demographic-research.org/Volumes/Vol13/13/

17. Enel, C., Pison, G. & Lefebvre, M. (1993). De l'accouchement traditionnel à l'accouchement moderne au Sénégal. *Cahiers Santé*, *3*, 441–446

18. Guyavarch, E. (2003). *Démographie et santé de la reproduction en Afrique sub-saharienne. Analyse des évolutions en cours*. Une étude de cas: l'observatoire de population de Bandafassi (Sénégal). (Paris: Thèse de doctorat, Muséum national d'histoire naturelle)

19. Garenne, M. & Fontaine, O. (1988). Enquête sur les causes probables de décès en milieu rural au Sénégal. (In J. Vallin, et al. (Eds.), *Mesure et analyse de la mortalité, nouvelles approches* (pp. 123–141). PUF, Paris: Cahier de l'ined n°119)

20. Desgrees du Lou, A., Pison, G., Samb, B. & Trape, J. F. (1996). L'évolution des causes de décès en Afrique : une étude de cas au Sénégal avec la méthode d'autopsie verbale. *Population*, *4*(5), 845–882

21. Pison, G., Langaney, A. (1985). The level and age pattern of mortality in Bandafassi (Eastern Senegal): Results from a small-scale and intensive multi-round survey. *Population Studies*, *39*(3), 387–405

22. Trape, J. -F., Pison, G., Preziosi, M. P., Enel, C., Desgrees du Lou, A., Samb, B., Lagarde, E., Molez, J. F., Simondon, F. (1998). Impact of chloroquine resistance on malaria mortality. *C.R Academy of Sciences Paris Sciences de la vie*, *321*, 689–697

23. Hill, A. (1989). La mortalité des enfants : niveau actuel et évolution depuis 1945. (In G. Pison, et al. (Eds.), *Mortalité et Société en Afrique* (pp. 13–34), PUF, Paris: Cahier de l'ined)

24. Sénégal (1970). Rapport de l'Enquête démographique nationale de 1970–71

25. Rutstein, S. O. (1984). *Infant and child mortality: Levels, trends and demographic differentials* (124 p). Comparative studies n 24, World Fertility Survey. (Voorburg, Netherlands: International Statistical Institute)

26. Sow, B., Ndiaye, S., Gaye, A. & Sylla, A. H. (2000). *Enquête sénégalaise sur les indicateurs de santé (ESIS) 1999*. Ministère de la santé, Groupe SERDHA and Demographic and Health Survey. (Calverton, Maryland: Macro International)

27. Claquin, P., Floury, B. & Garenne, M. (1987). Rapport d'évaluation de la couverture vaccinale des enfants de 12 à 23 mois en République du Sénégal au 1er juillet. Dakar, 76 p.

28. Evaluation du Programme élargi de vaccination (PEV) au Sénégal, juin 1990, OCCGE-Muraz, Bobo Dioulasso, 197 p.

29. Pison, G. & Desgrees du Lou, A. (1993) *Bandafassi (Sénégal). Niveaux et tendances démographiques 1971–1991*. Dossier et recherches n 40, (Paris: Institut National d'Etudes Démographiques)

30. Pison, G., Gabadinho, A. & Enel, C. (2001). *Mlomp (Sénégal): niveaux et tendances démographiques 1985–2000* (pp. 1–181). Dossiers et recherches, n 103. (Paris: Institut National d'Etudes Démographiques)

31. Duthé, G. & Pison, G. (2003). L'influence du contexte socioéconomique et sanitaire sur la mortalité. Le cas d'une région pauvre en milieu rural ouest africain. Communication présentée à la 4èmeConférence africaine sur la population, Tunis, 8–12 décembre 2003

32. Levi, P. & Adjamagbo, A. (2003). *Tableau de bord des principaux indicateurs socio-démographiques dans la zone de Niakhar au Sénégal.* Dakar: IRD. Retrieved from http://www.ird.sn/activites/niakhar/indicateurs/index.htm

CHAPTER 4. MALARIA, CLIMATE CHANGE AND POSSIBLE IMPACTS ON POPULATIONS IN AFRICA

ANDREW KARANJA GITHEKO

Climate and Human Health Research Unit, Kenya Medical Research Institute, Kisumu, Kenya

Abstract. The historical records for Africa show warming of approximately 0.7°C over most of the continent during the twentieth century. The Intergovernmental Panel on Climate Change (IPCC), in its Third Assessment Report (2001) recorded that global warming of 1.4 to 5.8°C can be expected over the coming century. Malaria is the most climate sensitive vector-borne disease, affecting most of the African population. Both global warming and increased climate variability can increase malaria transmission. It is the areas where transmission is currently low, such as the highlands, that are most affected. In these areas protective genetic polymorphisms are infrequent, and immunity levels are low so that all ages are vulnerable.

Introduction

Malaria is probably the most climate sensitive vector borne disease [1]; and currently Africa accounts for 90% of global malaria mortality [2, 3]. Malaria transmission depends on mosquito vectors, and their distribution depends on breeding habitat availability, suitability and productivity. Breeding habitat availability is related to hydrology, topography and precipitation, while their suitability is a function of the presence of plant and predator species. Productivity of the breeding habitat is a function of temperature. The rates of mosquito larval stage development, the adult female mosquito blood feeding frequency, and the speed of parasite development in adult mosquitoes are all temperature dependent and in some cases the relationship is exponential. Simply put, rainfall increases mosquito habitats while temperature increases the rate of mosquito and parasite development: the result is increased malaria transmission.

Small increases in temperature dramatically reduce the time it takes for the mosquito stages of the parasite to develop into infectious sporozoites. The average life span of a female *Anopheles gambiae* is about 21 days. It takes the malaria parasite 56 days to mature in the mosquito at 18°C, which is therefore longer than the average life span of the mosquitoes. At 22°C it takes only 19 days and at 30°C only 8 days (**Fig. 1**). The average temperatures in the East African highlands lie in the critical range of 18–22°C.

M. Caraël and J.R. Glynn (eds.), HIV, Resurgent Infections and Population Change in Africa, 67–77.

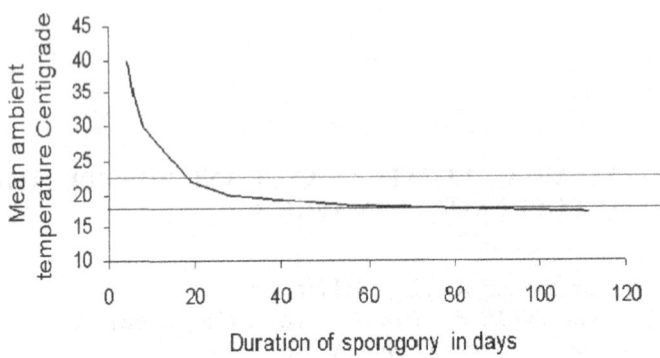

Fig. 1. The relationship between average ambient temperature and the time malaria parasites take to develop and become infectious in a female mosquito

Whereas malaria transmission is a function of vector density, disease outcome is a function of human immunity, depending on previous exposure and genetics. Malaria as a disease has a spectrum of pathologies ranging from asymptomatic infections to severe multi-organ and multi-system failure and death. The parasitological and clinical manifestations of malaria infections in a population are a function of transmission intensity and the duration of exposure. Severity of disease depends on the level of past exposure of individuals and populations. It depends on immunity due to repeated exposure over a lifetime, and genetically determined resistance due to natural selection following long-term population exposure. Climate changes exposing new populations and previously unexposed individuals to malaria therefore have major effects on disease incidence and severity.

Besides climate, the epidemiology of malaria is influenced by quality of health care, drug resistance, poverty, geographic location, land use and topography, among other factors. Land use changes following population expansion; and migration, such as deforestation, swamp reclamation and irrigation have created suitable breeding habitats and microclimates for *Anopheles gambiae*, the most efficient malaria vector in the world [4].

Here we examine the evidence for climate change and variability, its impacts on malaria morbidity and mortality in Africa, and how these vary depending on the underlying epidemiology of malaria in the area.

Malaria Epidemiology in Relation to Intensity and Duration of Exposure to Malaria

The level of malaria transmission is determined by the duration of and intensity of exposure to infections [5] (Table 1). In holo and hyper-endemic areas where transmission rates are very high, malaria mainly affects children under five years of age, with the greatest mortality occurring below the age of three years. Where transmission is less intense development of immunity is delayed and severe disease and mortality occurs in older children; and in areas of very unstable malaria (hypoendemic) all age groups are equally affected. In the highlands malaria epidemiology lies between meso and hypoendemic.

Table 1. Classifications of malaria endemicity as defined by spleen and parasite infection rates in children two to nine years old (except where otherwise specified) [5].

Classification	Spleen Rate (%)	Parasite Rate (%)
Holoendemic	> 75	>75 (in infants)
Hyperendemic	51–75	51–75
Mesoendemic	11–50	11–50
Hypoendemic	0–10	< 10

Malaria is a particular risk in pregnancy, particularly the first pregnancy, affecting both the mother and the foetus. Severe malaria-associated disease is more common in areas of low to moderate transmission such as the highlands of East Africa and other areas of seasonal transmission. In such areas severe disease in pregnant women has been associated with 20–30% maternal deaths and a high risk of spontaneous abortion, premature delivery and neonatal death [6]. An epidemic in Rwanda, at an altitude of 2300 m above sea level, in 1998 led to a four-fold increase in malaria admissions among pregnant women and a five-fold increase in maternal deaths due to malaria [7].

Certain gene polymorphisms such as sickle cell genotype and glucose-6-phosphate dehydrogenase (G6PD) deficiency confer protection against the severe form of malaria. Over time the frequency of these genotypes has increased in areas of intense transmission. For example in Western Kenya the prevalence of the sickle cell genotype was 26% in a malaria-holoendemic lowland area compared with 3% in an adjacent highland area. Similarly the prevalence of glucose-6-phosphate dehydrogenase deficiency was 7% in the lowlands and only 1% in the highlands [8]. Worldwide, more than 400 million people (90% being males) are affected by G6PD deficiency, in regions that are, or have been, endemic for malaria and in populations originating from these regions. Red blood cells with low G6PD activity offer a hostile environment to parasite growth and thus an advantage to G6PD deficiency carriers [9].

There are few molecular makers for immunity to malaria. However parasite density is a good indicator of a human population's level of immunity. Under very intense transmission in holoendemic areas the peak asexual parasite density is observed in children aged 6–11 months [10, 11]. At lower transmission rates the peak parasite density shifts to older children and in areas of unstable transmission parasite density may be equal across all age groups.

Studies have been undertaken across Africa to determine the relationship between all-cause mortality in children under five-years-old and estimates of malaria parasite prevalence [12]. It was observed that the unadjusted median mortality rates for children from birth to four-years-old living in areas with a parasitaemia prevalence of 25% was 13.7 per 1,000. This increased to 35.0‰ at a prevalence of 25–49‰ and 39.9% at a prevalence of 50–74%.

In areas of very low transmission intensity such as high altitudes, all age groups are susceptible to severe malaria. Under high transmission, severe malarial anaemia dominates and cerebral malaria is rare. As one moves towards lower transmission rates, cerebral malaria accounts for an increasingly large proportion of cases [13]. Malarial anaemia tends therefore to be relatively more important under high transmission settings and cerebral malaria tends to gain in importance under lower transmission settings. In a number of studies the total load of malaria morbidity, whether measured as non-severe malaria in the community or as severe malaria admitted to hospital, is low under stable low transmission conditions but is at its highest under moderate intensities [14]. In areas of low seasonal transmission, the prevalence of malaria infections is usually very low and the majority of people have no immunity to malaria. In these areas, during periods of hyper-transmission all ages are equally susceptible to infections and disease. At a high altitude of 2134 m, in Uasin Gishu district Western Kenya [15], no difference in re-infection rates between children and adults was found—an indication that malaria transmission was unstable at this high altitude. In the 1980s in the central highland plateau of Madagascar *Plasmodium falciparum* reemerged resulting in an overall parasite rate of 63.2%, which did not vary with age [16]. The full disease spectrum can be expected in all age groups in such a scenario.

Global Climate Change

Climate change includes a change in the mean meteorological parameters and a change in the frequency and amplitude of parameter variability. Climate change covers different aspects of climate, but we will here concentrate on the effects of global warming on malaria.

In 2001 the Intergovernmental Panel on Climate Change (IPCC), in its Third Assessment Report recorded that global warming of 1.4 to 5.8°C can be expected over the coming century [17]. Since the start of satellite records in 1979, both satellite and weather balloon measurements show that the global average surface temperature has increased significantly by +0.15 ± 0.05°C per decade. This difference occurs primarily over the tropical and sub-tropical regions [18]. The decade of the 1990s was the warmest recorded closely followed by the 1980s. According to the Climatic Research Unit and the UK Meteorology Office Hadley Centre the years 2003 and 2002 were the second warmest on record [19].

In addition to the general trend in warming, there has been substantial climate variability as a result of El Niños. The 1982–1983 El Niño event was classified as strong while that of 1997–1998 very strong. There were other weaker El Niño events in the early 1990s.

The General African Climate

The African climate is influenced by the Indian, Atlantic and Pacific oceans, the Mediterranean Sea, land cover, lakes and topography. The Inter-tropical Convergence Zone (ITCZ) primarily controls the main rainy seasons. While the tropical regions have two rainy seasons, the extreme north and south have only one distinct rainy season. The mean annual rainfall ranges from as low as 10 mm in the middle of the Sahara to more than 2000 mm in the tropical regions and other parts of West

Africa. Coefficients of rainfall variability are highest in the deserts and lowest in the wet tropical regions [20].

The African climate is generally warm (mean daily temperature >25°C); however, the extreme north and south regions experience some cooler weather (mean daily temperature <20°C). Similarly, while the low altitudes are warm, the higher altitudes are cool. The El Niño Southern Oscillation (ENSO) has a great influence on climate variability in Eastern and Southern Africa. These events are associated with floods and droughts [21]. Anomalous warming and precipitation particularly in the months of September, October and November in the Eastern African region follow this phenomenon.

Evidence of Climate Change in Africa

The most obvious and striking evidence of climate change in Africa has been the shrinking of glaciers on Mount Kilimanjaro, Mount Kenya and the Ruwenzori Mountains. In 1912 the glaciers of Mt Kilimanjaro measured 12 square kilometres; but in 1989 that figure was down to just 2.6 square kilometres—an 80% decrease [22]; while 92% of the Lewis Glacier, Mt. Kenya's largest glacier, has melted in the past 100 years [23]. In the Ruwenzori Mountains, since the 1990s the glacier area has decreased by about 75% [24]. The climatology of the African continent in the past century indicates that there have been two periods of warming; from the mid 1930s to 1940s and from the beginning of the 1980s to date [20]. The historical records for Africa show warming of approximately 0.7°C over most of the continent during the twentieth century and an increase in the frequency and intensity of climate variability [17].

Land use Change

The highlands of eastern and central Africa constitute about 23% of the total landmass of the region but house 51% of the population [25]. The highlands of these regions have a cool climate and until recently were free of intense malaria transmission. Due to their wet and cool climate they are agriculturally productive and human populations have thrived. The lack of malaria in the highlands was part of the reason why European farmers settled in the so-called White Highlands. For example the Boers who migrated from the Cape into the hinterland of Southern Africa in the mid-nineteenth century were successful largely because there was little malaria in the high veld [26].

As the population in the African highlands increases there is demand for more agricultural and settlement land. There are indications that forests and swamps are being converted to agricultural land, with a subsequent change in land cover and an increase in local temperature. For example, Afrane et al., (unpublished data 2005) showed that at a site in Western Kenya Highlands the houses in deforested areas were on average 1.7°C warmer than those in a forested area.

Malaria Epidemics and Climate Change

It is in areas where malaria transmission has been low or absent that climate change is expected to have its greatest effect. In these areas immunity is low in all age groups and the protective genetic polymorphisms are rare because there has been no selective pressure to maintain them in the population.

In Africa it has been estimated that the population at risk of epidemic malaria is 124.7 million. The 12.4 million cases of malaria per year due to epidemics result in an estimated 155,000–310,000 deaths, equivalent to 12–25% of annual worldwide malaria deaths [27].

About 17% of the total population in East Africa lives in highlands where there are risks of epidemics (Ameneshewa, personal communication). Climate change and variability affect the prevalence and distribution of malaria in the highlands of East Africa. It has been shown that 12–63% (mean = 36.1%) of the variance in the number of monthly malaria outpatients in a number of sites in the East African highlands is attributed to climate variability [28]. In Ethiopia it was shown that rainfall and minimum temperature could explain 85% of malaria incidence in areas of low and high transmission [29]; whereas in South Africa mean maximum daily temperature and rainfall were significantly associated with seasonal changes in malaria patient numbers [30]. In the highlands of western Kenya [31], it was found that epidemics occurred following anomalous monthly mean maximum temperatures just before and during the wet season. In a highland area of Rwanda malaria incidence increased by 337% in 1987, and 80% of this variation could be explained by rainfall and temperature [32]. A similar association has been reported in Zimbabwe [33].

Other epidemics in East Africa have largely been associated with El Niño. In the East African region El Niño events are characterized by heavy precipitation and anomalously warm seasons, which are associated with malaria outbreaks and epidemics [31, 34] (Fig. 2). Retrospective studies carried out on malaria in the highlands of Madagascar indicated strong correlations between the El Niño Southern Oscillation and both temperature ($r = 0.79$) and malaria ($r = 0.64$), suggesting that there might be an increased epidemic risk during post-Niño years [35]. During an El Niño in late 1987 malaria incidence in a high-altitude area in Rwanda increased by 337% over the three previous years; but the greatest impact was observed in children under two years of age, among whom incidence increased by 564% and case fatality rate by 501% [32]. Increased case fatality is associated with delayed treatment and/or drug failure. In Tanzania the risk of delivering a low birth weight baby in the first pregnancy in epidemic prone areas increased significantly approximately five months after a malaria epidemic caused by the 1997–1998 El Niño [36].

Malaria incidence in areas of unstable transmission is very sensitive to climate variability and can often result in epidemics[4]. During the great malaria epidemic in the highlands of Ethiopia (1,800 m), where the prevalence of parasitemia jumped from 3–12% to 40% during a period of El Niño (1958–1959), there was no significant difference in prevalence among the age groups. In many villages 50–75% of the village populations were sick with malaria and out of the estimated 3 million people affected 150,000 (5%) died [37].

It is to be expected that small changes in temperature and precipitation will support malaria epidemics at the current altitudinal and latitudinal limits of transmission[38].

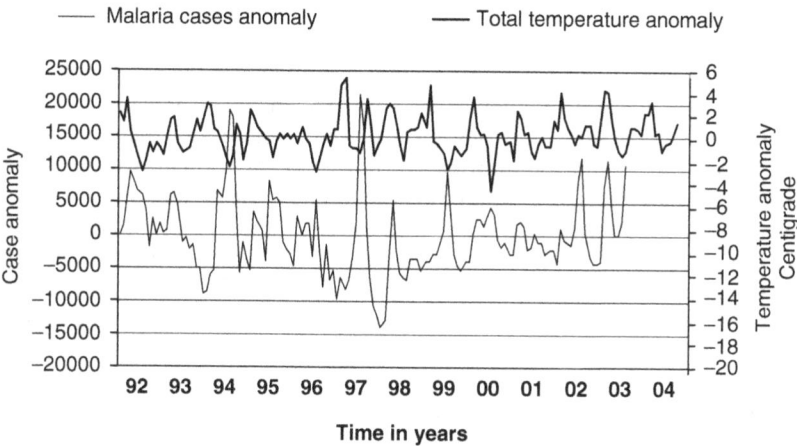

Fig. 2. Trends in temperature anomalies and in malaria case anomalies in the Kisii district in the highlands of Western Kenya (Merlin, Kenya 2003: unpublished data). Malaria infection prevalence in this area is about 10% (Githeko et al., unpublished 2005); and several epidemics have occurred in this area especially during El Niño episodes. For epidemics to occur, anomalously warm periods must coincide with rainfall periods. In 1998 the Kisii district was divided, so the data from 1999 onwards refer to a smaller area—hence the decrease in the number of malaria cases

Note. Anomalies are obtained by subtracting the long term mean of malaria and temperature data from the observed data. The anomaly is the value above or below the long-term mean

Rainfall in the Sahel/Guinea savannah fell by 20–30% from 1930–1950 to the present [39]. A greater than 80% fall in the prevalence of malaria has been observed in Northern Niger and Senegal from the early 1960s to 1990; and this has been linked to the disappearance of the major vector *Anopheles funestus* [40]. Flooding could facilitate breeding of malaria vectors and consequently malaria transmission in arid areas [41]; and this occurred in North Eastern Kenya during the 1997–1998 El Niño [42].

It has been shown in East Africa that malaria decreases with altitude. A rise in altitude of 154 m in humid areas is equivalent to a decrease in temperature of 1°C. In Tanzania the prevalence of malaria infections in the lowlands (200 m above sea level) is 79–90%, in the intermediate altitude (at 1,200 m above sea level) 27–46%, and in the highlands (1,700 m above sea level) 8–16% [43]. Thus an increase in temperature would change the prevalence of malaria in the highlands to that of lower altitudes. In the epidemic-prone highlands of East Africa anomalies in the mean monthly maximum of 2.2–4.5°C observed between January and March 1997 and 1.8–3.0°C in February–April 1998 were associated with 150–250 % increases in admissions for malaria treatment [44]. It has been projected using climate scenarios that there will be an estimated 5–7% increase (mainly altitudinal) in malaria distribution with surprisingly little increase in the latitudinal extents of the disease by 2100 [45].

Conclusions

Climate changes include both a change in the mean meteorological parameters and a change in the magnitude of departure from the mean. Whereas change in the mean temperature is a slow and long-term process, changes in the deviation from the mean can be large, abrupt, short lived, but frequent: climate variability is episodic. Although the effects of gradual warming in the African highlands may be slow enough to allow the human populations to develop immunity to malaria, climate variability such as the El Niño in East Africa and La Niña in Southern Africa can result in severe malaria epidemics resulting in high morbidity and mortality. In the 1990s when concerns arose in East Africa about malaria epidemics in the highlands, there were 4 El Niño events including the strongest El Niño on record [46].

In areas of moderate transmission such as the lower edge of the highlands, children less than nine years will be most affected. However as one moves to higher altitudes all age groups become victims. Pregnant women are particularly vulnerable during the first pregnancy. Even the unborn are victims of spontaneous abortions, which increase dramatically during epidemics.

It is worth noting that much of the controversy about climate change and increase in malaria transmission is due to the failure to distinguish between climate variability and climate change. Furthermore most scientists base their arguments on very coarse data such as mean monthly maximum temperature. Microclimate data need to be collected at much closer intervals (hourly) so as to detect changes occurring in mosquito breeding habitats and thus changes in malaria transmission. The most sensitive parameter, though rarely used, is degree–hour, which measures the total thermal energy in a microhabitat over time. There is a need to correlate microclimate data to the kinetics of blood digestion: the feeding frequency of mosquitoes and sporogonic development rates and aggregated data are not suitable for this type of analysis. This calls for a new level of sensitivity in assessing climate change and variability in relation to malaria transmission.

Acknowledgements

I am grateful for the access provided to me by Merlin Kenya to the malaria data from Kisii; and to the Kenya Agricultural Research Institute for the Meteorological Data. The assistance of Rosemary Owigar, an PhD student, is highly appreciated for organizing the meteorological data. This research is supported by the Kenya Medical Research Institute.

References

1. Githeko, A. K., Lindsay, S. W., Confalonieri, U. & Partz, J. (2000). Climate changes and Vector borne diseases: A regional analysis. *Bulletin of the World Health Organization*, 78, 1136–1147

2. Breman, J. G., Alilio, M. S. & Mills, A. (2004). Conquering the intolerable burden of malaria: What's new, what's needed: A summary. *American Journal of Tropical Medicine and Hygiene*, 71(Suppl 2), 1–15

3. D'Alessandro, U. & Buttiens, H. (2001). History and importance of antimalarial drug resistance. *Tropical Medicine and International Health, 11*, 845–848

4. Mouchet, J., Manguin, S., Sircoulon, J., Laventure, S., Faye, O., Onapa, A. W., Carnevale, P., Julvez, J. & Fontenille, D. (1998). Evolution of malaria in Africa for the past 40 years: Impact of climatic and human factors. *Journal of American Mosquito Control Association, 14*, 121–130

5. Molineaux, L. (1988). The epidemiology of human malaria as an explanation of its distribution including some implications for its control. (In W. H. Wernsdofer, & I. McGregor (Eds.), *Malaria. Principles and practice of malariology* (pp. 913–998). Edinburg: Churchill Livingstone)

6. Looareesuwan, S., White, N. J., Silamut, K., Phillips, R. E. & Warrell, D. A. (1987). Quinine and severe falciparum malaria in late pregnancy. *Acta Leiden, 55*, 115–120

7. Hammerich, A., Campbell, O. M. & Chandramohan, D. (2002). Unstable malaria transmission and maternal mortality: Experiences from Rwanda. *Tropical Medicine and International Health, 7*, 573–576

8. Moormann, A. M., Embury, P. E., Opondo, J., Sumba, O. P., Ouma, J. H., Kazura, J. W. & John, C. C. (2003). Frequencies of sickle cell trait and glucose-6-phosphate dehydrogenase deficiency differ in highland and nearby lowland malaria-endemic areas of Kenya. *Transactions of the Royal Society of Tropical Medicine and Hygiene, 97*, 513–514

9. Wajcman, H. & Galacteros, F. (2004). Glucose 6-phosphate dehydrogenase deficiency: A protection against malaria and a risk for hemolytic accidents. *Comptes Rendus Biologies, 327*, 711–720

10. Githeko, A. K., Brandling-Bennett, A. D., Beier, M., Atieli, F., Owaga, M. & Collins, F. H. (1992). The reservoir of *Plasmodium falciparum* malaria in a holoendemic area of western Kenya. *Transactions of the Royal Society of Tropical Medicine and Hygiene, 86*, 355–358

11. Bloland, P. B., Boriga, D. A., Ruebush, T. K., McCormick, J. B., Roberts, J. M., Oloo, A. J., Hawley, W., Lal, A., Nahlen, B. & Campbell, C. C. (1999). Longitudinal cohort study of the epidemiology of malaria infections in an area of intense malaria transmission II. Descriptive epidemiology of malaria infection and disease among children. *American Journal of Tropical Medicine Hygiene, 60*, 641–648

12. Snow, R. W., Korenromp, E. L. & Gouws, E. (2004). Pediatric mortality in Africa: *Plasmodium falciparum* malaria as a cause or risk? *American Journal of Tropical Medicine and Hygiene, 71*(Suppl 2), 16–24

13. Snow, R. W. & Marsh, K. (2002). The consequences of reducing transmission of *Plasmodium falciparum* in Africa. *Advances in Parasitology, 52*, 235–264

14. Tanser, F. C., Sharp, B. & le Sueur, D. (2003). Potential effect of climate change on malaria transmission in Africa. *The Lancet, 362*, 1792–1798

15. Marsh, K. & Snow, R. W. (1999). Malaria transmission and morbidity. *Parassitologia, 41*, 241–246

16. John, C. C., Koech, D. K., Sumba, P. O. & Ouma, J. H. (2004). Risk of Plasmodium falciparum infection during a malaria epidemic in highland Kenya, 1997. *Acta Tropica, 92*, 55–61

17. Lepers, J. P., Deloron, P., Andriamagatiana-Rason, M. D., Ramanamirija, J. A., & Coulanges, P. (1990). Newly transmitted *Plasmodium falciparum* malaria in the central highland plateaux of Madagascar: Assessment of clinical impact in a rural community. *Bulletin of the World Health Organization, 68*, 217–222

18. Intergovernmental Panel on Climate Change (IPCC) (2001a). Climate Change. In J. J. McCarthy, O. Canzianni, N. Leary, D. J. Dokken, & K. S. White (Eds.), *Third Assessment Report, Impacts, Adaptations and Vulnerability of Climate Change* (pp. 1023). Cambridge: University Press)

19. Intergovernmental Panel on Climate Change (1PCC) (2001b). Summary for Policy Makers. Working Group 1. Retrieved from http://www.ipcc.ch/pub/spm22-01.pdf

20. Climate Research Unit, UK. Retrieved from http://www.cru.uea.ac.uk/cru/info/ukweather/

21. Intergovernmental Panel on Climate Change (IPCC) special report (1998). Regional impacts of climate change: An assessment of vulnerability (pp. 517). (In R. T. Watson, M. C. Zinyowera, R. H. Moss & D. J. Dokken (Eds.), Cambridge: Cambridge University Press)

22. Nicholson, S. E. & Kim, J. (1997). The relationship of the Southern Oscillation to African rainfall. *International Journal of Climatology, 17*, 117–135

23. Hastenrath, S. & Greischar, L. (1997). Glacier recession on Kilimanjaro, East Africa, 1912–1989. *Journal of Glaciology, 43*, 455–459

24. Hastenrath, S. & Kruss, P. D. (1992). The dramatic retreat of Mount Kenya's glaciers between 1963 and 1987: Greenhouse forcing. *Annals of Glaciology, 16*, 127–133

25. Kaser, G. (1999). A review of the modern fluctuations of tropical glaciers. *Global and Planetary Change, 22*, 93–103

26. ACACIA retrieved from http://web.idrc.ca/en/ev-8082-201-1-DO_TOPIC.html

27. Githeko, A. K. & Clive, S. (2005). The history of malaria control in Africa: Lessons learned and future perspectives. (In K. J. Ebi, J. Smith, & I. Burton (Eds.). *Integration of public health with adaptation to climate change: Lessons learned and new directions*. London: Talyor & Francis)

28. Worrall, E., Rietveld, A. & Delacollette, C. (2004). The burden of malaria epidemics and cost-effectiveness of interventions in epidemic situations in Africa. *American Journal of Tropical Medicine and Hygiene, 71*(Suppl 2), 136–140

29. Zhou, G., Minakawa, N., Githeko, A. K., & Yan, G. (2004). Association between climate variability and malaria epidemics in the East African highlands. *Proceeding of the National Academy of Sciences, 101*(8), 2375–2380

30. Abeku, T. A., De Vlas, S. J., Borsboom, G. J., Tadege, A., Gebreyesus, Y., Gebreyohannes, H., Alamirew, D., Seifu, A., Nagelkerke, N. J. & Habbema, J. D. (2004). Effects of meteorological factors on epidemic malaria in Ethiopia: A statistical modelling approach based on theoretical reasoning. *Parasitology, 128*, 585–593

31. Craig, M. H., Kleinschmidt, I., Nawn, J. B., Le Sueur, D. & Sharp, B. L. (2004). Exploring 30 years of malaria case data in KwaZulu-Natal, South Africa: Part I. The impact of climatic factors. *Tropical Medicine and International Health, 9*, 1247–1257

32. Githeko, A. K., & Ndegwa, W. (2001). Predicting malaria epidemics using climate data in Kenyan highlands: A tool for decision makers. *Global Change and Human Health, 2*, 54–63

33. Loevinsohn, M. E. (1994). Climate warming and increased malaria in Rwanda. *The Lancet, 343*, 714–748

34. Freeman, T. & Bradley, M. (1996). Temperature is predictive of severe malaria years in Ziambabwe. *Transactions of the Royal Society of Tropical Medicine and Hygiene, 90*, 232

35. Kovats, R. S., Bouma, M. J., Hajat, S., Worrall, E. & Haines, A. (2003). El Nino and health. *The Lancet, 362*, 1481–1489

36. Bouma, M. J. (2003). Methodological problems and amendments to demonstrate effects of temperature on the epidemiology of malaria. A new perspective on the highland epidemics in Madagascar, 1972–89. *Transactions of the Royal Society of Tropical Medicine and Hygiene, 97*, 133–139

37. Uddenfeldt Wort, U., Hastings, I. M., Carlstedt, A., Mutabingwa, T. & Brabin, B. J. (2004). Impact of El Nino and malaria on birth weight in two areas of Tanzania with different malaria transmission patterns. *International Journal of Epidemiology, 33*, 1311–1319

38. Fontaine, R. S. Najjar, A. & Prince, J. S. (1961). The 1958 malaria epidemic in Ethiopia. *American Journal of Tropical Medicine and Hygiene, 10*, 795–803

39. Lindsay, S. W. & Martens, W. J. M. (1998). Malaria in the African highlands: Past, present and the future. *Bulletin of the World Health Organization, 76*, 33–45

40. Thomson, M. C., Connor, S. J., Ward, N. & Molyneux, D. (2004). Impact of climate variability on infectious disease in West Africa. *EcoHealth Journal, 1*, 138–150

41. Warsame, M., Wernsdofer, W. H., Huldt, G. & Bjorkman, A. (1995). An epidemic of *Plasmodium falciparum* malaria in Balcad Somalia, and its causation. *Transactions of the Royal Society of Tropical Medicine and Hygiene, 98*, 142–145

42. Connor, S. J., Thomson, M. C. & Molyneux, D. H. (1999) Forecasting and prevention of epidemic malaria: New perspectives on an old problem. *Parassitologia, 41*, 439–448

43. Lusingu, J. P., Vestergaard, L. S., Mmbando, B. P., Drakeley, C. J., Jones, C., Akida, J., Savaeli, Z. X., Kitua, A. Y., Lemnge, M. M. & Theander, T. G. (2004). Malaria morbidity and immunity among residents of villages with different *Plasmodium falciparum* transmission intensity in North-Eastern Tanzania. *Malaria Journal, 3*, 26–37

44. AIACC Project AF91 retrieved from http://www.aiaccproject.org/publications_reports/AIACC_Links_to_UNFCCC_NC.pdf

45. Tanser, F. C., Sharp, B. & le Sueur, D. (2003). Potential effect of climate change on malaria transmission in Africa. *The Lancet, 362*(9398), 1792–1798

46. STORMFAX retrieved from http://www.stormfax.com/lanina.htm#Table

CHAPTER 5. ECONOMIC CRISIS AND CHANGES IN MORTALITY DUE TO INFECTIOUS AND PARASITIC DISEASES IN ANTANANARIVO, MADAGASCAR

DOMINIQUE WALTISPERGER AND FRANCE MESLÉ
Research Unit, Population and Development,
Institut National d'Etudes Démographiques (INED), Paris, France

Abstract. Madagascar was severely affected by the economic crisis that hit sub-Saharan Africa in the 1980s. The crisis, exacerbated by a high degree of political instability, led to food shortages in the mid-1980s. The impact on mortality is not well known, owing to a lack of statistics for the whole island. Systematic analysis of the registers of the Municipal Hygiene Office (Bureau municipal d'hygiène: BMH) in Antananarivo is used to show the trend of mortality by cause in the capital since 1976. The food crisis substantially reduced life expectancy, which did not return to its 1976 level until 2000. Nutritional deficiencies and infectious diseases played a prominent role in the reduction in life expectancy. Mortality due to nutritional deficiencies fell as soon as the food supply improved, but mortality due to infectious diseases remains high, particularly among males aged 10–50, who are also particularly vulnerable to the increase in man-made diseases, including road accidents and alcoholism.

Introduction

Since independence (1960), the standard of living in Madagascar has steadily deteriorated. This socio-economic decline has been punctuated by political upheavals that have accelerated the process. Poor economic results have prompted leaders to embark on several structural adjustments, which eventually led to a severe food shortage that reached its height in the mid-1980s. An analysis of the death registers for the capital, Antananarivo, is used to evaluate the impact of the crisis on mortality [1, 2]. The role of infectious diseases and nutritional deficiencies is preponderant. However, since the mortality peak in 1986, at the height of the food shortage, infections have continued in recent years to contribute strongly to mortality, particularly among young adult males. After giving a brief overview of the economic and political context of the past 30 years, we analyse the trend in mortality by cause in Antananarivo to evaluate the role of different infectious and parasitic diseases, before looking more closely at two age groups: children aged 1–5, and adolescents and adults aged 10–50.

M. Caraël and J.R. Glynn (eds.), HIV, Resurgent Infections and Population Change in Africa, 79–99.
© Springer Science + Business Media B.V. 2008

Background

The declining standard of living in Madagascar is an extreme manifestation of the economic crisis that had a major impact on developing countries, particularly in Africa, in the 1980s. After the oil shocks of 1973–1974 and 1979, economic growth slowed sharply in industrialised countries. Public expenditure was cut and interest rates rose. Hastened by the increasing use of synthetic products, demand for commodities—the bulk of developing countries' exports—fell. Prices of non-oil commodities collapsed at the beginning of the 1980s, before rising again in 1984. Meanwhile, flows of official development assistance (ODA) stagnated between 1980 and 1984 [3].

The economic recession in developed countries had a disastrous impact on developing countries, which are highly dependent on the most advanced economies. Jacques de Larosière [4] estimated that a 1% decline in GDP growth in developed countries caused a 3% decline in developing countries. In developing countries, while average GDP growth was 3% p.a. between 1976 and 1980, it was negative between 1981 and 1985: −1.1% for a sample of 83 developing countries [3]. For one-fifth of those countries the total decline in GDP between 1980 and 1985 exceeded 20%.

A decline in GDP leads to higher unemployment and therefore lower household income. Women are forced to seek supplementary employment. Children are uncared for or abandoned. The slowdown in production pushes consumer prices up and therefore real wages down, which is particularly dramatic when wages are already low. The number of people living below the poverty line inevitably swells. Public spending is insufficient to counter this impoverishment. The result is a reduction in food rations, immunisation coverage and attendance at schools and health care.

There is a synergy between poor health care, poor hygiene and nutritional deficiencies [5]. Malnutrition weakens the immune system and leaves the body vulnerable to pathogenic infections that reduce appetite and/or, particularly with diarrhoea, cause loss of nutrients. In 1990–1992, 20% of the population of developing countries was deficient in the key micronutrients (iodine, vitamin A and iron); in sub-Saharan Africa the prevalence was 41% [5]. The situation has improved in Asia and Latin America, but has stagnated in Africa. In Mozambique, near Madagascar, 63% of the population is malnourished. Anaemia is common, due to malaria and to low consumption of animal products. Meat and milk are not eaten regularly but reserved for ceremonial occasions. In Madagascar per capita GDP fell by more than 30% in the space of 25 years [6]. Since 1995, the situation seems to have improved, but per capita income is still very low (**Fig. 1**). The governments in power in Madagascar in the 1970s and 1980s worsened the situation by introducing economic measures that exacerbated the crisis.

In 1972, after a student revolt and a general strike, Madagascar's president, Philibert Tsiranana, who had been in power since independence, was forced to resign. A transitional military government took over, followed by Didier Ratsiraka in 1975. The processing and marketing of rice were nationalised. Between 1975 and 1982, the price for rice paid to farmers fell by 25% while investments went mainly to industry.

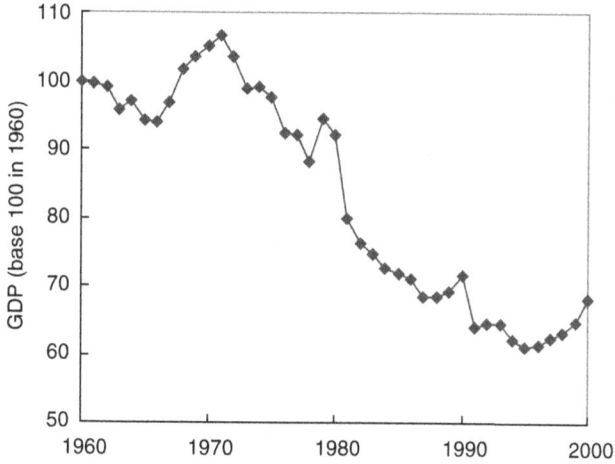

Fig. 1. Per capita gross domestic product (GDP) (in constant USD) in Madagascar since 1960

The policy undermined farmers' motivation and worsened the food shortage. In 1982 the situation was so bad that the government had to appeal to donors and introduced a structural adjustment programme, paving the way for the liberalisation of the farm sector. The state system that fixed the price of rice (85 Malagasy francs per kilogram at the beginning of 1985) coexisted with a black market where prices were much higher (200 Malagasy francs in August 1985). In 1985 the price paid to farmers was maintained, but caps on consumer prices were lifted. When the stocks collected by the state ran out in September, rice prices on the private market surged to more than 500 Malagasy francs per kilogram of rice by the end of the year [7]. The severe food shortage (and the sale of spoiled produce) reached its height in 1986. From 1986 onwards, nationalised companies were privatised and the production system reorganised. A buffer stock was created to cushion the impact of cyclical shortages. The state withdrew from commercial and financial activities in 1996.

Antananarivo, the capital of Madagascar, was not spared by the food crisis. Rice consumption fell by 20% between 1982–1983 and 1986–1987 [8]. The black market, which supplied 10 kg of rice per capita per year in the early 1980s, accounted for more than 50 kg four years later [9]. The increase in mortality was particularly acute in the capital. Before and after the food crisis of the mid-1980s, infant and child mortality in Antananarivo was significantly lower than in the country as a whole. However, this advantage almost completely disappeared in 1985 (**Fig. 2**). During the crisis period, although mortality rose nationwide, the increase was sharpest in the capital, closing the gap between Antananarivo and the rest of the country.

Mortality estimates for Antananarivo could be skewed by an inaccurate estimate of the city's population due to internal migration that may have taken place during the crisis. Unfortunately, apart from the two population censuses conducted in 1975 and

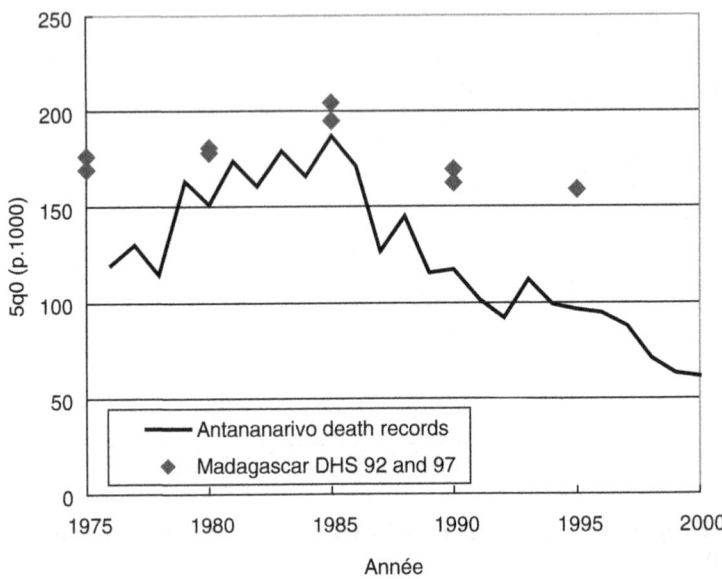

Fig. 2. Trend of the share of infant and child mortality
Source: [10, 11]; authors' calculations based on death records for Antananarivo

1993, there are no statistics available about such migration. However, large migratory flows into or out of the capital are unlikely to have occurred. Transport was so disorganised that travel was extremely difficult. Furthermore, such migration would have primarily concerned particular age groups, especially young workers. Overestimating or underestimating those age groups would have generated significant bias in mortality curves, but this is not the case. At most, the curves show a few random irregularities [2].

Database of Deaths in Antananarivo

The impact of the crisis on mortality is not easy to assess. There are no reliable, continuous data on mortality and causes of death for the country as a whole. Demographic and Health Surveys only make it possible to estimate infant and child mortality, and not even continuously. However, a recent project in Antananarivo has made it possible to gather information on deaths in the capital. Information from the Bureau municipal d'hygiène (BMH) death registers has been entered into a database to show the trend of mortality by cause since 1975. The quality of the data collected has been discussed in several previous publications [12, 2]. After a brief overview of the database, this paper will discuss its reliability.

The project, which was initiated in 1993 by Pierre Cantrelle, uses information from the BMH, which records deaths that occur in the city. The registers have been kept in their current form since 1975. The information in the registers consists of 14 items:

- death register number
- date of birth of the deceased
- sex of the deceased
- residential status of the deceased (resident or non-resident of Antananarivo)
- *fokontany* (district) of residence of the deceased if in Antananarivo
- *fivondronana* (*département*) of residence of the deceased if not a resident of Antananarivo
- date of death
- time of death
- date on which the death was notified
- place of death
- primary cause of death
- associated or external cause of death (in the case of an injury)
- occupation of the deceased or of the deceased's parents
- relationship of the person notifying to the deceased

All the information from the registers since 1976 has been entered into the database. In Antananarivo, it is almost impossible to bury someone without a burial permit. Cemetries are guarded and relatives must declare deaths to the BMH to obtain a burial permit. The infant and child mortality rates obtained from the database are comparable to those in the 1992 and 1997 DHS [1], which indicates good coverage of deaths by the registers. Furthermore, information on age at death improved over the period: in 1976, 55% of ages at death were known exactly. In 2000, the proportion was 80% [2]. On average there are 7500 deaths a year in a population of just over one million inhabitants.

In most cases, a doctor certifies the cause of death: a hospital doctor if the death occurred in hospital or a BMH doctor if the death occurred at home. All causes of death are coded by the same Malagasy doctor, Osée Ralijaona, according to the International Classification of Diseases, Ninth Revision (ICD-9), recommended by the WHO [13]. The accuracy of the diagnosis varies over the period, but the share of unknown or poorly defined causes never exceeds 20%, and for most years oscillates between 11% and 13% [2]. Beyond the specific problem with ill-defined causes, the diagnostic accuracy is not the same for all conditions. Some of them, such as accidents, maternal deaths or measles are easy to identify, while other diseases are more difficult to diagnose when there is no biological confirmation. This is especially the case for malaria, but also for tuberculosis. Consequently the diagnosis is probably more accurate for deaths which occur at the hospital.

The detailed causes are organised into eight main groups of causes, within which the main infectious and parasitic diseases are recorded separately (**Table 1**). Note that in this chapter we use "infectious diseases" to refer to the first group of diseases shown in the table, unless specifically stated otherwise. Many of the respiratory diseases and some of the others also have infectious origins.

To calculate mortality rates for five-year age groups, deaths were related to annual populations. Madagascar conducted its last two censuses in 1975 and 1993 [14, 15]. Given the lack of data on births and migration, annual populations were calculated

Table 1. Groups of causes of death used and corresponding codes from the International Classification of Diseases, Ninth Revision (ICD-9).

Cause of death	ICD-9 codes, detailed list
Infectious and parasitic diseases	001–139
Infectious intestinal diseases	*001–009*
Tuberculosis	*010–018*
Measles	*055*
Malaria	*084*
Other infectious and parasitic diseases	*020–139 (except 055, 084)*
Respiratory diseases	460–519
Pneumonia, bronchopneumonia, influenza, acute respiratory infection	*480–487*
Other respiratory diseases	*460–479, 488–519*
Nutritional deficiencies	260–269
Tumours	140–239
Diseases of the nervous system	290–379
Cardio-vascular diseases	390–459
Diseases of the digestive system	520–579
Other diseases	240–259, 270–389, 580–779
Maternal deaths	*630–679*
Injuries	800–999

by interpolating age-sex specific population data for Antananarivo for the years between 1975 and 1993 and by extrapolating those figures for the years 1994 to 2000 based on the same rate of increase. This type of estimate does not make it possible to take into account major fluctuations in migration. However, if there had been major migration flows, the annual age-specific mortality rates would show significant irregularities, particularly at the ages traditionally most likely to migrate, namely young adults. This was not found: the mortality curves obtained are fairly regular, with only a few random irregularities. These mortality curves were therefore simply smoothed[1] after age ten by referring to the United Nations model life tables [16, 17]. Cause-specific mortality rates were then calculated by applying the distribution of the various causes of death to the adjusted mortality rates for all causes for each age group. Standardised mortality rates were then calculated on the basis of the population structure from the 1993 census.

Impact of the Crisis on Mortality

Previous studies have demonstrated the extent of the health crisis that occurred concomitantly with the economic crisis [1, 2]. This paper includes the main findings of those studies, focusing specifically on the impact of the crisis on infectious disease mortality.

---

[1] The smoothing method used is based on a linear regression applied to survivors (logits(lx)) aged 15 and over. Mortality before age ten has not been adjusted. For more details, see [2].

Overview

Between 1976 and 1986, life expectancy in Antananarivo fell by 13 years for males and by 8 years for females. In 1986, average life expectancy was only 44.7 years for males and 53.0 years for females. After rising fairly rapidly in the late 1980s, life expectancy gains slowed, especially for males. In 2000, males had only just recovered the life expectancy level of 1976 and females had exceeded it by slightly more than two years (**Fig. 3**).

The Excess Mortality Due to the Crisis Varies with Age and Cause

A comparison of mortality rates during the crisis years (1984–1988) with a previous period (1976–1978) shows an increase in mortality that affected all ages, but to varying degrees (**Fig. 4**).

Infants aged under one year were the least affected during the famine years, probably because of breast-feeding and immunisation programmes conducted in the early 1980s. By contrast, mortality increased by more than 50% between ages one and four; and the most dramatically between ages five and nine. Mortality in the later age group increased by 2.5 times for boys and by almost 3 times for girls. Children in that age group, between early childhood and adolescence, are probably less protected by mothers than very young children and less able than older children to find food for themselves.

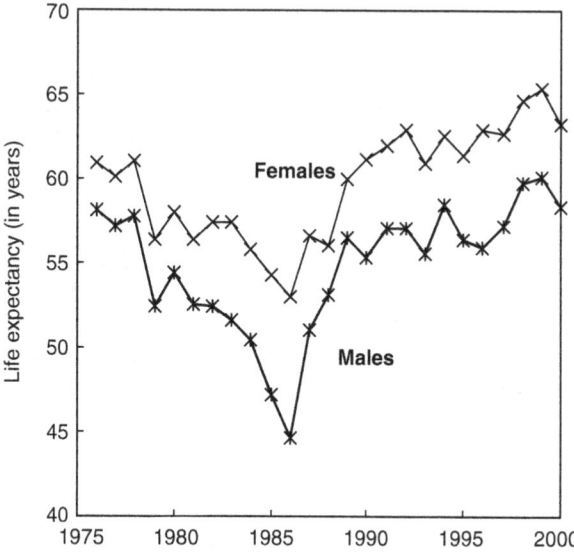

Fig. 3. Life expectancy at birth by sex. Antananarivo, 1976–2000

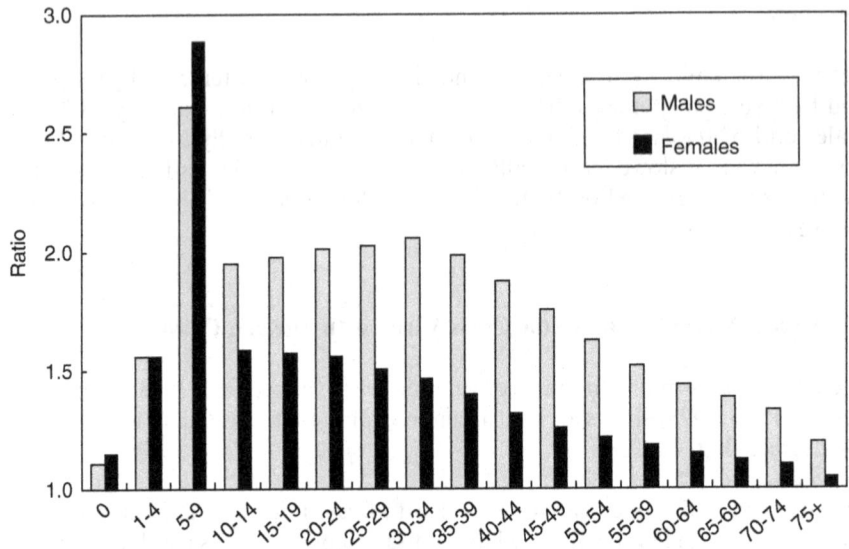

Fig. 4. Ratio of age-specific mortality between 1984–1988 and 1976–1978, Antananarivo

From age ten onwards, the effects of the crisis on female mortality decreased steadily with age. This is not the case for males, for whom the excess mortality due to the crisis remains very high—at around a two-fold increase—between ages ten and 40. Surprisingly, young men appear particularly vulnerable to crisis. After age 40, excess female mortality gradually disappears, but increased male mortality remains until the oldest ages.

The increase in mortality during the crisis varies with cause of death. Between 1976–1978 and 1984–1988, the most dramatic increase was in mortality due to nutritional deficiencies, which was multiplied by 4.5 among males and by 3.2 among females (**Fig. 5**).

Infectious and respiratory diseases were the next most sensitive to the crisis. Mortality due to infectious diseases was multiplied by almost 2 for males and by 1.6 for females, and mortality due to respiratory diseases was multiplied by 1.8 and 1.4 respectively. The crisis had a much smaller impact on the other main groups of causes of death, for most of which mortality increased moderately for males and remained stable for females.

Life Expectancy Changes by Age and Cause

The mortality ratios in the previous paragraphs are shown independently of mortality levels, and the causes or age groups for which mortality increased the most in relative terms are not necessarily those that account for the biggest change in life expectancy. To break down the change in life expectancy, it is preferable to determine the positive

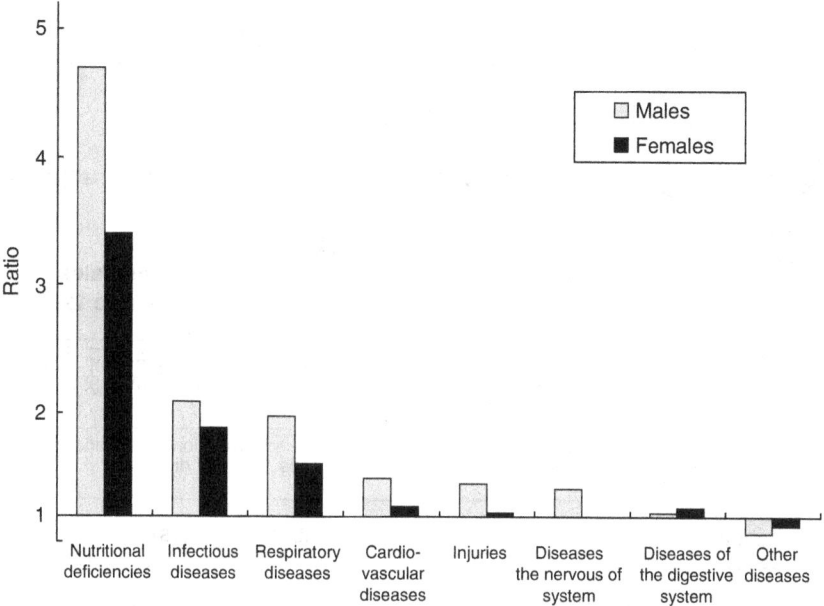

Fig. 5. Ratio of cause-specific mortality ratios between 1984–1988 and 1976–1978, Antananarivo

or negative contribution of each cause to life expectancy by age.[2] **Fig. 6** illustrates the contribution of each cause during the two periods.

Between 1976–1978 and 1984–1988, infectious diseases and nutritional deficiencies predominate in the decline in life expectancy, with the biggest impact due to infectious diseases, which cost males 3.5 years of life expectancy and females 2.7 years, compared with 2.5 and 1.8 years respectively for nutritional deficiencies. Mortality due to those two causes alone accounts for more than 70% of the fall in male life expectancy and for 80% of the decline in female life expectancy. Among males, the increase in mortality due to respiratory diseases also played a significant role, causing a decline of 1.5 years. For both sexes, the rise in mortality between ages one and four alone was responsible for a decrease of 2.0 years in male life expectancy and 2.2 years in female life expectancy, mainly generated by higher mortality due to nutritional deficiencies and infectious diseases. Conversely, the increase in mortality between ages five and nine only reduced life expectancy by 0.5 years because the extremely high relative mortality observed at those ages during the crisis (**Fig. 4**) was acting on a fairly low background risk of death, which reduces its impact on overall life expectancy. At adult ages, the crisis had a smaller effect on female mortality. By contrast, it had a very clear impact on male mortality, with men, like the youngest children, mainly succumbing to infectious diseases and nutritional deficiencies.

---

[2] We have used the algorithm suggested recently by Evgueni Andreev and his co-authors [18].

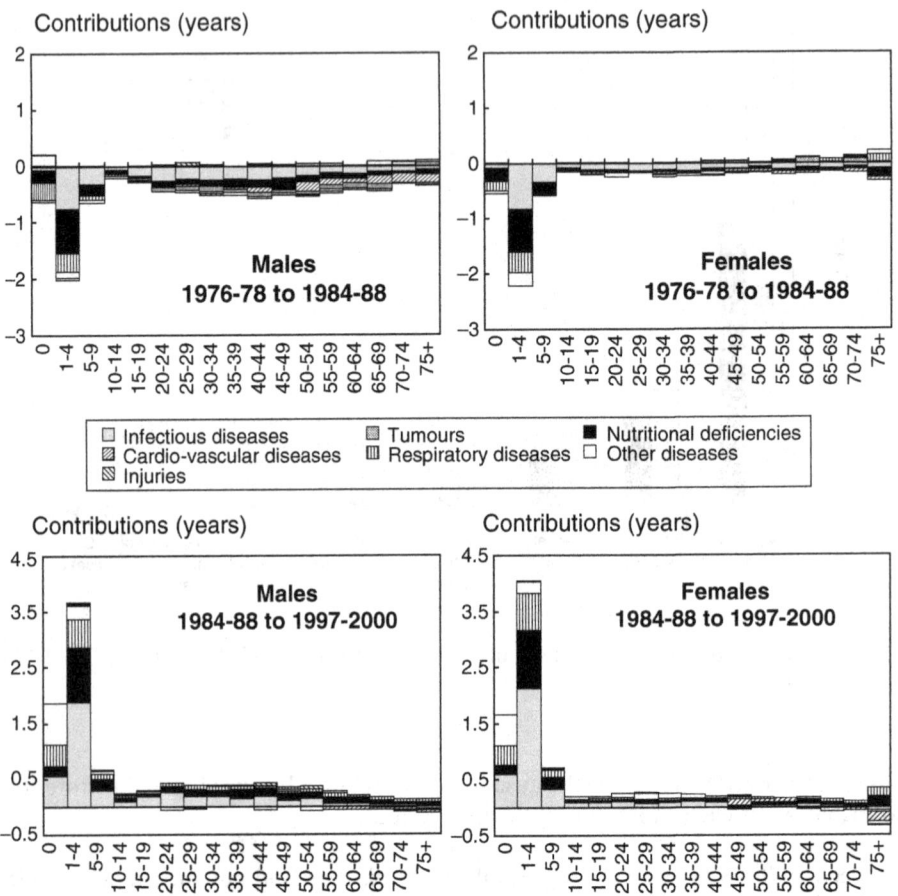

Fig. 6. Age-specific contributions of the main causes of death to changes in life expectancy between 1976–1978 and 1984–1988 and between 1984–1988 and 1997–2000
Source: [2]

The table reverses completely in the second period, with a drop in mortality for all ages and all causes, for both males and females. The decrease in mortality between ages one and four makes the biggest contribution to life expectancy, with a gain of 3.7 years for males and 4.0 years for females. That gain can be attributed mainly to the decline in mortality due to nutritional deficiencies and infectious diseases, including respiratory diseases.

Infant mortality was also reduced considerably by the decrease in the same three causes and in "other diseases", a group dominated at that age by perinatal diseases and congenital disorders. This was not simply a recovery after the severe crisis of the mid-1980s: children aged under five appear to have benefited from health programmes, which mainly targeted infectious diseases, implemented in the past two decades. This is particularly true for children aged under 1, who suffered less than older children from nutritional deprivation and who were the primary beneficiaries of health programmes.

Conversely, after age five, the gains are very small and just offset the losses in the previous period. Only adult women in Antananarivo attained a lower mortality rate than 20 years earlier. There is no sign of any fundamental improvement in health.

Infection: Trends Vary with Disease and Age

At all ages, the trend in mortality due to infectious diseases therefore played a key role in changes in life expectancy. However, the category "infectious diseases" covers various diseases, and the trend of each disease warrants more detailed examination. This is presented below, focusing on two age groups: children aged one–four, for whom the changes in mortality had a major impact on life expectancy, and males aged 10–49, who were the worst affected by the food shortage.

At Ages One–Four, Intestinal and Respiratory Diseases Predominate

Among young children, regardless of the period under consideration, infectious diseases are the primary cause of mortality (**Fig. 7**). However, the crisis clearly reduced the share of infectious diseases in total mortality. In 1976–1978, infectious diseases accounted for more than half of mortality. During the crisis, despite a large increase in total mortality, the share of infectious diseases fell below 50% because of the sharp rise in mortality due to nutritional deficiencies, whose share of total mortality rose from less than 20% to more than 25% in 1984–1986. As living conditions improved, and especially since the health programmes introduced after measles and malaria epidemics, infectious diseases declined faster than other causes of death, to below 40% in the last period. However, the crisis of the mid-1980s did not radically alter the ranking of causes of death for either boys or girls. At those ages, nutritional deficiencies were already the second cause of death in the mid-1970s and remained so at the end of the 1990s. Respiratory diseases are the third cause of death. The category "respiratory diseases" mainly consists of infectious diseases, such as pneumonia and acute infections of the upper respiratory tract, which further raises the share of infectious diseases in mortality at those ages.

For a more accurate estimate of the share of mortality due to infectious diseases, infectious respiratory diseases should be added to the traditional childhood infectious diseases included in the first group of causes of death. That has been done in **Fig. 8**, which shows annual mortality trends at ages one–four across all causes and due to infectious diseases (including respiratory diseases). The parallel between the two trends is striking: the increase in mortality among young children until 1985–1986 can be attributed to the increase in mortality due to infectious diseases, and the considerable decline in mortality at ages one–four in the 1990s is ascribable to the decrease in infectious diseases. **Fig. 8** shows the steady increase in mortality due to infectious diseases since the end of the 1970s, in line with the deterioration in the economic situation. Mortality due to infectious diseases then fluctuated at a very high level in the 1980s, but at those ages mortality in 1986 was not higher than in previous years.

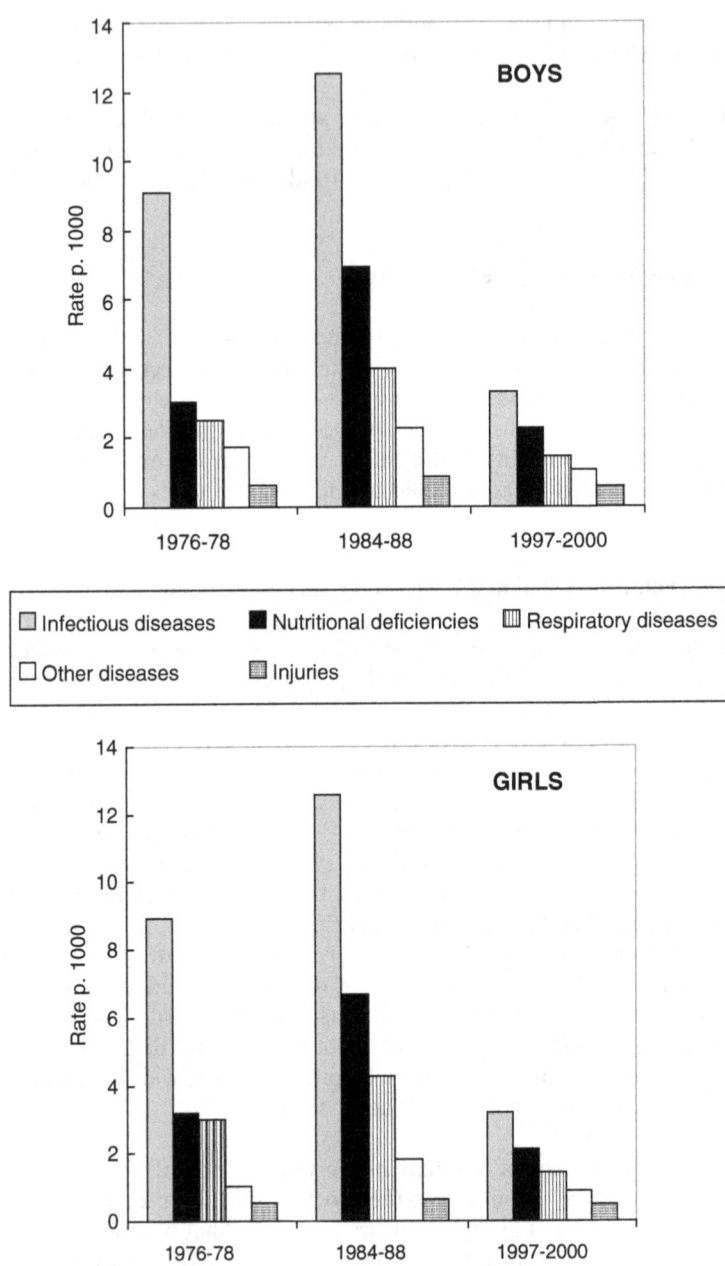

Fig. 7. Mortality rates at ages one–four for the main causes of death during 3 periods: 1976–1978, 1984–1988 and 1997–2000

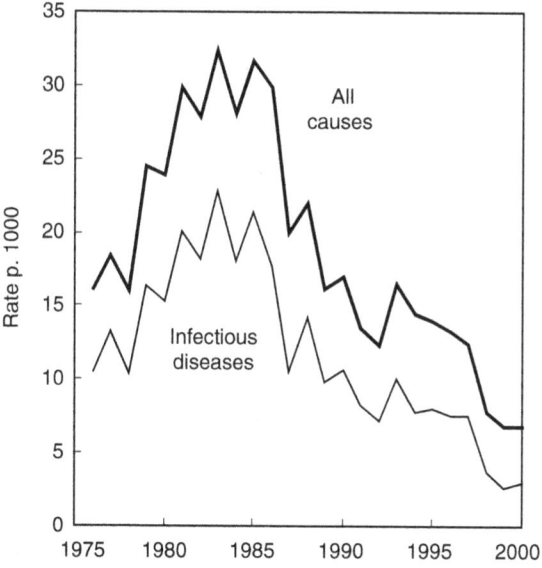

Fig. 8. Annual mortality rates across all causes and due to infectious diseases (including respiratory diseases) at ages one to four, both sexes

The mortality trend for the whole group of infectious diseases conceals different disease-specific trends (**Fig. 9**). Throughout the period, infectious intestinal diseases, especially diarrhoea, had the biggest impact: mortality peaked in 1986 at the height of the food crisis, before falling fairly quickly in 2000 to seven times lower than the 1976 level.

Until 1985, measles was the second-biggest killer among infectious diseases. Children's poor nutritional status coupled with insufficient immunisation coverage contributed to fatalities due to measles. In 1983, during a severe epidemic, measles caused almost one death in four among children aged one–four. That epidemic was followed by three other outbreaks (in 1985, 1988 and 1993) of decreasing severity. Extended vaccination programmes conducted in 1985 and 1987–1991 brought the situation under control. Since 1995, measles appears to be on the way to being eradicated.

Pneumonia, influenza and other acute infectious respiratory diseases were the third cause of death due to infectious diseases at the beginning of the period. Mortality due to infectious respiratory diseases began to increase at the beginning of the 1980s, before the crisis reached its peak, and began to decline in 1986, falling more sharply from 1995 onwards. In the most recent years, however, mortality due to infectious respiratory diseases has been rising slightly.

Compared with those three major groups of infectious diseases, mortality due to malaria has little impact on that age group. However, the trend is worrying.

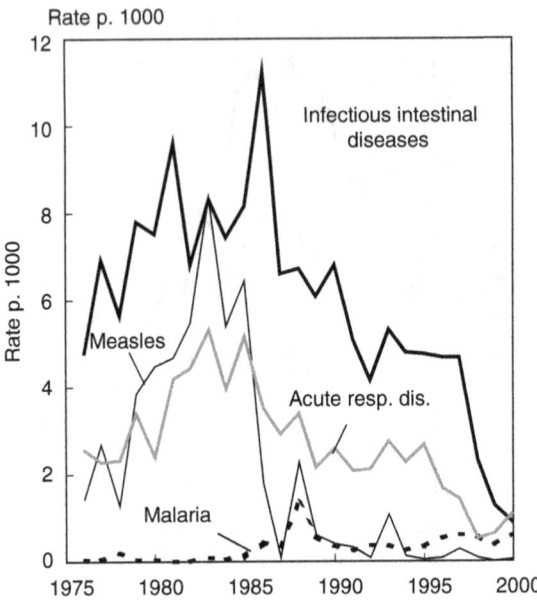

Fig. 9. Annual mortality due to the main infectious diseases at ages one to four, both sexes

Considered under control at the beginning of the 1970s, malaria reappeared in 1985. In 1988, a major epidemic broke out. In that year, more than 6% of deaths in that age group were due to malaria. Measures taken at the time (malaria programme in 1988–1997) halted the epidemic, but malaria was still endemic in the 1990s, and mortality remains significant.

At ages one–four, diarrhoea was the only infectious disease for which mortality was highest in 1986. For other diseases, mortality was highest in the early 1980s. It is likely that the increase in those diseases weakened children's immunity, making them more vulnerable to the food crisis of 1986. In that year, most deaths were attributed to nutritional deficiencies alone, which would not have caused as many deaths if children's general state of health had been better. This is an example of the synergy between malnutrition and infection, which, by mutually facilitating each other, cause a sharper deterioration in the population's state of health. However, the recent decline in mortality due to infectious diseases among young children holds out the hope that the vicious circle has been broken.

At Ages 10–49, Infectious Diseases Re-Emerge

The state of health of people aged 10–49 is altogether different. Among both males and females, the crisis altered the ranking of causes of death for many years **(Fig. 10)**. The share of infectious diseases, which accounted for only 15% of mortality in

1976–1978, more than doubled in 1984–1988 (33%), and, was still very high in 1997–2000, at just below 30%. Despite a sharp decline in the 1990s, mortality due to the group of infectious diseases still has not returned to its level of the 1970s and remains the leading cause of death among males and the second cause of death among females, just behind cardio-vascular disease. At the height of the crisis, mortality due to nutritional deficiencies increased dramatically, but fell again just as quickly. Conversely, among males, in recent years an increase in diseases of the nervous system, probably related to an increase in alcoholism has been observed. Between 1976 and 2000, mortality due to mental disorders and alcoholism increased more than fourfold for males aged 10–49. After the acute effects of the crisis, young men appear to have had difficulty coping, with the gradual deterioration of their health related to an increase in man-made and degenerative diseases, and have been unable to reduce the impact of infectious diseases.

As demonstrated in the previous section, after age ten, males suffered much more from the crisis than females. This is particularly true of mortality due to infectious and parasitic diseases (**Fig. 11**). Among males, we observe a very high mortality peak in 1986 at the height of the food crisis. Among females, infectious disease mortality also increased in that year, but did not peak until two years later.

Different infectious diseases have a different effect in men and women. Excess male mortality during the crisis period was particularly high for infectious intestinal diseases. In 1986, mortality due to those diseases was three times higher for males than for females (**Fig. 12**). Male mortality due to infectious intestinal diseases rose sharply again in 1995–1996 during another food shortage, caused by Cyclone Geralda. That second flare-up confirmed the greater vulnerability of males during subsistence crises. At the end of the 1990s, mortality due to infectious intestinal diseases increased again, this time for both sexes, probably due to the effect of the cholera epidemic that has been rife for several years in the north of the country.

The contrast between the sexes is even more striking with respect to mortality due to tuberculosis. Among males mortality due to tuberculosis began rising in 1984 and peaked in the next two years, before declining rapidly in the late 1980s. During the 1990s, however, mortality began slowly but steadily increasing again. The crisis had less impact on female mortality due to tuberculosis. By contrast, in recent years, the trend is just as unfavourable as for males. A tuberculosis programme introduced in 1994 has not yet curbed the insidious spread of the disease. The persistence of tuberculosis may be partly linked to the spread of HIV, but this cannot be the only explanation, since the prevalence of HIV is still below 2% in Madagascar (1.1 % among pregnant women in 2004 [19]).

Mortality due to respiratory infections (pneumonia, influenza and upper respiratory tract infections) also increased more for males than for females during the time of food restriction, in a similar trend to tuberculosis. In the most recent years, however, the trend for those respiratory infections has been much more favourable, and they are gradually decreasing.

At adult ages, malaria is the only cause of death that affects males and females in equal measure. The peak in mortality due to malaria in 1988 was at the same level

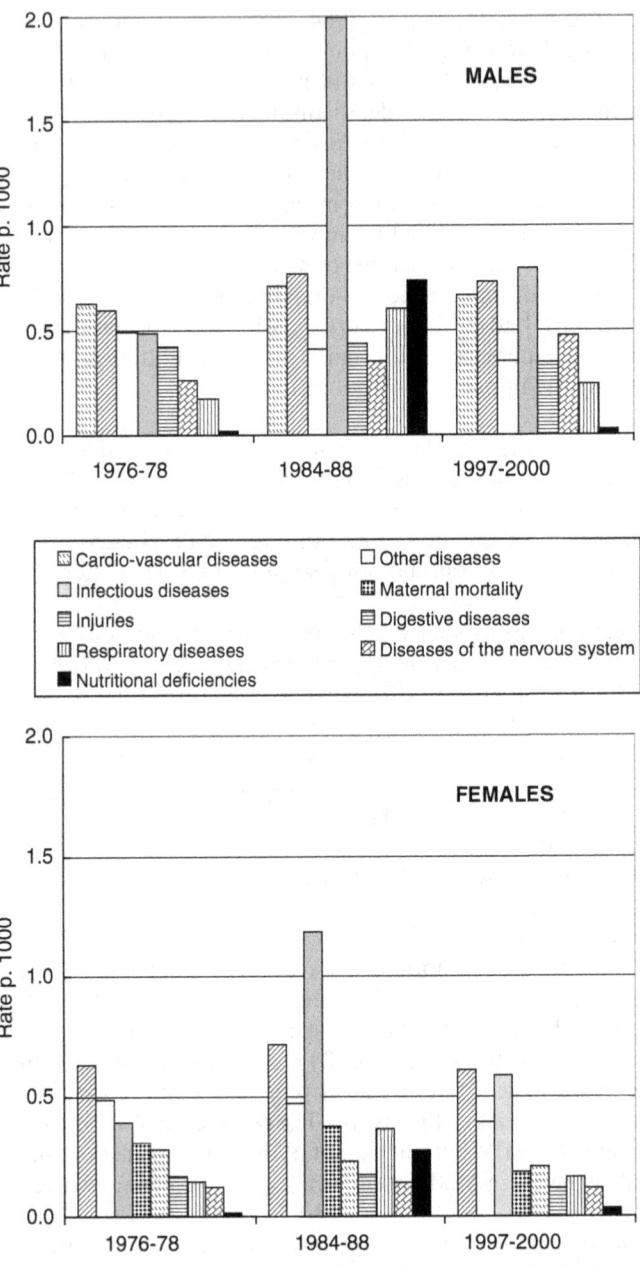

Fig. 10. Comparative mortality rates at ages 10–49 for the main causes of death during three periods: 1976–1978, 1984–1988 and 1997–2000 (Causes are ranked in 1976–78 order which is different for males and females)

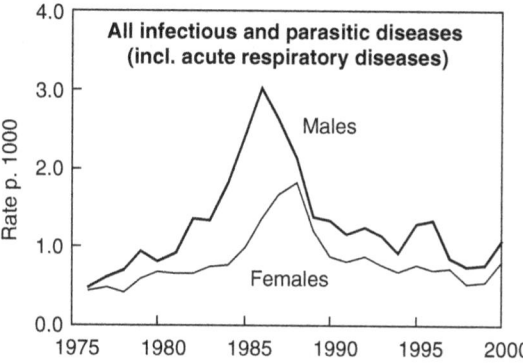

Fig. 11. Sex-specific annual mortality due to infectious diseases (including acute respiratory diseases) at ages 10–49

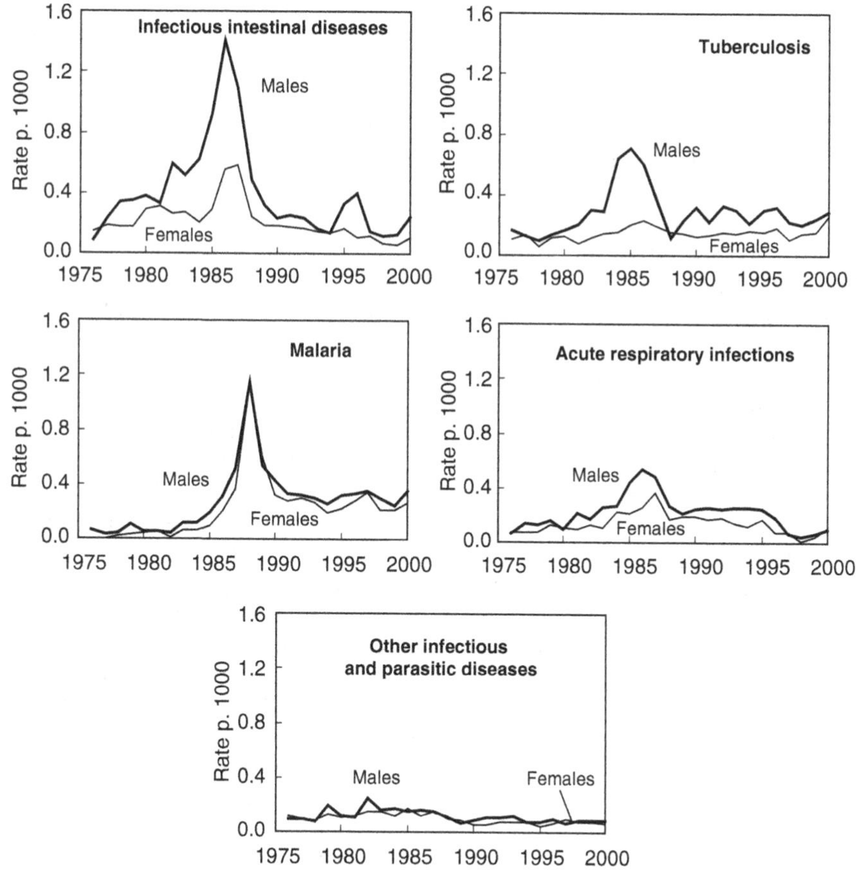

Fig. 12. Sex-specific annual mortality due to the main infectious diseases, at ages 10–49

for both sexes. The peak in female mortality due to infectious diseases observed in 1988 can be attributed to this sharp increase in malaria. In the following years, mortality due to malaria returned to a less alarming level, without however returning to the level of the first years of observation. Since 1995, mortality due to malaria has remained fairly constant, but much higher than in the 1970s.

Conclusion

Between 1976 and the beginning of the 1990s, the socio-economic situation in Madagascar deteriorated almost continuously, simultaneously with a health crisis that, in the space of ten years (1976–1986), reduced life expectancy at birth for residents of Antananarivo by approximately ten years. Since 1990, although the economic situation has not really recovered, its harmful effects on health have diminished, probably as a result of the implementation of health programmes, the formation of a buffer stock of rice ready for distribution in case of shortage, and the lifting of import taxes on food products when there are shortages.

Across all ages, mortality due to infectious and parasitic diseases increased until the mid-1980s, peaking at the height of the food crisis. It was not until the early 1990s that mortality due to those diseases returned to its original level (1976), before declining further. As the coding of the cause of death was undertaken by the same medical doctor for the whole period, these trends cannot be related to changes in coding practice. It is of course possible that according to the period some causes of death were more likely to be notified. For example, when shortage was at its maximum, the link to nutritional starvation was perhaps more frequent than in a period of larger food availability. This could result in some underestimation of infectious disease mortality during the crisis but does not fundamentally question the observed trends.

An examination of age-specific trends shows an almost across-the-board reduction in childhood diseases, apart from the peak during the crisis. This decline began in the 1970s for whooping cough, but is more recent for respiratory infections, diarrhoea and measles. The downward trend in childhood diseases reflects the effectiveness of health programmes: measles immunisation campaign in 1985, stepped up in 1987–1991; diarrhoeal disease programme (IEC campaigns on breastfeeding, oral rehydration therapies) implemented in 1988–1989. In Antananarivo drinkable water is available for a large part of the population. The water supply system, in place for several decades, was not jeopardized during the crisis. The water quality which is often a decisive determinant in infectious diseases, especially diarrhoea, is probably not a key factor in this specific context. The decrease in mortality due to diarrhoeal disease does not necessarily indicate a reduction in the frequency of diarrhoea, but that diarrhoea is less often fatal. According to the 1997 DHS [11], 28% of children aged under three in the capital had had at least one episode of diarrhoea in the fortnight prior to the survey.

By contrast, health programmes have proved less effective against malaria and tuberculosis, particularly among young adults. Action (chloroquine distribution in schools and public places, home insecticide spraying), against malaria from 1988 to 1997 and action against tuberculosis (prevention and therapy programmes) conducted from 1987 to 1991 and in 1994 succeeded in averting severe epidemics, such as those observed previously.

In 1962, WHO experts considered that malarial infection had been eradicated in the highlands [20]. Insecticide treatment, epidemiological monitoring and distribution of chloroquine were discontinued. When the disease reappeared in the mid-1980s, dispensaries lacked anti-malarial products and the population's purchasing power made them unaffordable anyway. As a result, the 1988 epidemic caused a great many deaths.

With regard to tuberculosis, immunisation coverage is satisfactory for children in the capital (96% in 1997 according to the DHS) [11], but not for older cohorts that did not benefit from the extended vaccination programme in their infancy. Given the overcrowding in the capital (more than three people per room on average, according to the 1993 census) tuberculosis could have devastating effects on the adult population. although it is potentially treatable and not too expensive [21].

There has been a similar lack of action on other respiratory infections. Famine-induced lower immunity probably accounted for the increase in mortality due to respiratory diseases in the 1980s. The environment also fosters the development of respiratory diseases. A recent study [22] showed that 85% of urban households use firewood for heating and daily cooking. Most homes do not have chimneys (smoke exits via the windows), which exposes household members to almost constant smoke inhalation. No education campaign has ever been conducted on this issue. In any case, without active assistance from the public authorities, households cannot afford to replace firewood with alternative fuels.

Even if they make a smaller contribution to mortality, many other infectious diseases continue to cause deaths in Madagascar. The cholera epidemic that broke out in the northwest of the island in 1999 is probably responsible for the increase in mortality due to infectious intestinal diseases in the past few years. Despite quarantining, the first cases of cholera in children in the capital were observed in a hospital between April and July 1999 [23]. Plague is still present. It had disappeared completely from the capital in the mid-1960s, but reappeared in 1979 in the poorest districts [24]. Since the early 1990s, between 50 and 100 suspected cases have been reported annually. In 1996, 147 suspected cases of plague were reported [25]. AIDS is also a threat, even if the prevalence of HIV is still low (less than 2%) [19, 26].

Poor nutritional status, endemic in Antananarivo, makes the population vulnerable to outbreaks of inadequately controlled infectious diseases and to the re-emergence of diseases that were thought to have disappeared. During the worst starvation years, the impact was especially important for children between one and ten and for young male adults. The male excess mortality is not specific to the Malagasy situation. It was also described by Kari Pitkänen during the Finnish Great Famine. He suggested that men might suffer from a biological disadvantage which makes them less resistant to infectious diseases at the same time as having very poor working conditions. The same phenomenon was observed during the famines which sucessively affected the Berat region in India in 1896–97 and 1899–1900 [27].

In Antananarivo, the reason for the male excess mortality from nutritional deficiencies during the starvation period remains unclear. It appears that this excess mortality goes with a higher male mortality due to tuberculosis, other infectious respiratory diseases, infectious digestive diseases and injuries (including suicide). It is not known if men are more severely starved or if they are less resistant to starvation. Two assumptions can be made. First male activities which are usually more physical, require more calories and will produce a more rapid energy consumption for the same amount of food intake. Second, women who are bearing children may benefit from a nutritional priority, even during a period of crisis. Health programs run by NGOs give a systematic priority to mothers and children. This is apparent from statistical data collected, for example by DHS surveys: the nutritional status of children and women is measured, but not that of adult men.

What is sure is that, whatever the sex considered, even if progress resumed in the 1990s, the battle against infectious diseases will never be won unless the economic situation improves enough to provide the population with adequate food.

References

1. Michel, G., Waltisperger, D., Cantrelle, P. & Ralijaona, O. (2002). The demographic impact of a mild famine in an African city: The case of Antananarivo, 1985–7. (In T. Dyson & C. O Grada (Eds.), *Famine demography. Perspectives from the past and present* (pp. 204–217). Oxford: Oxford University Press)

2. Dominique, W. & France, M. (2005). Economic crisis and mortality. The case of Antananarivo, 1976–2000. *Population-E, 60*(3), 199–230

3. UNDIESA (1996). *World Economic Survey 1986.* (New York: United Nations)

4. De Larosière, J.. (1986). Address before the Economic and Social Council of the United Nations, 4 July 1986. (Washington, DC: IMF)

5. Michael, L. (2001). *Nutrition in developing countries.* (Rome: FAO)

6. World Bank (2001). *World development indicators on CD-ROM.* (Washington, DC: World Bank).

7. Paul. D. A., et al. (1990). *Macroeconomic adjustment and the poor. The case of Madagascar* (Monograph 9). Cornell Food and Nutrition Policy Program. (Ithaca, New York: Cornell University)

8. World Bank (1989). Poverty Alleviation in Madagascar. *Country Assessment and Policy Issues.* (Washington, DC: World Bank)

9. Rachel, R. & Roubaud, F. (1996). La dynamique de la consommation dans l'agglomération d'Antananarivo sur longue période (1960–1995) et les stratégies d'adaptation des ménages face à la crise. *Economie de Madagascar, 1*(October), 9–39

10. Centre National de Recherche sur l'Environnement (1992). *Madagascar 1992, enquête nationale démographique et sanitaire.* (Antananarivo/Calverton: CNRE/Macro International)

11. Institut national de la Statistique. Direction de la démographie et des statistiques sociales (1998). *Enquête démographique et de santé, Madagascar, 1997.* (Calverton: Macro International)

12. Dominique, W., Cantrelle, P. & Ralijaona, O. (1998). *La mortalité à Antananarivo de 1984 à 1995.* Documents and Manuels du CEPED, n° 7. (Paris: CEPED)

13. World Health Organisation (1977). *World health manual of the international statistical classification of diseases, injuries, and causes of death, 1975.* (Geneva: WHO)

14. Institut National de la Statistique et de la Recherche Economique (1980). *Recensement général de la population et des habitats 1975. Données démographiques milieu urbain.* Antananarivo

15. Institut national de la Statistique (1997). Direction de la démographie et des statistiques sociales. *Recensement général de la population et de l'habitat, août 1993. Rapport d'analyse, Etat de la population.* Vol. II, tome 1. Antananarivo

16. United Nations (1982). *Model Life Tables for Developing Countries.* (New York: Department of International Economic and Social Affairs)

17. *MORTPAK-LITE* (1988). The United Nations software package for mortality measurement. Interactive software for the IBM-PC and compatibles. Population studies, 104. (New York: United Nations, Department of International Economic and Social Affairs)

18. Evgueni, A., Shkolnikov, V. & Begun A. Z. (2002). Algorithm for decomposition of differences between aggregate demographic measures and its application to life expectancies, healthy life expectancies, parity-progression ratios and total fertility rates. *Demographic Research, 7,* 500–521

19. UNAIDS (2004) *AIDS epidemic update. December 2004.* Geneva: WHO)

20. Jean, M., et al. (1997). La reconquête des Hautes Terres de Madagascar par le paludisme. *Bulletin de la société de pathologie exotique, 90*

21. World Health Organisation (2001). *Progress in TB control in high-burden countries, 2001. Global DOTS expansion plan* (pp. 181–183). (Geneva: WHO)

22. Rabevohitra, F. (2001). *Impacts de l'utilisation des combustibles en bois and de la pollution atmosphérique à l'intérieur des maisons sur la santé à Madagascar.* Bako Nirina, July 2001

23. Raobijaona, H., et al. (1999). Premiers cas de choléra observés chez l'enfant à l'Hôpital général de Befelatana, Centre hospitalier universitaire d'Antananarivo. *Archives Institut Pasteur Madagascar,* 65(2), 71–74

24. Coulange, P. (1989). Situation de la Peste à Tananarive (de son apparition en 1921 à sa résurgence en 1979). *Archives Institut Pasteur Madagascar, 56,* 9–35

25. Ratsifasoamanana, L., et al. (1998). La peste: maladie réémergente à Madagascar. *Achives Institut Pasteur Madagascar, 64,* 12–14

26. UNAIDS/World Health Organisation (2004). *Report on the Global AIDS Epidemic, 2004.* (Geneva: WHO)

27. Tim, D. & O Grada, C. (Eds.) (2002). Introduction. (In *Famine Demography. Perspectives from the Past and Present.* Oxford: Oxford University Press)

CHAPTER 6. ECONOMIC AND ETHICAL ASPECTS OF CONTROLLING INFECTIOUS DISEASES

JOSEPH BRUNET-JAILLY

Institut de Recherche pour le Développement, Paris, France

Abstract. Controlling infectious diseases is expensive and decisions have to be made on how to spend the money. Cost effectiveness analysis provides a rational basis for making these decisions, even if the present state of the art in this domain does not escape criticism. A presentation of the methods currently available, of the results they have produced, and of the criticisms they deserve, is followed by a discussion of the economic and ethical justifications of adopting a cost-effectiveness approach. This approach is then illustrated by an application to the choice of the best strategy to face up to the HIV/AIDS and tuberculosis epidemics.

Introduction

Beyond the claim of the "right to health", often heard in the North, or of "health for all", a slogan popularised in the South, it is evident that controlling all diseases would require huge sums of money, much larger than those actually earmarked for it. It is also clear that societies as well as individuals want to meet other needs as well as health. Therefore, every attempt to control disease should be based on decisions made using the best available instruments. The available instruments fit into various categories: macroeconomic models incorporating health status variables for the labour force [1, pp. 190–195], [2, 3]; expanded national income estimates incorporating a (willingness-to-pay based) value for mortality reduction [4, 5]; cost-benefit comparisons allowing determination of the most beneficial use of additional resources [6]; and cost-effectiveness ranking assessing the consequences of different allocations (within the health system) of resources to the varied and multiple health interventions proposed by professionals. We will focus on this last method.

In the absence of a systematic and strict use of the best knowledge available in the field, and of the best available instruments, the evolution and results of the health system are entirely dependent upon supply dynamics. As a profit-making industry, the health system uses every opportunity to exploit a new product, a new market or a new production technology [7]. The technological change and the asymmetry of information between physicians and patients push towards expanding the supply of services and goods which are all supposed to prevent diseases or control them. With no assessment of the

M. Caraël and J.R. Glynn (eds.), HIV, Resurgent Infections and Population Change in Africa, 101–119.
© Springer Science + Business Media B.V. 2008

results obtained, the production of specific goods and services is endlessly growing, and exhibits economic rent, i.e. income originating in market inequities, for example in the discretionary power of health professionals to induce demand, as illustrated by the loose fit of health performance to health expenditure [8, pp. 40–44]. The market logic of this endless expansion is at the origin of the creation of inequalities by the supply of care itself: more attention is given to health problems arising among rich countries and patients, and other illnesses are neglected or "orphaned" [9, 10].

The question is not simply one of advocating more money to control diseases. Rather there are sensitive issues of prioritisation. The economic consequences of diseases, particularly the cost of treatment (and sometimes of prevention itself) and moreover the gap between what could technically be done and what could socially and economically be achieved, raise issues of choice, resource allocation among beneficiaries, and therefore selection of beneficiaries. These are the issues which will be addressed here.

As we shall see, considering two important cases, in some instances at least the most solid knowledge is surprisingly ignored. The two examples that we consider are the case of a recent deadly epidemic (HIV/AIDS), and that of a re-emerging disease (tuberculosis). In both cases, we will seek to make use of the best quantitative work, and see what is done with it, in practice. But, for an adequate understanding of the situation of the poorer countries, it is useful to begin with a few rough estimates.

Infectious Diseases in the Global Burden of Disease

Assessments of the global disease burden [11, 12] stem from the seminal idea that each illness or accident induces a given number of years of life lost, be it because of premature death (effect on mortality) or because of a temporary or permanent reduction of the capacity to lead a normal life (effect on morbidity). The simplest measure is the disability adjusted life years (DALY); other measures have been proposed and are also of use. Their relative merits are discussed in detail elsewhere (see the most accurate criticism in [13]; see also [14, 15] and an extensive discussion in [16]). Criticisms of DALYs include the following: 1) the main problem with this measure is its static character: health expectancies are calculated for a period (i.e. using current observed event rates), not for a cohort (that would allow for varying prevalence rates), as would be needed to account for large epidemics; 2) the estimates imply the choice of a target, the best expected survivorship, against which to compare the current conditions and their change; the target is, in practice, of an arbitrary nature (the maximum expectancy of life at birth for Japanese women in the early nineties); 3) the relative value of the various health-states has to be defined, and a choice has to be made between the valuation given by individuals, their relatives, the general public, or health care providers, for example, and between different valuation methods; 4) the method uses a valuation of health states at different ages, and the ethical ground of such an age-weighting has been questioned; 5) there is no built-in concern for equity in the DALY calculation.

Despite its approximate nature, the global burden of disease approach is preferred because it offers the only usable yardstick for comparing the combined impact of various diseases on mortality and morbidity, and of the various health interventions on these endpoints. It assembles the best information needed to make more rational public health choices. The competing approaches, notably cost-benefit analysis, use much more debatable monetary values of human life [6], or they adopt highly theoretical [3] or macro-economic formalizations [4, 5], that cannot help the decision-making process. In the global burden of disease approach, the arbitrary target is equivalent to an equity weight giving higher value to a year gained in a country where life expectancy at a given age is below standard [17, p. 5]; time discounting, giving higher value to a DALY gained in the immediate future than to one gained in a more distant future, allows the method to take into account the trade-off between health activities benefiting present vs. future generations [17, p. 3], [18, pp. 668–670]; age-weighting is a means of incorporating currently accepted judgements about the relative priority to be given to each age-group [18, p. 667], [19, p. 18]. Ethical arguments are inescapable [20] and of an intrinsically debatable nature: for example, not all ethicists consider that a handicapped patient should, when treated for a disease unrelated to the handicap, take priority over any other patient [13, p. 700]. Minimizing the DALYs probably is not what people consider in their everyday life decisions, but if we only want to ground collective strategies on individual decisions, the solution would be either to rely on market values, or to generate norms using surveys of representative samples of the population [17, p. 6], [20, p. 632].

Therefore, we use the disease burden framework. In this analytical framework, what burden do the infectious diseases have? [21]

Infectious diseases account for over half the total burden of disease in poor countries with high mortality rates (**Fig. 1**). In particular, they cause over 13 million deaths each year, and account for one out of every two children's deaths. In addition, a small number of infectious diseases are responsible for 90% of deaths: pneumonia, AIDS, diarrhoea, tuberculosis, malaria, and measles [24, pp. 3–4].

More specifically, HIV/AIDS alone accounts for one quarter of the burden in countries of the African region with the highest mortality rates, and 8% in the other (low mortality) African region; tuberculosis 2 and 3% respectively, malaria 9 and 12% respectively [24]. In sub-Saharan Africa, an estimated three million people became newly infected with HIV in 2003, and 2.2 million died (75 % of the three million deaths globally that year, almost one in five deaths (all ages) and one in two deaths of adults aged 15–59 [25]. We will focus on this infection and on tuberculosis.

These data point to the relative magnitude of the problems to be addressed, but take into account neither the existence (or absence) of effective interventions to help fight against these diseases, nor the cost of each of the proposed interventions.

Identification of the Most Cost Effective Programmes

For over ten years now, we have known not only that there are real possibilities of ranking health programmes according to their cost-effectiveness, but also that the systematic implementation of the programmes selected according to such rankings

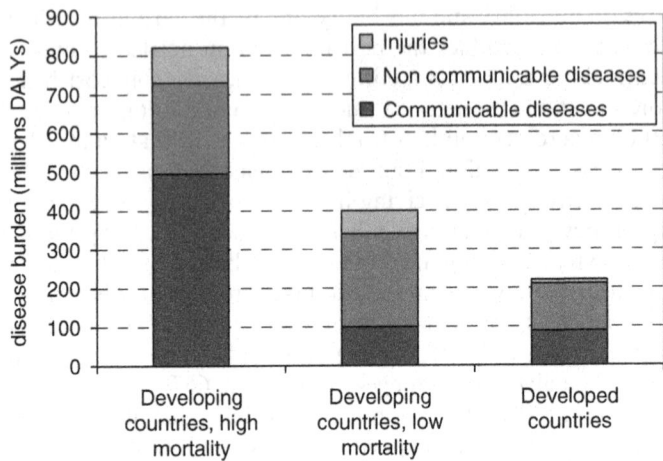

Fig. 1. Volume and structure of the disease burden for three groups of countries, 2001
Source: from [21, p. 81]
Note: "developing countries, high mortality" are all countries from WHO Afr-D, Afr-E, Sear-D, Emr-D regions ; "developing countries, low mortality" are all countries from WHO Amr-B, Sear-B, Emr-B and Wpr-B regions ; "developed countries" are all countries from WHO Amr-A, Eur-A, Eur-B, Eur-C and Wpr-A regions ; "high mortality" means child mortality within the fourth and fifth quintiles of the distribution, and high or very high adult mortality; countries with high child mortality are classified into high or very high adult mortality using the regression line of the regression of 45q15 on 5q0; [23, p. 182–183]

should help obtain results in the fight against the disease that would be of a quite different order of magnitude than those currently achieved. To quote WHO: "most of the 13 million deaths a year from infectious diseases can be prevented. Low-cost health interventions already exist to either prevent or cure the infectious diseases which take the greatest toll on human lives. And most of these interventions have been widely available for years" [21, pp. 6–7].

The interventions to be selected must not only be effective, as not all effective interventions can be carried out: the interventions to be selected must be chosen among the *most* cost-effective. If one does not explicitly operate such a selection, either by ignorance or deliberate choice, one would waste a portion of the resources by using them for interventions that are not the most effective for a given expenditure.

Effectiveness is often measured in DALY, as discussed above, and the cost is estimated in dollars. Interventions can thus be categorized according to their cost per DALY [26, pp. 6–7, pp. 54–57], [27]. But it may be necessary to take into account the level of resources in the country involved. Thus, the "macro-economics and health commission", established within the World Health Organization, has suggested, as a general rule of thumb, that interventions which cost *less than three* times the gross domestic product per capita for each DALY earned should be considered as having a high enough cost-effectiveness ratio that, if a country does not undertake them all with its own resources, the international community should seek the means to finance them. In the World Health Report 2002, interventions are considered *very* cost-effective if they cost *no more than one times* the gross domestic product per capita for each DALY gained [22, p. 108].

Rich countries are quite aware of the problem too: in the 1990s, the Organisation for Economic Co-operation and Development (OECD)[1], gathering 30 member nations sharing a commitment to democratic government and market economy, stated that medical innovations should be adopted if the marginal cost per year of life saved were *lower than twice* the gross domestic product per capita (and rejected if such cost exceeded *six times* the gross domestic product). [28] Thus, in spite of their ageing populations, in spite of the level of their health systems, rich countries estimate that one does not live on medical care alone: they discreetly set rules that help restrict the adoption of some medical innovations.

In the WHO special report on infectious diseases, this type of approach leads to establishing a list of recommended programmes: integrated care for sick children (notably pneumonia, diarrhoea, malaria, measles, malnutrition), immunization of children (diphtheria, whooping cough, tetanus, poliomyelitis, measles, and tuberculosis), "short course" therapy under direct observation (tuberculosis), impregnated mosquito nets, availability of essential drugs, strategies for preventing HIV/AIDS, and vitamin and mineral supplements [22, pp. 7–8]. Extensive applications of the same approach are now available [25, 27].

Economic and Ethical Importance of This Approach

The adverse consequences of the current definition of priorities following supply dynamics alone are widely recognized nowadays at the international level. Public funding of health, because it is focused on hospitals and other specialized services, which are accessed electively by the rich, subsidizes the consumption of health goods and services for the rich more than for the poor. In Côte d'Ivoire, at the beginning of the 1990s, "the subsidy to the poorest quintile is 64% lower than that which goes to the richest quintile" [29]. Comparable studies conducted by UNICEF under the 20/20 project led to similar conclusions for several other countries [30]. The same has now been observed in about 30 countries over recent years [31, p. 39—see **Fig. 2**], [32].

In 2001, 46 countries (including 31 African countries) had a per capita *government* health expenditure (at average exchange rates) of less than US$ 10; 18 countries (14 African) had a per capita *total* health expenditure of less than US$ 10 [33, pp. 144–147], making it difficult to ensure that even the most basic health needs are met. In 1997–2000, the total per capita health expenditure in low income countries was about US$ 21, compared to US$ 115 in middle income countries and US$ 2735 in high income countries [34]. Add to this the fact that "more money is not the solution when provided to governments that fail to make cost-effective use of resources.

---

[1] Organisation for Economic Cooperation and Development

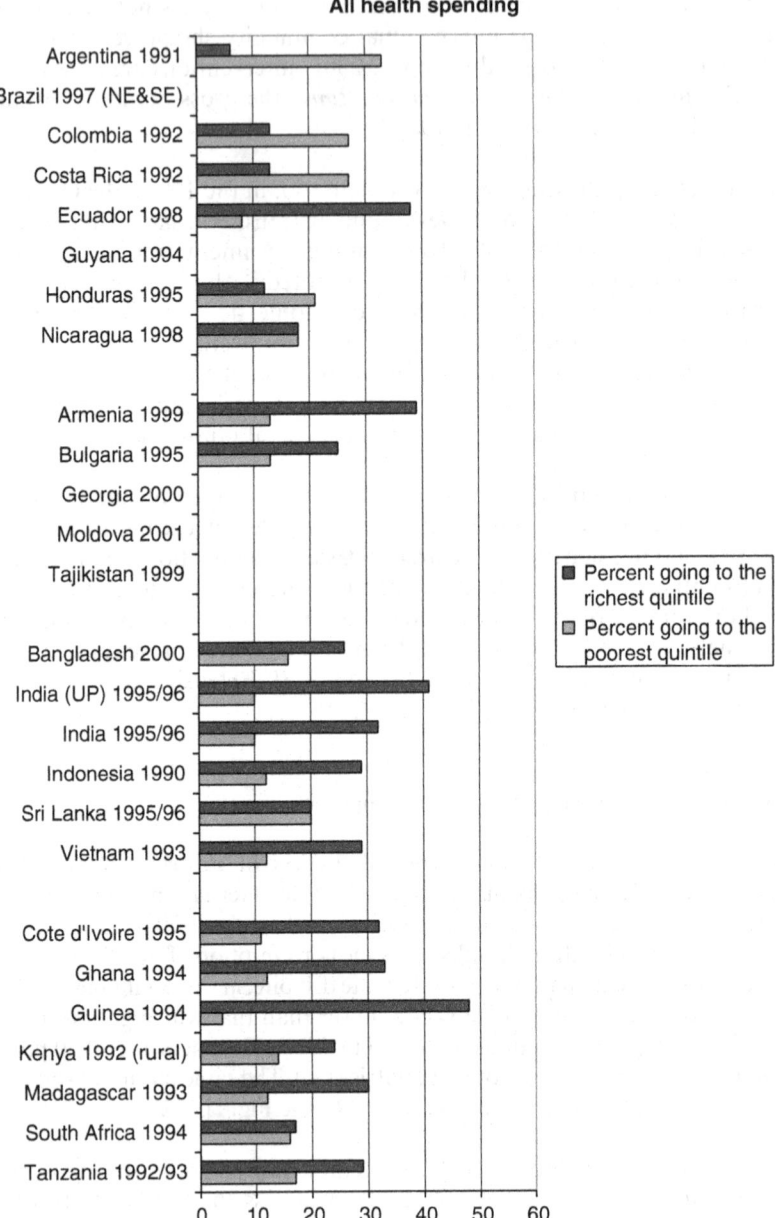

Fig. 2a. Percent of total health spending going to the first and the fifth quintiles

Primary level only

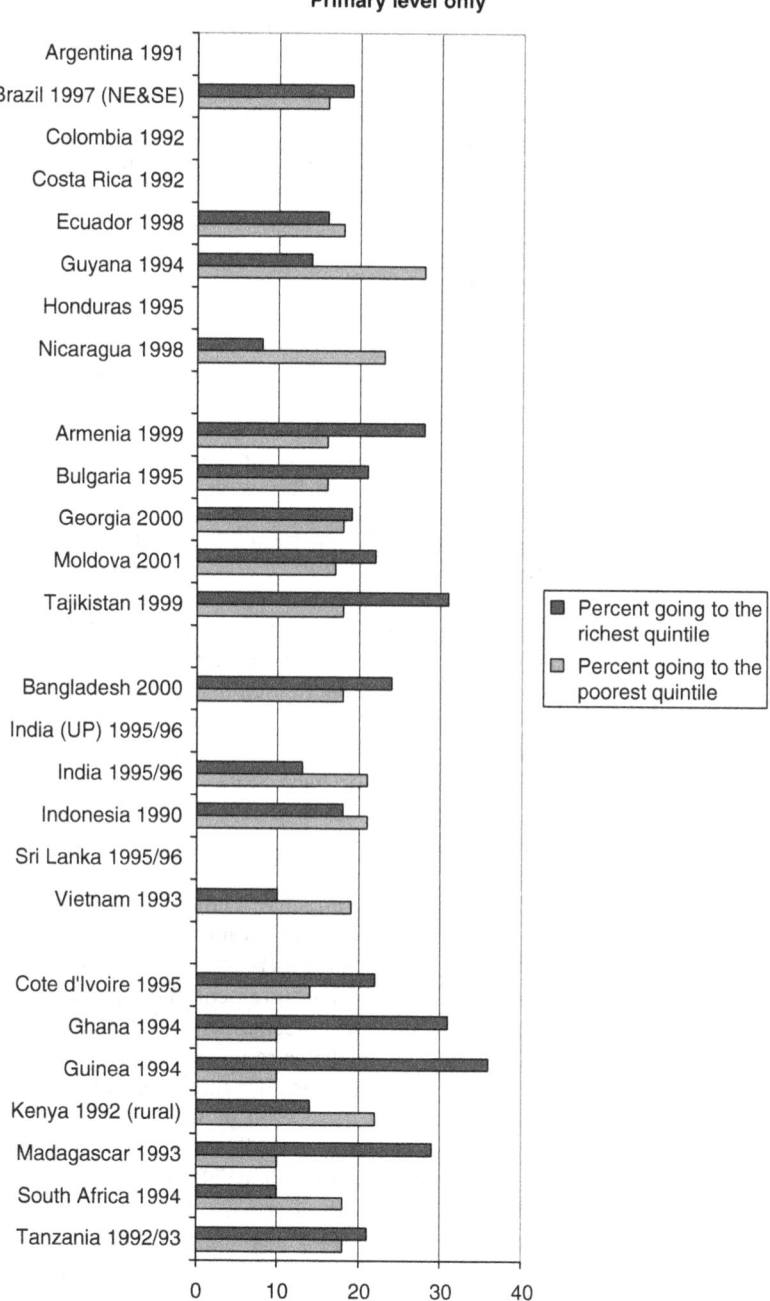

Fig. 2b. Percent of primary level health spending going to the first and fifth quintiles
Source: from [32]

In some developing countries, 60% or more of government health expenditures are devoted to meeting the operating costs of urban hospitals and expensive equipment" [21, p.12].

> Unfortunately, for a number of reasons, they [the most cost-effective interventions] are not being used. ... Government failure to prioritize, lack of cross-sectoral collaboration and the inability of weak health service delivery systems to reach the entire population—particularly the most vulnerable and difficult-to-reach—are contributing factors [21, pp. 6–7].

If, in individual countries, the limited available resources were allocated to the most effective interventions, then the health priorities, and health policies as a whole, would be quite different from one country to another, and from one continent to another. There would no longer be a universal health policy, as required by most WHO goals, for example [35, p. 6]:

> "The Initiative will advance the United Nations goals of promoting human rights as codified in the Universal Declaration of Human Rights, as expressed by the WHO Constitution in seeking the attainment of the highest possible standards of health, and clarified in the Declaration of Commitment of the United Nations General Assembly Special Session on HIV/AIDS in 2001 [35, p. 10]

and by most of WHO guidelines and toolkits (for an example see [36]). In practice, "country ownership", as a means to get a lot of external aid, is simply understood as an explicit approval of those international statements and guidelines. Were each country enabled to define its health priorities itself, it would be satisfied with doing what it could do best to treat its population, given its resources and external assistance: with an entire responsibility hanging on each State's own shoulders, and with external aid apportioned out according to measured results on the health status, all means might be used in a much more efficient manner.

Systematic recourse to best knowledge on cost effective medical interventions is therefore not a dangerous and unjustified drift towards economic thinking; it is a means to obtain the best result (in terms of mortality and morbidity) for the resources society devotes to health care; moreover, it is an ethical requirement [37], as it helps avoid the provision of care becoming, as it is nowadays, a mechanism to boost social inequalities, notably by concentrating the bulk of health care resources on specialized care, only available to a few people. As an example, consider the maternal mortality risk, ranging from 1 out of 16 in Africa to 1 out of 4000 in Western Europe [38]: but "the proportion of women with direct obstetric complications treated in emergency obstetric care facilities can be as low as 5 percent" [39, p. 79] as in Uganda, a country where each of the 12 referral hospitals and each of the 38 government district hospitals has an obstetrics and gynaecology service [40]; as these facilities are not accessed by those who need their care, they have no impact on the maternal mortality risk.

The Case of a Recent Disease: HIV/AIDS

What studies do we have at hand to select the most cost-effective interventions in the fight against HIV/AIDS? A recent synthesis [41] examined the results of

24 usable studies. The main findings are that cost-effectiveness varies greatly across interventions: from 1 $ per DALY gained by selective blood safety measures, or targeted condom distribution with STD treatment, for example, to 75 $ per DALY gained by single-dose nevirapine and short-course zidovudine for prevention of mother-to-child transmission, and up to several hundred dollars for other interventions such as home care programmes or highly active antiretroviral therapy (HAART) for adults. The conclusion is:

> The most cost effective interventions are for prevention of HIV/AIDS and treatment of tuberculosis, whereas HAART for adults, and home based care organised from health facilities, are least cost effective. For some interventions, such as prevention of mother-to-child transmission, tuberculosis treatment and home based care, there are particular strategies that provide the best value for money (best buy) [41, p. 1638].

The authors, who are perfectly aware of the scope and significance of this conclusion, underscore the full limitations of the rare studies available, and therefore of their comparativeness [42, 43, 44]. Then, after a reminder that ranking interventions according to their cost effectiveness is not enough to set public funding priorities, they turn to the role of all other determinants, but conclude that the essential factor remains cost effectiveness. The criticisms of this analysis point to an alleged "leverage effect" of HAART on HIV prevention, and an alleged potential to secure the future against disabling social and economic ills; they also contrast the narrow variables of cost-effectiveness analysis and "humanitarian considerations" [45, 46]. But, the authors of the review respond: "as a method for organizing evidence, cost-effectiveness remains the most comprehensive approach to assess clinical and social information on outcomes, dealing at the same time with resource availability" [47].

We do understand that the DALY-based approach does not take into account the indirect effects of AIDS-related young adult deaths: a sharply increasing number of orphans, severe loss of skilled work force, huge difficulties in raising and educating the children. ... Nevertheless, such indirect effects are by no means specific to the AIDS epidemic: maternal mortality, or road accident injuries, cardiovascular diseases, etc. have similar consequences; the scope only differs. We have to consider the scope, and to measure the dimensions of the problem, but with the same instrument that is applied to other diseases. Therefore, we need a single yardstick: and as long as we do not have a better summary measure of the burden of disease, we must use the DALYs.

Secondly, we consider a detailed study by the World Health Organization, extending the same method (cost-effectiveness analysis) to help assess whether the current mix of interventions is efficient, as well as whether a proposed new technology or intervention is appropriate [48]. The generalized cost-effectiveness analysis has been developed for use in the WHO "*Cho*osing *I*nterventions that are *Cost-E*ffective" (*CHOICE*) programme [49]. When applied to HIV/AIDS, it can take into account not only the main proposed types of interventions (antiretroviral treatment; treatment of sexually transmitted infections; education of sex workers; school education; communication–information–education; prevention of mother-to-child transmission; voluntary testing and counselling; highly active antiretroviral treatment), but also some twenty combinations of the above. Overall, about thirty control strategies are examined, and the coverage rates are included in the analysis whenever possible [50].

The results concerning the group of countries of the Africa region which have both high infant and child mortality rates and a very high rate of mortality among adults[2] are as follows: in this group of countries (Algeria, Angola, Benin, Bupkina Faso, Cameroon, Cape Verdé, Chad, Comores, Equatorial Guinea, Gabon, Gambia, Ghana, Guinea, Guinea Bissan, Liberia, Madagascar, Mali, Mauritania, Mauritius, Niger, Nigeria, Sao Tome and Principe, Malawi, Senegal, Seychelles, Sierra Leone, Togo), all treatment strategies using antiretroviral drugs are "dominated"; i.e. other strategies would use available resources more efficiently, producing a larger reduction of the disease burden. In other words, even if AIDS may require "heroic" efforts, and "although HAART has a role in these efforts, it is important that its provision not usurp funding that would otherwise be available for more clearly cost effective interventions, that might have greater effects" [51, p. 50].

Therefore, both reviews have the same conclusion: HAART is not the best use of money among available interventions against HIV/AIDS in low resource countries.

Does the actual strategy of international organizations in the field make use of the best knowledge at our disposal to-date? WHO turns away from the conclusions of its experts to launch a programme aimed at making antiretroviral drugs available to three million patients by 2005. But for what reasons, exactly? Because of "a unique combination of opportunity and political will" resulting in considerably increased funding, making it possible to undertake "major new investments in countries' health systems" [35, pp. 5–7], and allowing "countries to support effective systems of delivering chronic care" [52]: the *supply dynamics* are clearly apparent, whereas the real political commitment seems "only skin deep" [53].

The World Bank sounds more dubious:

> Much of the focus of the Global Fund and the President's Emergency Plan for AIDS Relief (PEPFAR)[3] initiative is on treatment, a very complex undertaking due to the need for continuous monitoring of patient adherence to the drug regimen, drug resistance awareness, and the need for treatment to be on-going over the patient's lifetime. This growing emphasis on treatment will put even greater demands on a chronically weak health system as well as increase the need to safeguard the appropriate balance among HIV/AIDS interventions, including ensuring a continuing and enhanced focus on prevention [53, p. 2].

The amounts of money involved are very large. "Bank funding for HIV/AIDS in Africa has grown exponentially, from commitments of less than US$5 million annually before 2001 to more than US$300 million committed in 2003 for all Multi-Country HIV/AIDS Program (MAP)[4] projects." [53, p. 5]; add the Global Fund (US

---

[2] The countries involved are: Botswana, Burundi, Central African Republic, Congo, Cote d'Ivoire, Democratic Republic of the Congo, Eritrea, Ethiopia, Kenya, Lesotho, Malawi, Mozambique, Namibia, Rwanda, Swaziland, South Africa, Uganda, Tanzania, Zambia, Zimbabwe (see [23]).

[3] The President's Emergency Plan for AIDS Relief, [54].

[4] Multi-Country HIV/AIDS Programmes, see [54].

$1.5 billion over two years), the US PEPFAR initiative (up to US $15 billion over five years), the Gates and Clinton Foundations, bilateral donors, and other development partners; and note that "a priority for the new funders is on anti-retroviral treatment" [53, pp. 7–8]. On the other hand, the Global Fund does not enter a discussion of priorities: "The Fund will pursue an integrated and balanced approach covering prevention, treatment, and care and support in dealing with the three diseases" [54], and therefore apparently takes no account at all of the best available knowledge. The sole priority now is to have the money paid out. And, as we cannot exclude the possibility that this "new" money is simply reallocated, and therefore no more available for its previous purposes in the health sector, the problem of finding a convincing justification of such "public health" choices is clearly enhanced.

The Case of a Re-emerging Disease: Tuberculosis

Unlike AIDS, tuberculosis is no longer examined by WHO in a way that makes it possible to rank the proposed interventions according to their cost-effectiveness: the risk-approach has been adopted by the CHOICE programme, and it excludes consideration of each disease in isolation. Ten years ago, only two interventions were clearly recommended: BCG vaccination, and case finding and treatment, concentrating on infectious cases [27, p. 19]; [27, Chap. 11]. Since then, the directly observed short-course therapy (DOTS) strategy was launched [57], and WHO has adopted a risk based approach, which precludes all forms of clear recommendations concerning individual medical interventions against individual infections. As a result, the issue of tuberculosis is not raised, for example, in the last World Health Reports, and the extensive work on cost-effectiveness analysis, as referred to in the preceding section, does not apply to this disease [22]. We are thus looking forward to the new edition of *Disease Control Priorities* [58], including a chapter by Christopher Dye and Katherine Floyd, who put together the pieces of a cost-effectiveness analysis to be developed in the final version of the book. For the present, the discussion focuses essentially on the weaknesses of technical knowledge about the efficiency of currently proposed interventions: surely this is important, but simply as the first step of the cost-effectiveness approach.

Tuberculosis worries anew because of co-infection with HIV, which considerably increases the risk of developing the disease [59, p. 1012]. The case fatality rate is high for undiagnosed cases, or those with drug resistance, or with HIV infection. Overall in Africa, 38% of new cases of tuberculosis are HIV infected [60, p. 4].

It is possible to treat latent tuberculosis infection, and some protection has been shown in controlled trials. It is comparatively cheap and has been recommended, particularly for HIV positive patients, but it is rarely done, because of the poor logistics and the condition of health facilities [61, p. 2182] and concern about drug resistance. In addition, the treatment seems to be only effective for a period of two to three years after its cessation and to have no effect on mortality [60, p. 9].

As far as immunization is concerned, some experts assess that, "despite the phenomenal number of BCG vaccinations given to children, there have been few assessments of BCG effectiveness at the population level" [60, p. 8]. A meta-analysis of over 1200 articles from international publications concluded that the overall protective value of BCG against all forms of TB was of the order of just 50%, but that protection against more serious infection was greater, being 64% and 78% against tuberculous meningitis and disseminated infection, respectively. However, it is difficult to speak of an overall protection of 50%, in view of the considerable heterogeneity in the results: BCG provides a good protection in some areas and none at all in other [62]. Moreover, the effect of immunization seems to ensure protection against more serious forms of the disease among children (meningitis and miliary tuberculosis); but even with high coverage rates it does not have any marked impact on transmission, and therefore on incidence [60, p. 6].

Short term treatment under surveillance,[5] applied to patients with smear positive pulmonary tuberculosis (i.e. having visited a health facility) would cure most of the cases found (85% is the current target of the WHO programme); but extensive coverage is needed if we want to reduce incidence by this means; 155 countries have officially implemented this type of programme; but "the central problem is that, even if DOTS programmes have expanded geographically, they have not reached beyond existing public health services" [60, p.11]. Indeed,

> population units nominally covered by DOTS do not necessarily provide full access to DOTS services. Access to health services varies widely, within and across countries, according to the number and distribution of health centres, travel time for patients, transportation infrastructure, the number and type of health care providers, out-of-pocket costs to patients, and others factors [64, pp. 13–14].

Therefore the DOTS programs are in fact dependent on passive case detection; and those countries which have not set up a passive detection system are not in a position to organize more active testing.

Where HIV prevalence is high, as in East and South Africa, aggressive programmes of chemotherapy against tuberculosis, perhaps including the active search for cases, would be necessary in order to reverse the growth in TB incidence. Mathematical modelling indicates that, even in the case of a major HIV epidemic, early tuberculosis detection and treatment are the most efficient means of reducing the burden of this disease [65]. The alternatives—i.e. prevention of HIV infection, treatment of latent tuberculous infection, and antiretroviral therapy—are less promising strategies for the next decade, even if HIV prevention is, in the long run, an important method. According to results obtained in South Africa for a given cohort, the treatment of AIDS patients with ARVs would be likely to reduce the incidence among AIDS patients to that observed just after seroconversion [66]; but, as discussed previously, is it the best use of the resources available, and is it ethically justified to apply that strategy to the entire population at risk? Moreover, many people get TB before they become eligible for ARVs.

---

[5] The five elements of the DOTS TB control strategy are:
- Sustained political commitment
- Access to quality-assured TB sputum microscopy
- Standardized short-course chemotherapy to all cases of TB under proper case-management conditions
- Uninterrupted supply of quality-assured drugs
- Recording and reporting system enabling outcome assessment (see [63])

The troubling uncertainties we are experiencing on these difficult issues leave room for hazardous extrapolations. Thus, the study just cited was immediately used to conclude that "HIV-1 control is required for effective tuberculosis control" and that "HAART can have a critical role in addressing the therapeutic nihilism surrounding the HIV-1 and tuberculosis co-epidemic in South Africa and other African countries" [66, p. 2063]. However, this conclusion is erroneous: further analysis demonstrates that large-scale use of antiretroviral drugs would, in fact, not be enough to guarantee control of tuberculosis, because of the induced extension of the period during which AIDS patients will remain likely to develop tuberculosis [67, see also 65].

Conclusion

As this discussion shows, the effects of every medical intervention must be described with a high level of accuracy and its cost effectiveness must be included in the analysis, if we want to get the best health impact of the resources that are allocated to the health system. But to choose the most cost-effective intervention is to choose the patients who will receive treatment, and this is also designating those who will not be cared for. To-date, in order to avoid facing this problem, public opinion is repeatedly called upon to contribute additional resources (an attitude which only dodges and defers the issue); and multiple actions are implemented according to all available means (including the professional and political power of promoters lobbying for each strategy); this attitude has no economic or ethical rationale.

It is perfectly true that the instruments at our disposal to-date which have been meant to enlighten our choices are defective; it is also true that these instruments have to be adapted to unprecedented and rapidly evolving problems, notably now the fact that, for several diseases already, the incidence, transmission, and resistance to drugs are affected by HIV-1 [61, p. 2185]. To take into account these reciprocal influences between AIDS and the other infections involved (essentially sexually transmitted diseases, tuberculosis, and malaria, but perhaps also helminthiases), models should incorporate all kinds of probabilities of co-infection and the best prescriptions based on methodically analysed clinical results: we can probably manage the complexity of the model, but we lack the data to run it. However this is no reason at all for neglecting or refusing to use the best instruments available to-date.

We do understand that the cost-effectiveness argument is called into question, and often on a peremptory note: "health economists should stop making an 'authoritarian' use of a mistaken version of the cost-effectiveness argument to legitimate delays and withdrawals from governments and donor organizations in launching of large scale programs for access to ART" [68, p. 254].

The cost-effectiveness stand definitely lacks the desired perfection we too wish it could have. Thus, the current studies unquestionably do not take into account the full dimensions of the problem: for example the devastating loss of capacity of social and economic reproduction, or the consequences with non-market goods and services. But although the extension of the measurement domain is desirable, it should be applied to all infections, which must be compared using a single yardstick.

In fact, the cost-effectiveness argument is not contested as much because it is erroneous, as because it has an exceptional characteristic, that of promoting a certain form of justice among care recipients in each country: this quality escapes the attention of some [69, 70, 71]; but it is essential. In the simplest terms possible, and contrary to most common opinion, it is profoundly unfair to treat patients of an individual infection, in the poverty context, as we would treat patients with the same infection in richer countries: this is because a "universal standard" for some will inevitably be held at the expense of other sick people who, poor and deserving of compassion as they too are, will not receive the basic treatments they need and could greatly benefit from. As an example, was it fair to establish in Côte d'Ivoire a programme of access to antiretroviral drugs while this country could not provide a caesarean section to every woman in parturition for whom this intervention was required [72]?

Selecting a disease and saying that patients suffering from it are entitled either to a universal standard or to a reasonably similar one [73, 74], without considering the cost-effectiveness of such interventions, and without comparing it to the cost-effectiveness of other interventions against other diseases, in the given content would amount to neglecting the shocking situation in which all those other patients who are not members of the selected group are found [75, 76, 77]. It is an injustice which favours a selected subsample of patients, while deliberately ignoring the entire sick population; therefore making a purely formal application of universal principles, and adopting de facto a "double standard" [78, 73, 79] that leads to tremendous discrimination. This was the strategy of all associations of persons living with HIV/AIDS, of non-governmental organisations, and of all the pressure groups that fought to obtain lower treatment prices. The result has been achieved, but the basic principles of equity in access to care have been discarded, and national and local health systems are less fair today than they were two decades ago.

A local fairness system can be implemented through decentralized use to the maximum extent possible of the cost-effectiveness criterion. Such decentralization helps gather the opinions of patients at risk to be deprived of treatment, and not at the time of illness, but when they are in a condition to behave as citizens [80]: the selection criteria in choosing the patients to be treated must be made explicit and adopted with full knowledge of the facts [81]. This is the only way to ensure respect for human dignity [71, 82].

For over ten years, all those who have been thinking about the future of our health systems know that the allocation of resources, the development of a fair health system, and arbitration between the rights and demands of competing groups are and will be "the important moral issues of the future" [83, p. 1855], [84]. Introducing some fairness in public health decisions is our priority, and we do not have the right to ignore the fact that we have an instrument which, albeit imperfect, is capable of providing data that would justify the decisions made. We do not need only evoke humanitarian considerations, we do not need only evoke the omitted impacts likely but not accounted for, we do not need only seek refuge behind political pressures [45, 46]: only activists of all walks of life are content with these arguments which are fit to impress politics and public opinion.

References

1. Brunet-Jailly, J. (1999). Peut-on faire l'économie du sida? (In Becker, C., Dozon, J. P., Obbo, C., Toure, M. (Eds.), *Vivre et penser le sida en Afrique* (pp. 179–199), Dakar/Paris: Codesria-Karthala-Ird)

2. Drouhin, N., Touzé, V. & Ventelou, B. (2003). AIDS and economic growth in Africa, a critical assessment of the "base-case scenario" approach. (In Moatti J. P., Coriat, B., Souteyrand Y., Barnett T., Dumoulin, J. & Flori, Y. A. (Eds.), *Economics of AIDS and access to HIV/AIDS care in developing countries, issues and challenges* (pp. 383–411). ANRS: Paris)

3. Bell, C., Devarajan, S. & Gersbach, H. (2004). *The long-run economic costs of AIDS, Theory and an application to South Africa.* Retrieved January from http://www1.worldbank.org/hiv_aids/docs/BeDeGe_BP_total2.pdf

4. Nordhaus, W. D. (2000). New directions in national economic accounting. *American Economic Review, Papers and Proceedings, 90*(2), 259–263

5. Jamison, D., Sachs, J. D. & Wang, J. (n.d.). *The effect of the AIDS epidemic on economic welfare in sub-Saharan Africa.* Paper n° WG1:13, Commission on Macroeconomics and Health, 14 p. + annexes. Retrieved January 2004 from http://www3.who.int/whosis/cmh/cmh_papers/e/papers.cfm?path=cmh,cmh_papers&language=english

6. Mills, A., Shillcutt, S. (2004). Communicable diseases. (In Lomborg, B. (Ed.). *Global crises, global solutions* (pp. 62–114). Cambridge: Cambridge University Press)

7. Schumpeter, J. A. (1934). *The theory of economic development.* (Cambridge, Massachusetts: Harvard University Press). (First edition: 1912)

8. WHO World Health Report (2000). *Health systems: Improving performance.* Retrieved from http://www.who.int/whr/2000/en/whr00_ch2_en.pdf

9. Yach, D., Hawkes, C., Gould, C. L., Hofman, K. J. (2004). The global burden of chronic diseases: Overcoming impediments to prevention and control. *JAMA, 291*, 2616–2622

10. Trouiller, P., Olliaro, P., Torreele, E., Orbinski, J., Laing, R. et al. (2002). Drug development for neglected diseases: A deficient market and a public-health policy failure. *The Lancet, 359*, 2188–2194

11. WHO (2001). National burden of disease studies, a practical guide, Edition 2.0, October 2001. Retrieved January from http://www3.who.int/whosis/menu.cfm?path=whosis,burden,burden_manual&language=english

12. Mathers, C. D., Stein, C., Ma Fat, D., Rao,C., Inoue, M., Tomijima, , N., Bernard, C., Lopez, A. D. & Murray, C. J. L.(2002), Global burden of disease 2000, Version 2 methods and results, *Global Programme on Evidence for Health Policy, Discussion Paper No. 50,* World Health Organization, October 2002. Retrieved January 2004 from http://www3.who.int/whosis/menu.cfm?path=whosis,burden,burden_gbd2000docs&language=english

13. Anand, S. & Hanson, K. (1997). Disability-adjusted life years, a critical review. *Journal of Health Economics, 16*, 685–702

14. Almeida, C., Braveman, P., et al. (2001). Methodological concerns and recommendation on policy consequences on the World Health Report 2000. *The Lancet, 357*, 1692–1697

15. Reidpath, D. D., Allotey, P. A., Kouame, A., Cummins, R. A. (2003). Measuring health in a vacuum, examining the disability weight of the DALY. *Health Policy and Planning, 18*(4), 351–356

16. Murray, C. J. L., Salomon, J. A., Mathers, C. D., Lopez, A. D. (Eds.) (2002). *Summary measures of population health, concepts, ethics, measurement and applications.* (Geneva: WHO). Retrieved January 2004 from http://whqlibdoc.who.int/publications/2002/9241545518.pdf

17. Williams, A. (1999). Calculating the global burden of disease, time for a strategic reappraisal? *Health Economics, 8*, 1–8

18. Richardson, J. (2002). Age weighting and time discounting, technical imperative versus social choice. (In C. J. Murray, J. A. Salomon, C. D. Mathers, A. D. Lopez (Eds.). *Summary measures of population health, concepts, ethics, measurement and applications* (pp. 663–676). Geneva: Geneva)

19. Murray, C. J. L. & Lopez, A. D. (n.d.). *Progress and directions in redefining the global burden of disease approach, a response to Williams,* Discussion paper n° 1. Retrieved December 2004 from http://www3.who.int/whosis/burden/discussion_papers.cfm?path=evidence,burden,burden_papers&langage=english

20. Richardson, J. (2002). The poverty of ethical analysis in economics and the unwarranted disregard of evidence. (In C. J. L. Murray, J. A. Salomon, C. D. Mathers, A. D. Lopez (Eds.). *Summary measures of population health, concepts, ethics, measurement and applications* (pp. 627–640). Geneva: WHO)

21. WHO: Report on infectious diseases, 1999. Retrieved January 2004 from http://www.who.int/infectious-disease-report/pages/textonly.html

22. WHO: World Health Report 2002, p. 81. Retrieved February 2004 from http://www.who.int/whr/2002/en/whr02_ch4.pdf

23. WHO World Health Report, 2003, pp. 182–183. Retrieved from http://www3.who.int/whosis/member_states/member_states_stratum.cfm?path=whosis,evidence,cea,cea_regions,member_states_stratum

24. WHO: Table DALY6 (2000b). Retrieved February 2004 from www3.who.int/whosis/menu.cfm?path=evidence, burden,burden_estimates,burden_estimates_2000V2

25. AIDS Epidemic Update December 2004. Retreived from http://www.unaids.org/wad2004/EPI_1204_pdf_en/Chapter3_subsaharan_africa_en.pdf

26. World Bank: World Development Report (1993). *Investing in health.* (Washington, DC: World Bank)

27. Jamison, D. et al. (1993). Disease control priorities in developing countries. (Oxford: Oxford Medical Publications)

28. Garber, A. M. (2001). Advances in CE analysis. (In A. J. Culyer & J. P. Newhouse (Eds.). *Handbook of health economics*, I. Amsterdam: Elsevier Science)

29. Demeny, L., Dayton, J. & Meyra, K. (1995) *L'incidence des dépenses sociales publiques en Côte d'Ivoire* (projet révisé, version provisoire) février

30. UNICEF (1999): *Country experiences in assessing the adequacy, equity and efficiency of public spending on basic social services,* document prepared for the Hanoi Meeting on the 20/20 Initiative. (New York: UNICEF)

31. World Development Report 2004, p. 39. Retrieved February 2005 from http://www-wds.worldbank.org/servlet/WDSContentServer/WDSP/IB/2003/10/07/000090341_20031007150121/Rendered/PDF/268950PAPER0WDR02004.pdf

32. Filmer, D. (2003). The incidence of public expenditures on health and education, Background note for World Development Report 2004, *Making services work for poor people.* Document n° 26950. (Washington, DC: World Bank). Retrieved February 2005 from http://www-wds.worldbank.org/servlet/WDSContentServer/WDSP/IB/2003/10/20/000160016_20031020130801/Rendered/PDF/269500Benefit11e0WDR20040Background.pdf

33. World Health Report 2004 (pp. 144–147)

34. World Development Report 2004, (pp. 256–257). Retrieved from http://econ.worldbank.org/files/30042_select.pdf

35. WHO (2004). *Treating 3 million by 2005, making it happen!* Retrieved February from http://www.who.int/3by5/publications/documents/en/treating3millionby2005.pdf

36. A public health approach for scaling up antiretroviral treatment: A toolkit for programme managers. Retrieved from http://www.who.int/hiv/pub/prev_care/en/arvtoolkit_frweb.pdf

37. Williams, A. (1992). Cost-effectiveness analysis, is it ethical. *Journal of Medical Ethics, 18*, 7–11

38. WHO-UNICEF-UNFPA (2001). *Maternal mortality in 1995, estimates developed by WHO, UNICEF, UNPFA.* (Geneva: World Health Organization)

39. PNUD (2005). *Investing in development: a practical plan to achieve the millenium development goals.* UN Millenium Project, Millenium Project-Earthcan, 2005. Retrieved January from http://unmp. forumone.com

40. Retrieved February from http://www.health.go.ug/hospital_services.htm; and http://www.health. go.ug/docs/hospitals.xls

41. Creese, A. K., Floyd, A. & Alban, L. (2002). Guinness: Cost-effectiveness of HIV/AIDS interventions in Africa : A systematic review of the evidence. *The Lancet, 359*(May), 1635–1642

42. Kumaranayake, L. (2002). Cost-effectiveness and economic evaluation of HIV/AIDS-related interventions, the state of the art. (In S. Forsythe (Ed.). *State of the art: AIDS and economics* (pp. 64–74). Toronto, Canada: International AIDS-Economics Network)

43. Walker, D. (2003). Cost and cost-effectiveness of HIV/AIDS prevention strategies in developing countries, is there an evidence base? *Health Policy and Planning, 18*(1), 4–17

44. Freedberg, K.& Yazdanpanah, Y. (2003). Cost-effectiveness of HIV therapies en resources-poor countries. (In J. P. Moatti, B. Coriat, Y. Souteyrand, T. Barnett, J. Dumoulin, J. Y. Flori (Eds.). *Economics of AIDS and access to HIV/AIDS care in developing countries, issues and challenges* (pp. 267–291), Paris: ANRS)

45. Piot, P., Zewdie, D., Türmen, T. (2002). HIV/AIDS prevention and treatment, Correspondence. *The Lancet, 360*, 86

46. Groemaere, E., Ford, N., Benatar, S. R. (2002). HIV/AIDS prevention and treatment, Correspondence. *The Lancet, 360*, 87

47. Creese, A., Floyd, K., Alban, A., Guinness, L. (2002). Author's reply. *The Lancet, 360*(July 6), 88

48. Balthussen, B., Adam, T., Tan Torres, T., Hutubessy, R., Acharya, A., Evans, D. B., Murray, C. J. L. (2003). *Generalized Cost-Effectiveness Analysis, A Guide.* Global Programme on Evidence for Health Policy. (Geneva: World Health Organization)

49. Retrieved from http://www3.who.int/whosis/menu.cfm?path=whosis,cea&language=english

50. WHO: WHO-CHOICE, Results, CEA summary results. Retrieved February, December 2004 from http://www3.who.int/whosis/cea/cea_data_process.cfm?path=evidence,cea,cea_results,cea_results_ summary&language=english

51. WHO: *Improving Health Outcomes of the Poor*, The Report of Working Group 5 of the Commission on macroeconomics and Health. Retrieved January 2004 from http://www3.who.int/whosis/cmh/ cmh_papers/e/papers.cfm?path=cmh,cmh_papers&language=english

52. Changing History, World Health Report (2004). Message from the Director General. Retrieved from http://www.who.int/whr/2004/en/overview_en.pdf

53. MAP_Interim_Review: Interim review of the multi-country HIV/AIDS program for Africa. Retrieved from http://www.worldbank.org/afr/aids/map/MAP_Interim_Review-04.pdf

54. Retrieved from http://www.usaid.gov/our_work/global_health/aids/pepfarfact.html

55. Retrieved from http://www.worldbank.org/afr/aids/map.htm

56. The Framework document of the global fund to fight AIDS, Tuberculosis and malaria. Retrieved from http://www.theglobalfund.org/en/files/publicdoc/Framework_uk.pdf

57. WHO: An Expanded Framework for Effective Tuberculosis Control, Geneva, WHA44/1991/ REC/1

58. Retrieved February 2004 from http://www.fic.nih.gov/dcpp/toc.html

59. Corbett, E. L., Watt, C. J., Walker, N., Maher, D., Williams, B. G., Raviglione, M., Dye, C. (2003). The growing burden of tuberculosis, global trends and interactions with the HIV epidemic. *Archives of Internal Medicine, 163*(May), 1009–1021

60. Dye, C. & Floyd, K. (2004) *Tuberculosis, DCP2.* Retrieved February from www.fic.nih.gov/dcpp. dcp2.html

61. Corbett, E. L., Steketee, R. W., O ter Kuile, F., Latif, A. S., Kamali, A., Hayes, R. J. (2002) HIV-1/ AIDS and the control of other infectious diseases in Africa. *The Lancet, 359,* 2177–2187

62. Fine, P. E. (1995). Variation in protection by BCG, implications of and for heterologous immunity [review]. *The Lancet, 346,* 1339–1345

63. Retrieved February from http://www.who.int/tb/dots/en/(accessed February, 2004)

64. WHO Report (2004). Global tuberculosis control, surveillance, planning, financing, WHO/HTM/ TB/2004.331. Retrieved from http://www.who.int/tb/publications/global_report/2004/en/

65. Currie, C. S. M., Williams, B. G., Cheng, R. C., Dye, C. (2003). Tuberculosis epidemics driven by HIV, is prevention better than cure? *AIDS, 17,* 2501–2508

66. Badri, M., Wilson, D. & Wood, R. (2002) Effect of highly active antiretroviral therapy on incidence of tuberculosis in South Africa, a cohort study. *The Lancet, 359,* 2059–2064

67. Williams, B. & Dye, C. Antiretroviral drugs for tuberculosis control in the era of HIV/AIDS, Science express. Retrieved 14 August 2003 from www.sciencexpress.org

68. Moatti, J. P., Coriat, B., Souteyrand, Y., Barnett, T., Dumoulin, J., Flori, J. Y. (2003). *Economics of AIDS and access to HIV/AIDS care in developing countries, issues and challenges.* (Paris: ANRS)

69. Boelaert, M., Van Damme, W., Meessen, B. & Van der Stuyft, P. (2002). The AIDS crisis, cost-effectiveness and academic activism. *Tropical Medicine and International Health, 7*(12),1001–1002

70. Farmer, P. A. (2001). The major infectious disease in the world, to treat or not to treat. *The New England Journal of Medicine, 345,* 208–210

71. Retrieved December 2004 from http://www.copenhagenconsensus.com/Files/Filer/CC/Press/UK/ copenhagen_consensus_result_FINAL.pdf

72. Brunet-Jailly, J. (1997). *Le sida et les choix de stratégie sanitaire : l'exemple de la Côte d'Ivoire.* Communication à la Xème Conférence sur les MST/SIDA en Afrique, Abidjan 7–11 Décembre 1997. Retrieved December 2004 from http://www.iaen.org/papers/index.php?search=1&view=search& open=brunet-jailly&submit=go&conjunction=any

73. Laurent, C. et al. (2004). Effectiveness and safety of a generic fixed-dose combination of nevirapine, stavudine and lamivudine in HIV-1-infected adults in Cameroon, open-label multicentre trial. *The Lancet, 364*(July), 29–34

74. WHO (2003). Scaling up antiretroviral therapy in resource-limited settings: treatment guidelines for a public health approach, 2003 revision. Geneva: World Health Organization. Retrieved from http:// www.who.int/hiv/pub/prev_care/en/arvrevision2003en.pdf

75. Brunet-Jailly, J. (2003). Une éthique de la recherche médicale immédiatement universelle: un moyen de protéger la recherche médicale des pays du Nord? *Autrepart, 28*(Septembre), 37–53

76. Brunet-Jailly, J. (2001). Quels critères pour une juste répartition des soins? *Esprit*, (Janvier), 98–113

77. Molyneux, D. H. (2004). "Neglected" diseases but unrecognised successes: challenges and opportunities for infectious disease control. *The Lancet*, published online July 13, 2004, http://image.thelancet.com/extras/03art7073web.pdf

78. An (2004). Is it churlish to criticise Bush over his spending on AIDS? Editorial. *The Lancet, 364*(July), 303–304

79. Kumarasamy, N. (2004). Generic antiretroviral drugs, will they be the answer to HIV in the developing world. *The Lancet, 364*(July), 3–4

80. Van Balen, H. & Van Dormael, M. (1999). Health services professionals and users. *International Social Science Journal, 161*, 313–326

81. Callahan, D. (1990). Rationing medical progress, the way to affordable health care. *N Engl J Med, 322*, 1810–1813

82. Horton, R. (2004). Rediscovering human dignity. *The Lancet, 364*, 1081–1085

83. Marseille, E., Hofman, P. B. & Kahn, J. G. (2002). HIV prevention before HAART in sub-Saharan Africa. *The Lancet, 359*, 1851–1856

84. Richardson, J. (2002). Evaluating summary measures of population health. (In C. J. Murray, J. A. Salomon, C. D. Mathers, A. D. Lopez (Eds.), *Summary measures of population health, concepts, ethics, measurement and applications* (pp. 147–159). Geneva: WHO)

Part II
HIV and its Impact

CHAPTER 7. HIV INFECTION IN YOUNG ADULTS IN AFRICA: CONTEXT, RISKS, AND OPPORTUNITIES FOR PREVENTION

MICHEL CARAËL
Faculté des Sciences Sociales, Université Libre de Bruxelles, Brussels, Belgium

JUDITH R. GLYNN
Department of Epidemiology and Population Health, London School of Hygiene and Tropical Medicine, London, UK

Abstract. Young adults in Africa are both the group with the highest incidence of HIV infection and the key target group for interventions. Each new generation of adolescents provides another opportunity for prevention, but these opportunities are being missed. In this article we review the contextual and proximate determinants of risk behaviour and HIV infection in young adults, and the effects of different control strategies.

Introduction

By the end of 2005, around 38.6 million people world wide were estimated to be infected with HIV/AIDS. The same year, there were globally an estimated 4.1 million new infections and 2.8 million deaths attributable to AIDS. By far the worst-affected region, sub-Saharan Africa, is home to around 24.5 million people living with HIV/AIDS [1]. Based on epidemiological studies carried out in the 1990s, it has been estimated that 90–95% of new cases of HIV infection in Africa are due to sexual transmission. Multiple sexual partners and sexually transmitted infections (STIs) were identified as the principal individual risk factors for HIV infection [2].

Some researchers have questioned the hypothesis that in sub-Saharan Africa the virus is transmitted predominantly by sex. For example, Packard and Epstein [3] and, more recently, Gisselquist et al. [4] have suggested that renewed attention should be given to the importance of transmission by blood and contaminated injection equipment. Among the numerous arguments refuting a prominent role for nosocomial transmission of HIV, the relative absence of HIV infections among children aged five to 14 found almost everywhere in Africa suggests that parenteral transmission of HIV does not play a major role [5]. In rural Uganda for example, the prevalence of HIV among children aged five to 12 was 0.4% as opposed to 8.2% among sexually active adults [6].

M. Caraël and J.R. Glynn (eds.), HIV, Resurgent Infections and Population Change in Africa, 123–154.
© Springer Science + Business Media B.V. 2008

In many parts of the developing world, the majority of new HIV infections occur in young adults but this is especially noticeable in Africa where the main mode of HIV transmission is heterosexual sex. As a result, in the continent, about six million young women and three million young men aged 15–24 are estimated currently to be living with HIV [1]. The reasons why young women are more vulnerable to HIV than young men are still not well understood, but unless new HIV infections among them are addressed it is unlikely that HIV control can be achieved in Africa. Whether prevalence stabilizes or declines depends largely on the risk behaviours of susceptible young people as almost all young people enter adulthood HIV-negative. Thus the age at sexual debut and the subsequent behaviour of young people should be the focus of HIV prevention programmes. Yet the very nature of adolescence—characterized by experimentation and risk-taking, but also procreation and parenthood—make youth particularly vulnerable to HIV.

Selected contextual determinants of young people's sexual risk behaviour will be discussed in the first part of this chapter, with special emphasis on how they increase the vulnerability of young people to HIV; the more proximate determinants of young people's sexual behaviour and the biological co-factors of HIV transmission will be discussed in the second section. The third section will briefly review HIV control programmes for young people and the effectiveness of program interventions.

Contextual Determinants

Demographic Change, Urbanization and Poverty

With a demographic growth rate of more than 3% and an age pyramid reflecting the slow decline of mortality in the under-fives, the more sexually active age-groups in developing countries account for a high proportion of the population, much higher than in industrialized countries. 51% of the African population is less than 18 years old, compared to 22% in industrialized countries. A high proportion of this age group is already sexually active [7]. It is estimated that those aged under 25 years account for more than two-thirds of all cases of STI and more than 60% of new cases of HIV infections [8, 1].

The urban populations of sub-Saharan Africa have increased by 600% in the last 35 years: a growth rate which has no precedent in human history. At the same time, sub-Saharan Africa has been undergoing a regression in all its development indices: it has the worst socio-economic parameters (in terms of levels of literacy, school enrolment, maternal mortality, infant mortality, life expectancy) and the most adverse levels of health cover (physician per inhabitant, access to health services) of any world region. From the end of the 1980s, health service reform and the principle of user-fee service and structural reforms imposed by the International Monetary Fund, have increased inequalities in the access to health and social services and decreased their quality [9, 10]. Public expenditure on health care has, on average, not exceeded 2% of the gross national product and the private health sector has played an increasing role, with a deepening of inequity in access. As a result, self-medication and drugs have become increasingly available through pharmacists, drug sellers and traditional healers. In the 1990s, sub-Saharan Africa recorded the world's highest youth unemployment. Youth unemployment accounted for as much as 80% of total unemployment. It is estimated that only 5–10% of new entrants into the labour market can be absorbed by the formal economy [11].

The growth of shanty towns around urban centres in Africa has gone hand-in-hand with an explosion in the number of unemployed and a considerable deterioration in urban services [12]. In 2003, sub-Saharan Africa had the highest rate of slum-dwellers, with 72% of the urban population living in slums. Although there are dramatic differences in income, quality of life and access to services in cities, generally the average level remains extremely low in Africa compared to other continents. In the last decade, 57% of the "poorest" persons (defined as those below the lowest quartile) and 34% of other groups living in urban areas had no access to essential services such as water, electricity or flush toilets. In Asia and Latin America, equivalent figures were about 12% and 2–6% respectively [13]. Access to these services can be used as a proxy to define relative poverty at household or community level.

The association between socio-economic status and HIV infection is not straightforward. It was noted that HIV infection was more common in better educated people of higher socioeconomic status in the early years of the epidemic, but it was postulated that this pattern would change as HIV spread in the population [14]. There is some evidence that this is so for associations with education, with a shift in some later studies and among younger adults towards lower risks of HIV with higher levels of education [15–17]. The pattern is less clear for other measures of socio-economic status and may vary by region and area [18]. Poverty in an urban environment has different implications for sexual behaviour than poverty in rural areas where social control is usually much stronger and where new social needs are less present.

A multivariate analysis of data collected in Kisumu, Kenya showed that there was a significant association between access to running water and electricity in the community and the lack of HIV infection. The authors also found that young women in the lowest socio-economic status group had a significantly younger age at first sexual intercourse and higher occurrence of Herpes infection [19]. In a national survey in South Africa, young people aged 15–24 living in poor informal settlements had more than double the HIV prevalence of those residing in wealthier urban areas—20% versus 9% [20]. In this age group, 79% living in informal urban settlements reported being sexually active as compared to 53% of those living in formal urban areas. In another large survey in South Africa, Pettifor et al. [21] showed that young people in poor informal urban areas had a much higher HIV prevalence rate than those living in urban formal areas: 17% versus 10%. HIV prevalence was three times higher among young women than among young men.

In another study in Nairobi, Kenya [22], the mean age at first intercourse of young women in the poor urban periphery occurred two years earlier than for young women living in wealthier urban areas. These women also reported significantly less knowledge about means of protection from HIV, more sexual partners and lower condom use than young women living in more residential districts. In a comprehensive study using data collected from young people from the KwaZulu-Natal Province in South Africa [23], economic disadvantage was found to significantly affect a number of sexual behaviours and experiences of young women and men. Low socio-economic status not only increases the risk of transactional sex among women, it also raises the risk among women of experiencing coerced sex and for men of having multiple sexual partners. Low socio-economic status was also associated with lower risk of secondary abstinence among women, lower age at sexual debut, lower condom use at last sex, and poorer communication with the most recent sexual partner. Low socio-economic status has more consistent negative effects on female than on male behaviours; it also increases the risk of early pregnancy.

An extensive review of the literature on the sexual behaviour of young people in South Africa, including qualitative studies and unpublished reports [24] found multiple links between poverty and various unsafe sexual behaviours. Poorer young people are reported to have less knowledge of HIV/AIDS and to begin having sex at younger ages. Poverty and lack of parental resources are cited as primary reasons for young women to trade sex for goods or favours or to engage in relationships that involve financial support. Condom use is reported to be consistently lower in these types of sexual encounters.

Migration and Mobility

The selected data above show how low socioeconomic status in the African urban context creates an unprecedented pressure on sexual mores and leads to unsafe sexual behaviours among young people, especially among young women. However, the explosive urban growth experienced by the African continent is largely due to immigration of young rural men and to a lesser extent, women, in search of work [25].

A system of migrant labour that separates individuals from their families and that prolongs absence of the regular partner for economic reasons is frequent in Africa. In a survey in five African countries, the proportion of married men not cohabiting with their spouse in the last 12 months varied from 11% in Tanzania to 43% in Côte d'Ivoire [26]. In rural Zimbabwe, among married men and women, 34% and 51% reported that their spouses lived away from home [27]. Non-cohabitation was more common in those aged under thirty and was closely associated with increased numbers of casual sexual contacts by men during their absence.

The demographic imbalance in the sex ratio which commonly results from this trend is an important determinant of a rapidly expanding HIV epidemic, since it creates a specific demand for transient sexual relations. This factor not only affects migrant receiving areas but also sending areas. For example, in KwaZulu–Natal, in a community where migration affects nearly two-thirds of the adult male population, a study in discordant couples showed that, in nearly 30% of cases, the infected person was the female partner who stayed home in the rural area [28].

Mobility and circulation are not restricted to rural-urban movements. In many African countries, wide differences exist within rural areas depending on how close any given place is to trading points; as in the rural districts of Manicaland, Zimbabwe where the HIV prevalence of women increased from 25% in traditional rural areas to 50% for those living close to highways in shopping centres; figures for men were

20% and 28% respectively [27]. Previous studies in Rwanda and Uganda had also reported similar disparities [29, 30]. Circulation of migrants between rural and urban or market settings is facilitated by roadways: often it is expressed by a greater degree of exposure to the highest levels of urban HIV prevalence and by an unravelling of traditional sexual behaviour, as has been shown in rural Senegal [31].

A study in Yaoundé, Cameroon revealed the importance of mobility as an independent behavioural risk factor. In men, HIV prevalence increased in relation to the length of time spent travelling outside the city. It rose from 1.4% in men staying at home to 3.4% in those absent from the city for less than one month, and to 7.6% in those away for more than one month [32]. Another study in Zimbabwe has also shown that migrant workers working on rural estates have more sexual risk behaviours leading to higher rates of HIV prevalence as compared to other sexually active men and women living in rural areas, 26.4% and 38.8% versus 20.9% and 29.7% respectively [27]. While the prevalence of HIV is generally higher in the cities, reflecting a looser degree of social control over sexuality and an individualization of sexual behaviour, in some provinces of South Africa, Zimbabwe or Kenya, there is no more major difference in HIV prevalence between urban and rural settings. Indeed, temporary mobility is not found exclusively in urban areas; in the rural setting, in large farms and agro-industrial concerns, it is common to see high concentrations of young men and women gathering for the harvest season.

The situation which provides the most tragic illustration of the effect of migration on the HIV epidemic is that in the southern pole of the African continent, where the dramatic economic migration of single men to the mines and other industries of South Africa has impinged, over generations, on marriage and sexual behaviour [33–36]. Most men in Swaziland and Lesotho work there under temporary contracts. Their monthly income allows them ready access to local female prostitution while their wives seek relationships with the few men remaining in the community.

Political Crisis and Conflicts

Since the 1980s, more than half of all African countries have been involved in armed conflict. As a result, prevention programs for STI, including HIV are usually interrupted, health services are disrupted and situations of risk increase tremendously. The number of refugees is estimated to be close to 10 million. Refugees, persons displaced because of conflict and war, and especially young women and children, are extremely vulnerable to sexual violence and STIs/HIV because of their destitution and powerlessness [37]. A study in Sierra Leone found that 9% of women displaced by armed conflict in 1997–1999 had been sexually assaulted by combatants. The study concluded that war-related rape and other forms of sexual violence were committed on a widespread basis among internally displaced persons [38]. Conflicts invariably disrupt access to basic necessities and fragment families, forcing people to become displaced as they flee in search of security and sustenance. Women and girls are particularly prone to the sexual predation of men who can control access to areas, food, shelter and protection.

Gender Inequality and Power Imbalance

The status of women is closely tied up with kinship systems and the different forms of subordination limiting their access to education, the market economy and other sources of independent income. In most patrilineal African societies, social restrictions concerning female sexuality are particularly strong and tend to limit the prospects of premarital and especially extramarital sexual relations. However, men are not submitted to such restraints or social conventions, permitting them to have numerous female partners [26]. Dominant versions of masculinity encourage young boys to "try out" their sexuality with a variety of female partners while young women are encouraged to remain virgins, although many do not (**Fig. 1**). Male domination in the area of sexuality is a decisive barrier to educating women about reproductive health and the main impediment to consistent condom use. For example, a study in South Africa found that women with low relationship control were 2.1 times more likely than other women to use condoms inconsistently and women experiencing forced sex 5.8 times [39].

In many societies of sub-Saharan Africa, gender power differences are particularly expressed in relationships between adolescent girls and older men with higher economic status. Older age and higher income allow men to have more power in reproductive and sexual decision making. In an extensive review of the literature on transactional and cross-generational sexual relations in Africa [40], the authors found evidence of a recent increase in these types of relationships, known as "commoditization" of sexual relationships. They also portrayed two types of analysis used in the literature: one underscores how adolescent girls can be coerced into sexual risk behaviours by external factors such as economic constraints, peer and parental pressures, and social norms of male dominance. The second sees adolescent girls as social actors who have learned that their sexuality is a valued resource and try to bargain the benefits of sexual relations with multiple partners, in a context of gender inequality. Indeed, the economic value of sexuality for adolescent girls is particularly important because they have fewer market opportunities than married women and less money than boys. Older men prefer adolescent girls because they are believed to be less risky for STIs, including HIV and they are less expensive than older women. The review emphasized that girls often appear to be able to negotiate relationship formation and continuance but that once in a sexual partnership they are less able to control the conditions of sexual intercourse including condom and contraceptive use.

A recent review of the literature on sexual violence in the context of HIV [41], in particular with regard to young women, has shown that forced sex occurs universally, and that its frequency is high in Africa. In several surveys, between 15 and 30% of women stated that their first episode of intercourse had been forced and at least 10% said that they had been raped. This violence is often part of a low female status which encompasses arranged early marriages, female genital mutilation, polygamy and wife inheritance. Domestic violence, generally associated with alcohol consumption, was reported by 16 to 50% of women questioned. In one study of high school students, girls of lower socioeconomic status reported experiencing eight times as much physical abuse and four times as much attempted and actual rape within relationships as did those of higher socioeconomic status [42]. Several studies show that young girls who have gone through the trauma of rape and violence later adopt a sexual behaviour far more at risk for STIs. A study in rural Uganda [43] showed that HIV-positive women were seven–ten times more likely to have experienced coercive sex.

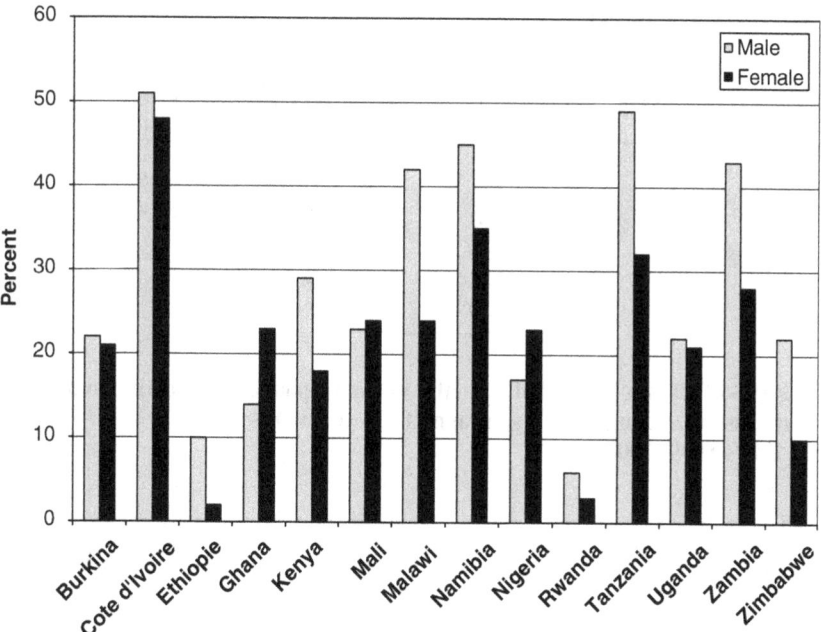

Fig. 1. Proportion of individuals who report having had pre-marital sex among men and women aged 15–19 in selected African countries
Source: **DHS 1999–2003.**

Proximate Determinants of HIV: Sexual Networks

Sexual Risk Behaviour in Young Men and Women

In surveys in 14 countries, pre-marital sex was reported by about 23% of young men and women aged 15–19, but with considerable variation between countries (**Fig. 1**). The proportion was higher among men than women in 8 countries surveyed, equal in four countries, and lower in Ghana and Nigeria. There were large differences among men and women: overall an average of 85% of sexually active men aged 15–24 years reported pre-marital sex in the last year, but this was only reported by 35% of sexually active women in the same age group.

The rate at which sexual partners is changed is a critical factor in the spread of a sexually transmitted virus. A constant feature of surveys on sexual behaviours is that most young women report having few sexual relations and most young men acknowledge more, although this asymmetry varies in its extent. For the 14 countries surveyed, the proportion of men aged 15–19 reporting more than one sexual partner in the last 12 months varied from 12% to 46% with a median of 21%. For young women, it was much lower: varying from 2% to 15%, with a median of 4%. The median M : F ratio of numbers of partners was six with the lowest ratio, 2.5 in Tanzania and the highest of 13 in Nigeria.

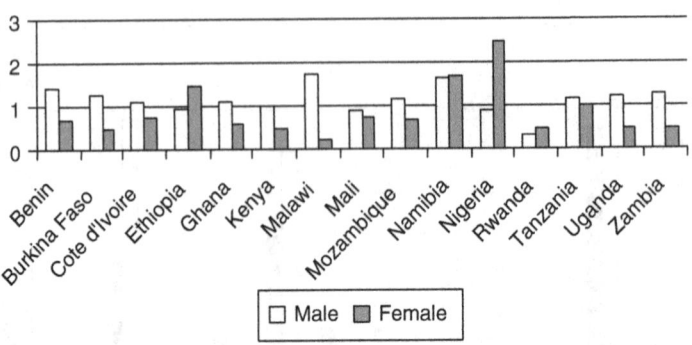

Fig. 2. Ratio of the proportion of sexually active respondents reporting multiple partners in the last year comparing age group 20–24 versus 15–19
Source: DHS 1999–2004

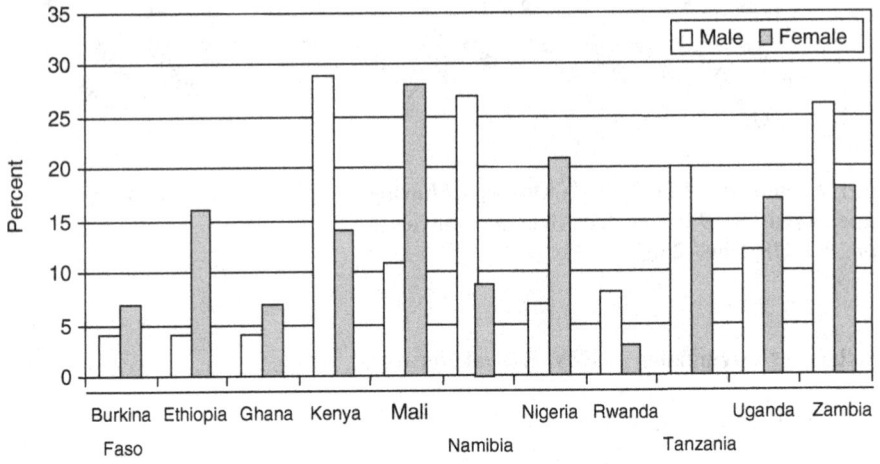

Fig. 3. Percentage of men and women reporting non-marital sex before age 15
Source: DHS

The peak rate of partner change among young men is usually in the age group 20–24 as shown in **Fig. 2**, where in 10 countries out of the 15 surveyed, the ratio of male respondents who reported more than one sexual partner in the age group 20–24 as compared to the age group 15–19 is higher than one. Among young women the ratio is less than one in 11/15 countries surveyed, showing that the peak age for partner change is commonly before age 20: this reflects an earlier age at first marriage or cohabitation in women than in men.

Age at first sex before 15 years, is reported by a substantial proportion of young people as illustrated in **Fig. 3**. The median proportion of young women who report sex before age 15 is around 15% with a range from 3% to 28%. In six out of 11 countries for which recent data are available, more men than women had had first sexual relations before age 15. These figures show indirect evidence that, in these countries, a substantial proportion of young men initiate sexual intercourse with female sex workers.

Surveys in three African countries have shown that an early age at the time of first sexual intercourse is correlated with an increased number of premarital sexual partners compared to those whose first episode of sexual intercourse occurred later [44]. This study also concluded that both men and women who experience their first episode of sexual intercourse at an early age will have more divorces and more extramarital sexual partners, later in life. This effect was more marked in men but was also significant in young women. In a cross-sectional study in four African cities (the "Four Cities Study", in Kisumu, Kenya; Ndola, Zambia; Yaoundé, Cameroon; and Cotonou, Benin) an earlier age at first sexual intercourse was associated with a higher number of sexual partners and a longer period of premarital sexual activity. After having adjusted for current age, HIV infection was associated with an earlier age at the time of first sexual intercourse in two cities with a high HIV prevalence, Ndola and Kisumu, but this effect was considerably reduced after having adjusted for the total number of sexual partners [45]. Similar findings have recently been shown in Zimbabwe [46].

Commercial Sex

The results of simulations with mathematical models suggest that patterns of sexual behaviour whereby men have sex with a small group of highly sexually active women and some contacts with low activity women, lead to high level HIV epidemics [47]. When men marry late and premarital relations for young women are barely tolerated, as is the case in the cultures of Ethiopia, Rwanda and Burundi, many young sexually active men tend to rely on commercial sex workers. Because of this pattern, in those cities, it has been suggested that HIV can be transmitted far more rapidly in the general population than in, for example, Kinshasa or Yaoundé, where control on young women is less strict and sexual relationships more diversified [48].

In sub-Saharan Africa, in 23 countries for which national data are available, the proportion of young men aged 15–24 reporting commercial sex in the last 12 months varied from around nine to 16%, according to the region and to the definition of commercial sex (**Table 1**). Although the question of the definition of commercial sex in different cultural contexts is still unsolved (commercial versus transactional sex), it is striking that the peak prevalence of male contacts with female sex workers in all

Table 1. Proportions of Young Men 15–24 Reporting Sex in Exchange for Gifts, Favours or Money in the Last 12 Months.

Regions in Africa	Median	Lowest	Highest
Western Africa* (N = 9)	10.1	3	13.2
Central Africa* (N = 5)	16	8.5	19.3
Eastern & Southern Africa** (N = 9)	8.9	1	15.5

* Definition used was "sex in exchange for gift, favour or money".
** Definition used was "sex in exchange for money" (DHS 1995–2003).

regions is among the age group 20–24 followed by a decline in older age groups. The explanation for this general trend is straightforward: in the age group 15–19, many young men are not yet sexually active. After age 20–24, many young men are married and have less commercial/transactional sex: the average age at marriage for men ranges from 23 to 26 years. The proportion of men aged 25–49 who report female sex worker contacts/transactional sex corresponds typically to 0.7 of the proportion of those aged 15–24 years in the same populations.

A few countries seem to display a different age pattern, with men reporting more commercial sex in the age group 25–29. Gabon and Côte d'Ivoire are countries hosting a large number of single migrant workers who may continue to have commercial sexual contacts at older ages. In Lesotho, a majority of men are seasonal migrants to South Africa; hence, nuptiality patterns are atypical. In Zimbabwe, age at first sex for women and men is the oldest in sub-Saharan Africa (median age for women = 19.1); hence the peak of sexual activity occurs in the 25–29 age group. In Cameroon, 60% of young males and females report pre-marital sex and 20% of men report sex with a female sex worker in the last 12 months, a much higher proportion and a different pattern than other African countries.

A multivariate analysis of socioeconomic determinants of male contacts with sex workers was conducted in six study sites in sub-Saharan Africa, in the early 1990s [49]. Among the variables included in the analysis, age was identified as the main covariate of commercial sex in most sites. In the majority of sites, but not in Côte d'Ivoire and Kenya, increased education, urban residence and some occupational categories were also significant predictors of sex worker contacts. Other determinants of "demand" for sex workers included marital status (widowed, divorced or single), non-cohabitation with regular partner and migration, and prolonged postpartum abstinence.

Male clients of sex workers usually also have non-commercial sexual contacts. Among the men who were clients of sex workers in the Four Cities Study, approximately one-third reported also having had sexual relations with adolescent girls [50]. In a study in Cotonou, Benin, it was estimated that the number of men who visit sex workers was close to 20,000 or 13% of the male population. Twenty-seven percent of clients were married and a further 52% had a regular girlfriend [51]. In Nyanza Province, Kenya, the majority of clients of sex workers were married and had extramarital partners in addition to sex workers. Most clients had visited three–five different sex workers in the previous year [52].

Female sex workers and their male clients have very high risks of HIV infection in most urban areas of Africa [53]. Women involved in non-commercial sexual relationships are often unaware that their partner may link them to a larger network of sexual contacts and associated risks of HIV/STDs.

Transactional Sex

From qualitative studies in sub-Saharan Africa, which were recently reviewed [40], it appears that the exchange of gifts of money for sex is relatively common among adolescents throughout Africa. For example, the proportion of unmarried sexually

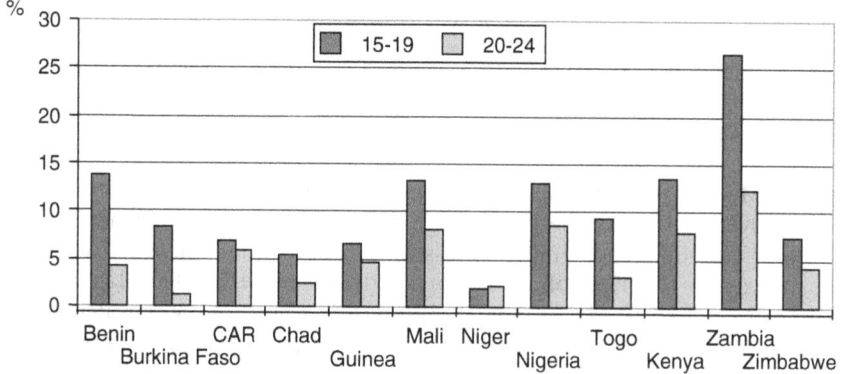

Fig. 4. Proportion of sexually active women reporting sex in exchange for money or gifts, in the last 12 months
Source: DHS 1994–99. In Zimbabwe and Central African Rep (CAR) the time period is the last 4 weeks

active young girls aged 15–19 reported as having recently received money or gifts in exchange for sex, was 13% in Zimbabwe (within the past four weeks), and 31% in Uganda (last sexual encounter). The results of National population surveys in 12 African countries conducted during the 1990s are illustrated in **Fig. 4**. Here the proportion of sexually active women reporting exchange of sex for money or gifts was recorded in the last 12 months. The percentages ranged from 2% to 27% among the 15–19 age group and were higher among this age group than among women aged 20–24 in all countries except Niger. In multivariate analysis, younger age, marital status, and living in urban areas were the only factors significantly associated with transactional sex [54]. The distinction between exchanges of sex for money and receiving gifts that are a normal part of a dating relationship is not always clear. Indirect evidence suggests that money or gifts are often part of a power relation—even in the absence of large age differences—that favour unsafe sex practices [55, 56].

Among the women who reported non-spousal partnerships in the last 12 months in Kisumu and Ndola—two cities with high HIV prevalence—around 40% reported at least one relationship with sex in exchange for money, compared with 6% of women in Cotonou and 14% in Yaoundé, where HIV prevalence was much lower.

Age Differences Between Partners

Age differences in partnerships and sexual networks promote spread of HIV infection between generations. Age mixing between young women and older men, whether inside marriage or outside it, is one of the critical factors driving the spread of HIV in Africa [55–57]. In addition, the transactional component to these sexual relations makes unsafe behaviour more likely.

A study in rural Uganda [56] showed that HIV-1 infection was more common in women with older male sexual partners, whether married or not. Among women aged

15 to 19 years, the adjusted risk of HIV infection doubled among those reporting male partners 10 or more years older compared to those with male partners zero to four years older; among women 20 to 24 years of age, the RR (relative risk) was 1.24. The attributable fraction of prevalent HIV infection in women aged 15 to 24 years associated with partners ten or more years older was 9.7%.

A study in Manicaland, Zimbabwe [55] observed another trend: the youngest women tended on average to have the greatest age difference from their partners, at about eight years. This difference gradually lessened to four years when the women had reached the age of 24. Half of all men aged 30–34 were HIV infected compared to only 3% of men aged 19–20. Among 15–19-year-old women, HIV prevalence rose in clear relation to the age of their most recent partner. HIV prevalence among teenage women whose last partner was less than five years older than themselves was about 16%; among women with partners 10 or more years older, prevalence was twice as high. The authors conclude that a one-year increase in age difference between partners was associated with a 4% increase in the risk of HIV. Young men reported more partners than did women but with infrequent coital acts and greater use of condoms.

In Kisumu, Kenya, similar trends in HIV seropositivity were found but only among married women: no woman aged 15–19 who was married to a man less than four years older than herself was infected with HIV, compared to half of those who had husbands ten years or more older than themselves [58]. In Burkina Faso, having had a first male partner aged more than 24 years was significantly and independently associated with a greater risk of HIV infection among women [59].

How prevalent is a large age difference between partners? Study results highlight the age differences between partners depending on whether sexual relations are marital or extramarital. Clearly polygyny is an important factor that explains age differences between married partners. In the Four Cities Study, the age differences between spouses were 5–7 years. But occasional sexual partners of married men tended, on average, to be 7–8 years younger than themselves. In Cotonou and Yaoundé, around 14% of casual sexual relations took place with women ten or more years younger than their male partners; this figure was 9 to 11% in Kisumu and Ndola. The older the married man, the greater was the age difference with their occasional partners [57].

In the Zambian national survey, sexual partners of married men were on average six years younger but among those who reported that they had occasional partners in addition to their wife, approximately one quarter said they had partners ten years younger than themselves [60]. Similar figures have been reported in Zimbabwe and Tanzania. A review of the literature on age asymmetry and HIV prevalence, and a study in Kenya, also found evidence of a significant relationship between larger age difference and unsafe behaviours, including non-discussion of HIV and non-use of condoms [40, 61].

Early Marriage for Young Women as a Risk Factor for HIV

In sub-Saharan Africa, less than 1% of young men sexually active before 20 are married compared to 60% of young women [7]. In countries with large HIV epidemics, early marriage paradoxically represents a significant risk factor for young women. In Carletonville, South Africa, among women aged 15–24, HIV seropositivity was 63% among those who were married compared to 37% among those who were sexually active and non-married [8]. In Kisumu and Ndola, among the 15–19 age groups, rates of HIV infections were respectively 33% and 22% for married women and 27% and 17% for non-married women. These differences are explained by the fact that, compared to other women of the same age, those who get married early are already more sexually experienced by about a year; they report having had sexual intercourse more often in the previous week—50% in Kisumu and Ndola, compared to 11% and 2% among sexually active unmarried women—and use condoms less often. They are also less likely to be educated, more often from the countryside and know less about HIV/AIDS [62]. In addition, the male partners of single adolescent women are on average three–five years younger than those of married adolescent women. In Kenya, age differences between married partners were 10.2 years for young women married before the age of 15, 7.7 years for women married between 15–19, and six years for women married after age 20 [58].

Studies also show that men who marry at a young age are more likely to be HIV-infected than those who remain single. In Kisumu, 26.3% of married men aged 20–24 were sero-positive compared to 8.3% of single men. In Ndola, the corresponding figures were 28.6% and 9.7% [63]; however, some of these infections will have come from transmission within marriage.

The institution of polygamous marriage contributes to age differences and HIV risk. In Kisumu, where 18% of married young girls aged 15–24 are in a polygamous union, the HIV prevalence was 46% among young girls in a polygamous marriage compared to 35% among those in a monogamous marriage. Male spouses of a polygamous union were on average six years older than those in a monogamous union [58].

In women in high prevalence areas both high rates of premarital infection and transmission within marriage are important sources of HIV infection. In a study in Kisumu and Ndola it was estimated that more than half the infections in women were acquired pre-maritally, that at least one quarter of cases of HIV infection in recently married men were acquired from extra-marital partnerships, and that for both men and women, less than one half of HIV cases were acquired from their spouse [58].

Biological Susceptibility of Girls to HIV

Epidemiological Evidence

During the nineties, the relative proportion of young women and young men infected with HIV in Africa was unclear, as virtually no data were available for young men. Most data were derived from HIV sentinel surveillance systems based on pregnant women attending antenatal clinics. Recent population or community surveys show that in most countries of sub-Saharan Africa, the HIV prevalence among young women aged 15–24 is two to four times higher than that for young men of a similar age (**Fig. 5**). This pattern is even more striking among the age group 15–19: for example, in population surveys, HIV prevalence was 23% for women and 3.5% for men in

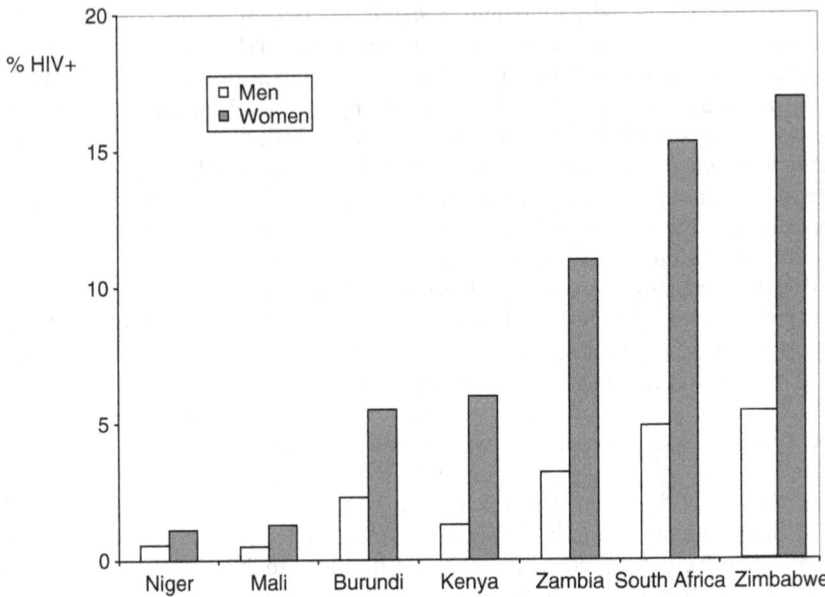

Fig. 5. HIV prevalence among 15–24 year-olds in selected sub-Saharan countries, 2001–2003
Source: **DHS+**

Kisumu, Kenya; 15.4% and 3.7% in Ndola, Zambia; 19.6% and 2.5% in Carletonville, South Africa [59, 60], 19% and 1.8% in the rural district of Rakai, Uganda [66]. The magnitude of this difference at young ages and its consistency across a range of different settings including urban and rural areas makes it likely that it reflects biological as well as behavioural differences between men and women.

The gradient in HIV seropositivity with increasing age seems to be much steeper for young women than for young men. In Kisumu, for example, it increases from 6% at age 15 to 33% at age 19 for women as compared to 0 to 9% for men. This steep growth rate of HIV infection cannot be explained solely by a greater risk of exposure to HIV associated with the number and risk profile of sexual partners unless extreme assumptions are made about under-reporting by the women [58]. The probability of HIV transmission appears to be high among young women from the time of first sexual intercourse. In Ndola, 25% (2/8), and in Kisumu 27% (3/11), young women who reported having had only one sexual partner and only 1–5 episodes of sexual intercourse were already infected by HIV. In men with equivalent sexual histories no HIV infections were found (0/4 and 0/11 respectively) ("Four Cities Study," unpublished data). Even if under-reporting of sexual partners by young women is taken into account, this strongly suggests a differential probability of HIV sexual transmission between the sexes at young ages.

In studies of discordant couples, virus transmission was estimated to be about 0.001–0.003 per sex act and two to three times higher from men to women than from women to men [67]. However, one study in Uganda found no difference in HIV transmission between male to female and female to male [68]. Studies among HIV discordant couples, where, by definition, the transmission has not occurred at the time of HIV sero-conversion, may not give a realistic measure of the probability of transmission in other situations and particularly at young ages. For example, one study in Thailand among female sex workers and their clients, estimated the probability of female-to-male transmission of HIV-1 per sexual contact to be 0.056, more than 50 times higher than probabilities in discordant couples [69]. Clearly, the probability of HIV transmission per sexual act is not constant and is enhanced by biological factors that may be different between sexes at different ages. A recent study among HIV-discordant couples in Uganda found that the rate of HIV transmission per sexual act varies with stage of infection, viral load, presence of genital ulcer diseases and younger age of the index partner [70].

STIs as Co-Factors of Susceptibility to HIV

It is well established that the presence of reproductive tract infections is strongly associated with susceptibility to HIV, even after adjustment for sexual behaviour. The prevalence of genital ulcer disease (chancroid, syphilis, or herpes) is associated with an increased relative risk of HIV infection, ranging from 1.5 to 7.0 in both men and women [71].

Population studies show that the prevalence of STIs among women aged 15–19 is high, and much higher than among men: for example, in Ndola, Zambia, and Kisumu, Kenya, the prevalence of selected STIs in young women is 10–15 times higher than in men (**Fig. 6**). The susceptibility of young women to *Herpes simplex* virus infection type 2 (HSV-2) is extremely high: for example, in a study in Carletonville in South Africa [65], after a few episodes of unprotected sexual intercourse with a single sexual partner, around 40% of women aged 15–19 already had

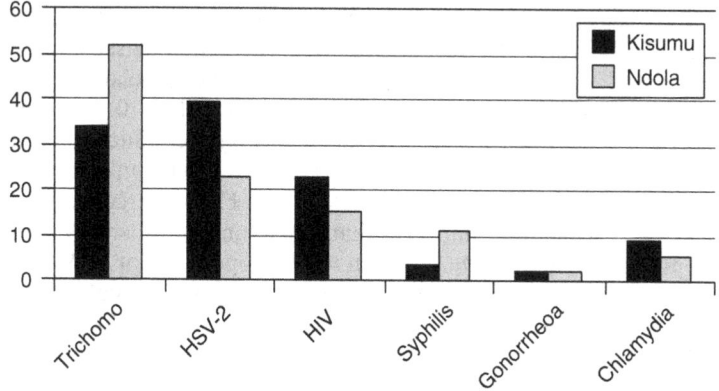

Fig. 6. Percentage of selected STIs among women aged 15–19 years
Source: Adapted from (64)

antibodies to HSV-2. This proportion rose to 80% for women reporting having had four sexual partners. For men, the equivalent figures were 16% and 22% respectively. The high prevalence of HSV-2 in young women will increase their probability of acquiring HIV. HSV-2 has become the primary cause of genital ulceration in most African countries and increasing evidence demonstrates a synergetic link between HIV and genital herpes. More than 30 epidemiologic studies have demonstrated that prevalent HSV-2 is associated with a 2- to 4-fold increased risk of HIV-1 acquisition [72, 73]. A recent meta-analysis of longitudinal studies found that HSV-2 infection increased the risk of HIV acquisition 3-fold in both men and women in the general population, and that the relative risk was even higher following recent HSV-2 infection [74]. It is likely that HSV-2 infection also increases the infectiousness of HIV-positive subjects, although the evidence for this is less clear. In a multivariate analysis of risk factors for HIV concordancy among married couples, the only significant factor explaining positive concordancy was HSV-2 seropositivity in one or both spouses [75].

In females, early sexual activity has been associated in some studies with an increase in prevalence rates of STIs and pelvic inflammatory diseases, raising the possibility that the physiological and immunological immaturity of the female genital tract may also be a risk factor for HIV [76]. It remains difficult to establish to what degree the young age at first sex for women contributes to their susceptibility to HIV. The "Four City Study" clearly raises the possibility of an aggregate of social and biological factors [77]. The high HIV and other STI prevalence among young women is not necessarily associated with a high degree of sexual activity as shown before: it reflects factors of social and biological vulnerability such as the lack of STI symptoms in young women, greater difficulty in recognising them, and greater difficulty in gaining access to the appropriate treatments.

Male Circumcision

The transmission of HIV from female-to-male and from male-to-female may be affected by the circumcision status of the male partner. In most studies, uncircumcised men have higher rates of HIV infection than their circumcised counterparts. A systematic review of 15 studies conducted in Africa on the association between male circumcision and HIV infection [78] showed a relative risk of 0.4. For example, a recent prospective cohort study of nearly 2,300 adult men conducted in Pune, India found that, after adjusting for socio-demographic and behavioural factors, circumcision was strongly protective against acquisition of HIV-1: circumcised men were 6.7 times less likely to acquire infection than uncircumcised men [79]. In Kisumu, Kenya, 24.9 per cent of uncircumcised men were seropositive for HIV compared to 9.6 per cent of circumcised men; there were no differences in sexual behaviour, condom use or STI prevalence between the two groups, suggesting that circumcision is an independent factor [80]. In a study in Uganda, no uninfected male partner of an infected female acquired HIV if he was circumcised, even if the female had a high viral load [81]. Male circumcision may protect against acquisition of HIV infection chiefly because of the removal of the foreskin which contains a high density of HIV-specific cellular targets.

Summary of Risk Factors for Young Women

In summary, the high susceptibility of young women to HIV infection is multifactoral and the phenomenon is not yet well understood. Several factors appear to interact:
- High biological susceptibility, linked to the immaturity of the genital tract, the role of genital ulcers and in particular infection with genital herpes virus.
- Behavioural factors, including early age at the time of first sexual intercourse and marriage, transactional sex, sexual relations with an older partner and forced coitus. The practical effect of these factors is greater difficulty in refusing sex and/or negotiating protected sexual intercourse.
- Contextual factors, influencing HIV exposure and susceptibility: poverty, inequalities of power between men and women, standards of masculinity, the inferior status of young women, and their low levels of access to information and services.

Systemic problems such as poverty, conflicts and food crisis are contributing to the tide of the HIV epidemic and are clearly increasing the vulnerability of young people to HIV infection. Poverty, low education, and lack of parental guidance and support influence young people's sexual behaviours by reducing access to information about safe sex practices or by inhibiting their ability to put such knowledge into practice. The gap between what young people know and how they act is sustained by social and economic realities that constrain their individual actions. Socioeconomic development should be the key to altering the determinants of sexual risk behaviours. The programmatic implications of these findings call for combined efforts to improve educational opportunities and to tackle unemployment; and to provide a shift in social norms to promote a healthy lifestyle for young people, especially young women, which includes HIV-protective behaviours. The assumption is that integrated, comprehensive approaches will be more effective in reducing risk for HIV infection than individual interventions and programmes. In the short term, the range of information and services provided to young women and their older partners should aim to reduce early exposure to sexual activity, including promotion of delaying first sex and teaching negotiation skills. Increased access to school education has also been shown to be associated with delayed first sex and increased condom use.

Another aim should be to reduce the likelihood of HIV transmission per sexual act. This calls for increased access to condoms, to increased recognition of early symptoms of STI, and better access to treatment for young people. Here also, cultural and religious sensitivities are major obstacles.

Finally, reducing age difference between partners and transactional sex will require deep changes in community norms and values. Patterns of sexual mixing as discussed before are mostly driven by economic forces and by young women's strategies to increase their social status [82]. Providing women with skills and opportunities that reduce dependence on men for financial support should be core components of prevention programmes. Several micro-credit studies targeting women indicate that economic empowerment translates into increased self-esteem, improved social networks, increased control over household decision-making, and increased bargaining power [83].

HIV Control Programmes for Young People

From Reproductive to Sexual Health

Young people's health has been a low priority due to the pressure for palliative/curative care in adults and the efforts taken to reduce high child mortality and morbidity. Youth were not considered as producers and this age group was seen as relatively healthy or affected only by minor diseases, such as STIs. Furthermore, one of the great obstacles to sexual and reproductive health programmes in sub-Saharan Africa and elsewhere has been the denial of young people's sexuality and the belief that sexual education and services would encourage experimentation and promiscuity—despite strong evidence to the contrary. That is why early efforts to target young people focussed on women and children, reproductive health, modern contraception and pregnant and parenting young people.

At the international level there has been a growing consensus that reproductive health interventions targeting young people should receive high priority. There have been numerous international summits on this topic since 1994, with government commitments, such as the International Conference of Population and Development in Cairo and follow up meetings; but even in 2001, at the United Nations General Assembly Special Session on HIV/AIDS, and in the declaration of the Millennium Development Goals, the concept of sexual health education was barely mentioned, because of lack of consensus among States.

In many sub-Saharan African countries, the policy environment needed to develop effective national HIV/STI prevention programmes for young people has considerably improved: most of the strategies and policies to strengthen the national response are in place, although often resulting in a large number of overlapping policies emanating from different ministries [84]. Policies may have an impact directly, for example by facilitating access to information and services that are essential for prevention, or indirectly by decreasing young people's vulnerability by affecting the environments in which they live, learn and earn.

However, beyond rhetoric, when it comes to implementation of these strategies, policy has not resulted in much change to existing structures in the last decade: only a fraction of young people have access to basic prevention and care services. For example, although STI services have a much higher profile than previously, at country level, they remain programmatically disjointed and disorganized: they are not widely provided through stand-alone public sector programmes, or firmly integrated into maternal and child health or family planning services [85]. As a result, they are not reaching those who most need them: only one in four African countries reported that at least 50% of STI patients are appropriately diagnosed, counselled and treated [84].

With the exception of Ethiopia, Uganda and Mauritius, life-skills based education is not yet incorporated in primary and secondary schools. Some sort of AIDS education is given in 60% and 80% of African countries in primary and secondary school curricula respectively, but this education consists mainly of medical or biological information. Fewer than one in four young people at high risk of HIV have access to information on risk reduction [84, 85].

In most of sub-Saharan Africa, prevention of mother to child transmission of HIV programmes cover less than a few percent of pregnant women. Only around 12% of people who want to be tested for HIV are able to access voluntary counselling and testing services. Around 30% of sex workers are covered by outreach prevention programmes [84, 86]. In sum, most programmes in African countries are still inadequate, at pilot stages in urban areas and dominated by a "project" mentality.

As a result of this poor coverage of basic interventions, comprehensive knowledge of HIV/AIDS among young people is still low in most African countries. For 18 countries where data were available after 2000, fewer than 50% of women aged 15–24 were able to both identify ways of preventing the sexual transmission of HIV and reject major misconceptions about HIV transmission or prevention. These percentages were higher for young men, and in urban settings as compared to rural ones. To the question "Can a healthy looking person have HIV virus" in 5 of the 21 countries surveyed fewer than 50% of young women responded correctly that this was true. In 12 countries where trends in knowledge were available, only three countries (Côte d'Ivoire, Malawi, and Mozambique) showed significant improvement [7]. Condom use in sexual relationships of risk for HIV has considerably increased over the years; however, in most countries, these changes are occurring against a backdrop of high HIV prevalence that limits its effectiveness. In only seven of 17 countries surveyed did more than 50% of men aged 15–24 report using a condom in the last sexual intercourse of risk (with condom use ranging from 30% in Ethiopia to 88% in Botswana). Condom use at last high-risk sex was low among young women in all countries (median below 30%); it was only above 50% in 2 of the 17, Burkina Faso and Botswana [7].

These results clearly show that either effective prevention programmes are not in place in most countries or that the coverage of the activities is so low as to have little impact at the population level, or both.

Effective HIV Prevention Interventions for Young People

HIV Prevention in Question

There has been a growing scepticism about the effectiveness of HIV prevention programmes for HIV, including programmes targeting young people. Indeed, more than 20 years into the HIV epidemic, despite recent increases in HIV/AIDS-related international and national funding, few countries in the world have been able to successfully reverse their HIV epidemics, although many countries have kept their national HIV prevalence at low levels.

The success of Uganda, where HIV prevalence among young women aged 15–19 years declined from 32.2% in 1991 to 10.3% in 1997, has not yet been replicated elsewhere [87, 88]. In sub-Saharan Africa, declining trends of HIV among women aged 15–24 years are usually used as a proxy for demonstrating recent change in HIV incidence. Declining HIV trends in this age group have been reported in several cities such as Cotonou, Lusaka, Addis Ababa, and Nairobi or in some regions of Tanzania [89], Malawi and Rwanda but in many other settings the HIV epidemic shows no signs of declining HIV incidence attributable to behavioural changes [90]. This questions the outcomes of past and current interventions, whether improvements in knowledge, attitudes, skills or reduction in risk behaviours, although it is clear that relationships between these factors and reduction in HIV incidence are complex and non linear [91].

Evaluation of Effectiveness of Interventions

Over the past decade, pressure for rapid and visible action against HIV epidemics has led many national AIDS programmes to consider evaluation of interventions as a low priority. It was assumed that what is effective was known. The pressure was to spend external funds on much-needed activities, and investment in evaluation was perceived as a research activity, far from programmatic concerns. As a result, not much has been learned about what works in prevention despite efforts to document "best practices" in HIV prevention [92]. Observational data at national level, from the few countries that have documented behavioural change and declines in HIV infection, are often difficult to interpret. For example, documented declines in HIV prevalence in Uganda have been attributed to a variety of interventions—from communication strategies to condom promotion—but it is still not clear which interventions produced the behavioural changes and the type and magnitude of these changes. In addition, it is likely that it was the specific combination of intervention strategies—including involvement by high-level political and other community leaders, behavioural change communication, and condom promotion—that produced significant changes [93]. Most of what has been learned has been documented in research projects, which makes it difficult to assess to what extent programmes can replicate findings on a large scale, in different contexts.

A large community randomised trial in Mwanza, Tanzania assessed a package of interventions in young people, including in-school sexual and reproductive health education, youth-friendly reproductive health services, community-based condom promotion and distribution, and other community activities to create a supportive environment for youth [94]. The intervention had no impact on biomedical outcomes, including HIV incidence [95]. In this trial the restriction to young people may have limited the impact, but another large trial of information and education, in Uganda, targeting a wider age range, also found no effect on HIV incidence, even when coupled with improved management of STIs [96]. Other trials are in progress, but these demonstrate the difficulty of assessing specific interventions against a background of other national and community interventions.

There has been increased recognition that the evaluation of the effectiveness of interventions aimed at prevention should necessarily entail the use of designs other than randomized controlled trials, and various types of evidence will need to be considered together [97]. Indeed, most interventions in HIV prevention are multifaceted and the pathways to impact are complex, reflecting the complexity of the relationship between risk behaviours and HIV [98].

One of the critical weaknesses in measuring the effectiveness of behavioural intervention is that nearly all behavioural outcomes are self-reported, which raises questions about their validity. This was recently demonstrated by the results of the community randomized trial in Mwanza, Tanzania, where both behavioural and biological outcomes were assessed and compared. Evaluation results showed that the intervention had a significant impact on knowledge, reported attitudes, and reported behaviours but not on HIV or other STIs [99]. This may mean that the interventions had more impact on reported than on actual behaviour, or that the limited age range and time frame of the intervention has not (yet) had a chance to impact on the larger sexual networks in the community.

Despite these challenges, several recent reviews of prevention interventions in developed and developing countries, covering adults and young people, have tried to assess their effectiveness by looking at intermediate variables, such as knowledge, intentions, communication, and changing norms that can indicate progress towards behavioural change [100–102]. In some studies, but not all, young people who received HIV risk reduction interventions had improved skills in negotiating lower risk sexual encounters, increased frequency of communications with sexual partners about safer sex, reduced sexual frequency, and increased reported condom use compared with comparison groups, making the case for some efficacy of HIV prevention.

We analyze below in more detail the evaluation of selected interventions addressing prevention of HIV among young people in sub-Saharan Africa, recognizing that most of the interventions reviewed have multiple components.

Mass Media

Mass media whether TV, radio, soap operas, posters, billboards and print materials have the potential of reaching young people in great number. The evidence in the published literature on the effectiveness of communication programmes is sparse. Media programmes may have multiple media components, and may also be part of more comprehensive youth HIV prevention programmes, such as LoveLife, and Soul City in South Africa, which include national mobilization, social marketing and mass media campaigns, life-skills training, peer education and outreach, and sometimes linkages with schools and community-based organizations. Out of 15 media interventions addressing HIV-related behaviours among youth evaluated in a recent review, 11 were from Africa [103]. Significant improvements in knowledge and interpersonal communication were noted but no evidence of improved skills or access to health services. Whereas the media interventions reported mixed or limited results with regard to delaying first sex and partner reduction behaviours, condom use showed significant increases in six of eleven studies reporting on this outcome. According to the authors, this suggests that the role of media programmes in addressing HIV prevention among youth extends beyond providing access to information to promoting adoption of HIV-preventive behaviours. In addition, the compelling dose-response data suggest that increasing exposure to the campaigns, through frequent broadcasts, employment of multiple media channels, or extended campaign duration, contributes to significant gains in knowledge and behaviour change. They also found that behavioural change communication is most effective when it works in support of the larger national strategy to combat HIV/AIDS. For example, the success of a condom social marketing programme in Tanzania that led to increased condom use, relied heavily on an extensive mass media campaign [104].

School Based Education

Coverage, sustainability, and the opportunity to intervene before risk behaviours become established mean that schools are an important venue for HIV preventive interventions. Schools, especially at primary level, are attended by most young people and provide opportunities to achieve high coverage of young people around the time of sexual initiation.

One review assessed 11 published and evaluated school-based HIV/AIDS risk reduction programmes for youth in Africa [105]. The objectives varied, with some interventions targeting only knowledge, others attitudes, and others behaviour change. Ten of the 11 studies that assessed knowledge reported significant improvements. All seven that assessed attitudes reported some degree of change towards an increase in attitudes favourable to risk reduction. In one of the three studies that targeted sexual behaviours, sexual debut was delayed, and the number of sexual partners decreased. In one of the two that targeted condom use, condom use behaviours improved.

Another recent review of sex and HIV education in schools [106] identified 22 programme evaluations in developing countries, including 12 in Africa. None of the interventions conducted in Africa increased sexual activity and eight out of 12 significantly delayed sex or reduced frequency of risk behaviours or increased condom use. Some programmes had a positive impact on more than one outcome. For example, an intervention in Tanzania both reduced the number of sexual partners among boys and increased reported condom use among both boys and girls [99]. The authors concluded that teacher-led curriculum-based interventions have particularly strong evidence of a positive impact on multiple behaviours. Effectiveness was less obvious for peer-led and non-curriculum based interventions. These studies provide strong evidence that some, but not all, programmes can increase knowledge about HIV/AIDS, perception of HIV risk, perceptions of peer norms regarding sex and condom use, self-efficacy to refuse sex, self-efficacy to use condoms, intentions to abstain from sex or to use a condom, and communication with parents or other adults about sex and condoms.

Community Based Interventions

Community interventions directed at both youth and adults are an essential component of HIV prevention planning for young people. However, identification of key stakeholders and accessible structures for broader interventions can be problematic. Furthermore, poverty, lack of education and other resources can mean that those youth who are most in need of interventions are often the most difficult to reach. Hierarchies of gender, age and power within communities can further interact to limit young women's access to such interventions. A recent review summarized the results of 25 evaluations of interventions [107], including 18 from Africa, using community members to target young people with information about HIV transmission and prevention. Although the weak quality of most evaluation designs was a problem, the authors found conclusive evidence of improvement in knowledge on HIV, in building communication skills and reducing sexual risk behaviours for interventions implemented through existing youth serving organizations or centres. Of

5 interventions aiming at delaying first sex, only one documented positive results. The authors also found plausible evidence of effectiveness in raising awareness and increasing community responsiveness for AIDS programme activities linked with social networks, including parents or as part of community-wide festivals or events. Overall, programmes have worked with peer-educators, trained professionals, community volunteers, government officials and other stakeholders as implementers, yet clear guidance has yet to be developed as to the relative merits and appropriateness of each strategy in differing settings.

Facility Based Intervention

Increasing young people's access to health services should become a central component of any HIV prevention strategy. Health services and supplies (e.g. antibiotics, condoms) are important for primary prevention, skills building and risk reduction. If facilities are user-friendly for youths, they can provide or refer for voluntary counselling and testing for HIV, STI care and treatment, and reproductive health. They can link to a range of service providers, public and private, government and NGO, include outreach and social marketing, and can channel young people towards other services that they require (e.g. schools and youth clubs). Increasing access also requires addressing young people's health seeking behaviours especially in ensuring that they seek services, thereby generating demand.

Diagnosis and treatment of STIs also has the potential directly to reduce HIV transmission at community level, although the evidence from intervention studies so far is mixed, in particular for young people [108]. However, a number of studies, targeting commercial sex workers give additional evidence of the efficacy of STI management for HIV prevention. For example, interventions among sex workers in Kinshasa and Abidjan, involving STI treatment and condom promotion resulted in a 50% reduction in HIV incidence among the sex workers (109–111). In addition, these interventions have the potential of decreasing HIV/STIs among their male clients (111–112) and therefore the general community.

A recent review shows that health services with regular screening have reported increases in condom use and reductions in STI and HIV prevalence among female sex workers. Such successful services generally include a strong peer education and empowerment component, emphasize consistent condom use, and provide effective treatment for both symptomatic and asymptomatic STIs [113].

Increased STI service utilization by young people after an intervention in schools with peer educators has been demonstrated in a study in Nigeria [114]. In Tanzania, multi-component interventions did not result in higher numbers of adolescents seeking STI treatment but this may have been the result of the successful treatment of symptomatic STI [115]. A study that evaluated the impact of three youth-friendly service projects in Lusaka, Zambia reported encouraging results: better clinic experience for adolescent clients and increased service use levels at some clinics. The findings also suggest that community acceptance of reproductive health services for youth may have a large impact on the health-seeking behaviours of adolescents [116].

For two major factors that may play a critical role in increasing HIV incidence among young women and in explaining gender differences in HIV infection, operational research is still in development. HSV-2 control for HIV prevention is far from being operationalized: several trials are in progress to measure the effect of anti-herpes treatment (either episodic or suppressive) on HIV acquisition or transmission and on the effects of a vaccine. Two randomized trials testing the efficacy of male circumcision in preventing HIV transmission or acquisition are currently underway in Kenya and Uganda, and one was recently completed in South Africa. All three studies are assessing whether circumcision protects against HIV acquisition among adult men; and the Uganda trial will also test whether male circumcision also protects female partners. The South African trial reported a 60% reduction in HIV incidence in circumcised men [117]. Whether male circumcision before puberty is acceptable and feasible as an added procedure within the remit of other preventive actions depends mainly on cultural factors, although its acceptability appears to be high among men and women, in South Africa, Kenya and Botswana [118–121].

Conclusion

Around the world, young people account for half of all new HIV infections, 2.1 million each year, with girls and young women especially at risk (1,122). The majority of young people with new infections are from sub-Saharan Africa. Half are poor, and one fourth live on less than US$1 per day. Many are sexually active, often without the power, knowledge or means to protect themselves. Challenges are enormous with socioeconomic development already hampered by AIDS mortality, and the region facing 14 million orphans.

There is enough evidence that behavioural interventions for young people, especially with multiple components can achieve behavioural change if scaled up at population level, beyond research projects. However, evaluation reviews also call for careful attention to characteristics and contexts of interventions, sustainability in efforts, with a dose-response effect in most successful interventions. Unfortunately most interventions with proven efficacy have not been taken to scale nor made available to the majority of young people in need of them. Institutional reasons vary from one country to another but generally include competing demands for scarce resources, lack of political commitment beyond declarations, lack of engagement of other sectors than health, lack of decentralization at community and district level, and lack of human resources in health and education sectors [90]. Analyses suggest that if the successes achieved in some countries in prevention of HIV transmission had been expanded to a global scale by 2005, about 29 million new HIV infections could be prevented by 2010, the majority in sub Saharan Africa [123], even in the absence of any progress in new technologies such as vaccine or microbicides.

Vulnerability factors highlighted in the paper have shown that structural factors including unemployment, poverty and gender norms can greatly influence the environment in which sexual behaviours of young people occur. Despite the difficulty of evaluating their effects, a relatively small number of intervention studies demonstrate the potential of structural interventions to increase HIV prevention (124–126). The broad agenda to reduce vulnerability factors is still often perceived as conflicting with risk reduction approaches and targeted interventions [127], although both should be increasingly recognized as complementary. Indeed, in recent years, greater attention has been paid to the possibilities of altering social and economic conditions in order to effect HIV prevention. UNAIDS and many international agencies have emphasized the links between environmental factors and HIV. Many Poverty Reduction Strategy Programs in Africa have factored HIV into their plans and increased their domestic funding to combat HIV/AIDS [128]. At the international level, increased funding has been made available through the Global Fund, the World Bank and bilateral donors [90]. As a result, prevention programmes should be scaled up and greater access to anti-retroviral treatment should lead to decrease in AIDS morbidity and mortality, and offer new possibilities for HIV prevention. Turning the tide of the HIV epidemic will not only demand increased resources and expansion of effective programmes, but also requires targeting of young people with appropriate interventions and tackling sexuality issues that remain particularly sensitive not only at the central political level but at the community level as well [129].

Bibliography

1. UNAIDS (2006). Report on the global AIDS epidemic. (Geneva: UNAIDS)

2. Wasserheit, J. N. (1992). Epidemiological synergy: Interrelationships between HIV infection and other sexually transmitted diseases. *Sex Transmitted Diseases, 19*, 61–67

3. Packard, R. M. & Epstein, P. (1991). Epidemiologists, social scientists, and the structure of medical research on AIDS in Africa. *Social Science and Medicine, 33*, 771–794

4. Gisselquist, D., Rothenberg, R., Potterat, J. & Drucker, E. (2002). HIV infections in sub-Saharan Africa not explained by sexual or vertical transmission. *International Journal of STD & AIDS, 13*, 657–666

5. Schmid, G. P., Buve, A., Mugyenyi, P., et al. (2004). Transmission of HIV-1 infection in sub-Saharan Africa and effect of elimination of unsafe injections. *The Lancet, 363*, 482–488

6. Kengeya-Kayondo, J. F., Malamba, S. S., Nunn, A. J., et al. (1995). HIV-1 seropositivity among children in a rural population of south-west Uganda: Probable routes of exposure. *Annals of Tropical Paediatrics, 15*, 115–120

7. DHS Demographic and health surveys (1995–2004). (Washington: Macro International. HIV/AIDS indicators database).Retrieved from Measuredhs.com

8. WHO (1995). Global prevalence and incidence of selected curable sexually transmitted diseases: overview and estimates. (Geneva: WHO)

9. Lurie, P., Hintzen, P. & Lowe, R. A. (1995) Socioeconomic obstacles to HIV prevention and treatment in developing countries: The roles of the International Monetary Fund and the World Bank. *AIDS, 9*, 982–984

10. World Bank reports (1992–1996). Public expenditure reviews. (Washington: World Bank)

11. ILO (2004). Global employment trends for youth 2004. (Geneva: ILO)

12. Adjamagbo, A., Delaunay, V. (1998). La crise en milieu rural ouest Africain: Implications sociales et conséquences sur la fécondité. Niakhar (Sénégal), Sassandra (Côte-d'Ivoire), deux exemples contrastés. (In F. Gendreau (Ed.), *Crises, pauvreté et changements démographiques dans les pays du sud* (pp. 339–355). Paris: Estem)

13. Hewett, P. & Montgomery, M. R. (2001). Poverty and public services in developing-country cities. Policy Research Division working papers. (New York: The Population Council)

14. Over, M. & Piot, P. (1993). HIV infection and sexually transmitted diseases. (In D. T. Jamison, W. H. Mosley, A. R. Mensham & J. L. Bobadilla (Eds.), *Disease control priorities in developing countries* (pp. 455–527). Oxford: Oxford University Press)

15. Hargreaves, J. R. & Glynn, J. R. (2002). Educational attainment and HIV-1 infection in developing countries: A systematic review. *Tropical Medicine and International Health, 7,* 489–498

16. Gregson, S., Mason, P. R., Garnett, G. P., Zhuwau, T., Nyamukapa, C. A., Anderson, R. M., et al. (2001). A rural HIV epidemic in Zimbabwe? Findings from a population-based survey. *International Journal of STD & AIDS, 12*(3), 189–196

17. Glynn, J. R., Caraël, M., Buvé, A., Anagonou, S., Zekeng, L., Kahindo, M., Musonda, R. M. & the Study Group on Heterogeneity of HIV Epidemics in African Cities. (2004). Does increased general schooling protect against HIV infection? A study in four African cities. *Tropical Medicine and International Health, 9,* 4–14

18. Wojcicki, J. M. (2005). Socioeconomic status as a risk factor for HIV infection in women in East, Central and Southern Africa: A systematic review. *Journal of Biosocial Science, 37,* 1–36

19. Hargreaves, J. R. (2002). Socioeconomic status and risk of HIV infection in an urban population in Kenya. *Tropical Medicine and International Health, 7,* 793–802

20. Nelson Mandela/HSRC Study of HIV/AIDS. (2002). South African national HIV prevalence behavioral risks and mass media: Household survey 2002 South Africa, Private Bag X9182. (Cape Town, 8000: Human Sciences Research Council Publishers)

21. Pettifor, A. E., Rees, H. V., Steffenson, A., et al. (2004). HIV and sexual behavior among young South Africans: A national survey of 15–24 year olds. (Johannesburg: Reproductive Health Research Unit, University of the Witwatersrand)

22. Zulu, E., Ezeh, A. C. & Nii-Amoo Dodoo, F. (2002). Slum residence and sexual outcomes: Early findings of causal linkages in Narobi, Kenya. Nairobi: African Population and Health Research Center, 2000. *and also* Zulu, E. M., Dodoo, F. N., Chika-Ezee, A. (2002). Sexual risk-taking in the slums of Nairobi, Kenya, 1993–8. *Population Studies, 56,* 311–323

23. *Hallman,* K. (2004). Socioeconomic disadvantages and unsafe sex behavior among young women and men in South Africa. Policy research paper n° 190. (New York: The Population Council)

24. Eaton, L., Flisher, A. J., Aaro, L. E. (2003). Unsafe sexual behaviour in South African youth. *Social Science and Medicine, 56,* 149–165

25. UN population division (2001). The world urbanization prospect: The 1999 revision. (New York: UNP)

26. Caraël, M. (1995). Sexual behavior. (In J. Cleland & B. Ferry(Eds.), *Sexual behavior and AIDS in the developing world* (pp. 75–123). London: Taylor & Francis)

27. Coffee, M. P., Garnett, G. P., Mlilo, M., et al. (2005). Patterns of movement and risk of HIV infection in rural Zimbabwe. *JID, 191,* 159–167

28. Lurie, M. N., Williams, B. G., Zuma, K., et al. (2003). Who infects whom? HIV-1 concordance and discordance among migrant and non migrant couples in South-Africa. *AIDS, 17,* 2245–2252

29. Van De Perre, Ph., Le Pollain, B., Caraël, M., et al. (1987). HIV antibodies in selected adults from a rural area in Rwanda, Central Africa. *AIDS, 4,* 212–216

30. Serwadda, D., Wawer, M. J., Musgrave, S. D., et al. (1992). HIV risk factors in three geographic strata of rural Rakai District, Uganda. *AIDS, 6,* 983–989

31. Lagarde, E., Pison, G. & Enel, C. (1995). A study of sexual behavior change in rural Senegal. *Journal of Acquired Immune Deficiency Syndromes*, 1–6

32. Lydie, N., Robinson, N. J., Ferry, B., Akam, E., et al., (2004). Mobility, sexual behavior, and HIV infection in an urban population in Cameroon. *Journal of Acquired Immune Deficiency Syndromes*, 35, 67–74

33. Hunt, C. W. (1989). Migrant labor and sexually transmitted diseases: AIDS in Africa. *Journal of Health and Social Behaviour*, 30, 353–373

34. Moody, T. D. (1988). Migrancy and male sexuality on the South African gold mines. *Journal of South African Studies*, 14, 228–256

35. Romero-Daza, N. (1994). Multiple sexual partners, migrant labor, and the making for an epidemic: Knowledge and beliefs about AIDS among women in Highland Lesotho. *Human Organization*, 53, 192–205

36. Timaeus, I. & Graham, W. (1989). Labor circulation, marriage and fertility in Southern Africa. (In R. J. Lesthaeghe (Ed.), *Reproduction and social organization in sub-Saharan Africa* (pp. 365–400). Berkeley: University of California Press)

37. Hankins, C., Friedman, S., Zafar, T., et al. (2002). Transmission and prevention of HIV and STIs in war settings: Implications for current and future armed conflicts. *AIDS*, 16, 2245–2252

38. Amowitz, L. L., Reis, C., Lyons, K. H., et al. (2002). Prevalence of war-related sexual violence and other human rights abuses among internally displaced persons in Sierra Leone. *JAMA*, 287, 513–521

39. Pettifor, A. E., Measham, D. M., Rees, H. V. & Padian, N. (2004). Sexual power and HIV risk, South Africa. *Emerging Infectious Diseases*, 10, 1996–2004

40. Luke, N. & Kurz, K. M. (2002). Cross-generational and transactional sexual relations in sub-Saharan Africa. AIDSMark project. (Washington, DC: International Center for Research on Women). *See also*: Luke, N. (2003). Age and economic asymmetries in the sexual relationships of adolescent girls in sub-Saharan Africa. *Studies in Family Planning*, 34, 67–86

41. Garcia-Moreno, C. & Watts, C. (2000). Violence against women: Its links with HIV/AIDS prevention. *AIDS*, 14(3), S253–S266

42. Whitefield, V. J. (1999) A descriptive study of abusive dating relationships amongst adolescents. Unpublished master's dissertation, University of Cape Town

43. Quigley, M. A., Morgan, D., Malamba, S. S., et al. (2000). Case–control study of risk factors for incident HIV infection in rural Uganda. *Journal of Acquired Immune Deficiency Syndromes*, 23, 418–425

44. White, R., Cleland, J. & Caraël, M. (2000). A multi-country analysis of associations between pre-marital sex and extramarital sex. *AIDS*, 14, 2323–2331

45. Auvert, B., Buve, A., Ferry, B., et al. (2001). Ecological and individual level analysis of risk factors for HIV infection in four urban populations in sub-Saharan Africa with different levels of HIV infection. *AIDS*, 15, S15–S30

46. Pettifor, A. E., van der Straten, A., Dunbar, M. S., Shiboski, S. C. & Padian, N. S. (2004). Early age of first sex: A risk factor for HIV infection among women in Zimbabwe. *AIDS*, 18, 1435–1442

47. Anderson, R. M., May, R. M., Boily, M. C., Garnett, G. P. & Rowley, J. T. (1991). The spread of HIV-1 in Africa: Sexual contact patterns and the predicted demographic impact of AIDS. *Nature*, 352, 581–589

48. Caraël, M. & Piot, P. (1998). HIV infection in developing countries. *Journal of Biosocial Science*, (Suppl 10), 35–50

49. Deheneffe, J. C., Caraël, M., & Noumbissi, A. (1998). Socio-economic determinants of sexual behaviour and condom use. (In *Confronting AIDS: Evidence from the developing world* (pp. 131–46). Washington: The World Bank)

50. Morison, L., Weiss, H., Hayes, R., Buve, A., et al. (2001). The role of commercial sex work in the HIV epidemics in four cities in Sub-Saharan Africa. *AIDS, 15*(Suppl 4), 61–69

51. Lowndes, C. M., Alary, M., Meda, H., et al. (2002). Role of core and bridging groups in the transmission dynamics of HIV and STIs in Cotonou, Benin, West Africa. *Sexually Transmitted Infection, 78*(Suppl 1), 69–77

52. Voeten, H., Egesah, O. B., Ondiege, M., et al. (2002). Clients of female sex workers in Nyanza Province, Kenya: A core group in STD/HIV transmission. *Sexually Transmitted Disease, 29*(8), 444–452

53. UNAIDS (2004). Report on the global AIDS epidemic. (Geneva: UNAIDS)

54. Chatterji, M., Murray, N., London, D. & Anglewicz, P. (2004). The factors influencing transactional sex among young men and women in 12 sub-Saharan African countries. Policy paper. (New York: Policy project)

55. Gregson, S., Nyamukapa, C. A., Garnett, G. P., et al. (2002). Sexual mixing patterns and sex-differentials in teenage exposure to HIV infection in rural Zimbabwe. *The Lancet, 359*, 1896–1903

56. Kelly, R. J., Gray, R. H., Sewankambo, N. K., et al. (2003). Age differences in sexual partners and risk of HIV-1 infection in rural Uganda. *Journal of Acquired Immune Deficiency Syndromes, 32*, 446–451

57. Ferry, B., Carael, M., Buve, A., et al. (2001). Comparison of key parameters of sexual behavior in four african urban populations with different levels of HIV infection. *AIDS, 15*, S41–S50

58. Glynn, J. R., Caraël, M., Buve, A., et al. (2001). Why do young women have a much higher prevalence for HIV than young men? A study in Kisumu, Kenya and Ndola, Zambia. *AIDS, 15*, S51–S60

59. Lagarde, E., Congo, Z., Meda, N., et al. (2004). Epidemiology of HIV infection in urban Burkina Faso. *International Journal on STD & AIDS, 15*, 395–402

60. Central Statistical office, Ministry of Health, Zambia (2004). Measure evaluation. Zambia sexual behaviour survey 2000. North Carolina, USA

61. Luke, N. (2005). Confronting the sugar daddy stereotype: Age and economic asymmetries and risky sexual behaviour in urban Kenya. *International Family Planning Perspectives, 31*, 6–14

62. Shelley, C. (2004). Early marriage and HIV risks in sub-Saharan Africa. *Studies in Family Planning, 35*, 149–160

63. Glynn, J. R., Carael, M., Buve, A., et al. (2002). HIV risk in relation to marriage in areas with high prevalence of HIV infection. *Journal of Acquired Immune Deficiency Syndromes, 33*, 526–535

64. Buve, A., Carael, M., Hayes, R. J., et al. (2001). Multicentre study on factors determining differences in rate of spread of HIV in sub-Saharan Africa: Methods and prevalence of HIV infection. *AIDS, 15*, 5–14

65. Auvert, B., Ballard, R., Campbell, C., et al. (2001). HIV infection among youth in a South African mining town is associated with herpes simplex virus-2 seropositivity and sexual behaviour. *AIDS, 15*, 931–934

66. Konde-Lule, J. K., Wawer, M. J., Sewankambo, N. K., et al. (1997). Adolescents, sexual behavior and HIV-1 in rural Rakai district, Uganda. *AIDS, 11*, 791–799

67. Mastro, T. D. & de Vincenzi, I. (1996). Probabilities of sexual HIV-1 transmission. *AIDS, 10*(Suppl A), S75–S82

68. Gray, R., Wawer, M., Brookmeyer, R., et al. (2001). Probability of HIV-1 transmission per coital act in monogamous, heterosexual, HIV-1-discordant couples in Rakai, Uganda. *The Lancet, 357*, 1149–1153

69. Mastro, T. D., Satten, G. A., Nopkesorn, T., Sangkharomya, S., Longini, I. M. Jr. (1994). Probability of female-to-male transmission of HIV-1 in Thailand. *The Lancet, 343*, 204–207

70. Wawer, M. J., Gray, R. H., Sewankambo, et al. (2005). Rates of HIV-1 transmission per coital act, by stage of HIV-1 infection, in Rakai, Uganda. *Journal of Infectious Diseases, 191*, 1391–1393

71. Royce, R. A., Sena, A., Cates, W., et al. (1997). Sexual transmission of HIV. *New England Journal of Medicine, 336*, 1072–1078

72. Corey, L., Wald, A., Celum, C. L. & Quinn, T. C. (2004).The effects of herpes simplex virus-2 on HIV-1 acquisition and transmission: A review of two overlapping epidemics. *Journal Acquired Immune Deficiency Syndromes, 35*, 435–445

73. Weiss, H. (2004). Epidemiology of herpes simplex virus type 2 infection in the developing world. *Herpes, 11*, 24–35

74. Freeman, E. E, Weiss, H. A., Glynn, J. R., Cross, P. L., Whitworth, J. A., Hayes, R. J. (2007). Herpes simplex virus 2 infection increases HIV acquisition in men and women: Systematic review and meta-analysis of longitudinal studies. *AIDS* (in press)

75. Freeman, E. E. & Glynn, J. R. (2004). Factors affecting HIV concordancy in married couples in four African cities. *AIDS, 18*, 171521

76. Duncan, M. E., Tibaux, G., Pelzer, A., et al. (1990) First coitus before menarche and risk of sexually transmitted disease. *The Lancet, 335*, 338–340

77. Caraël, M. & Holmes, K. (Eds.) (2001). The multicentre study of factors determining the different prevalences of HIV in sub-Saharan Africa. *AIDS, 15*, 1–4

78. Weiss, H. A., Quigley, M. A. & Hayes, R. J. (2000) Male circumcision and risk of HIV infection in sub-Saharan Africa: A systematic review and meta-analysis. *AIDS, 14*, 2361–2370

79. Reynolds, S. J., Shepherd, M. E., Risbud, A. R., et al. (2004). Male circumcision and risk of HIV-1 and other sexually transmitted infections in India. *The Lancet, 363*, 1039–1040

80. Auvert, B., Buve, A., Lagarde, E., et al. (2001). Male circumcision and HIV infection in four cities in sub-Saharan Africa. *AIDS, 15*, S31–S40

81. Gray, R., Azire, J., Serwadda, D., et al. (2004). Male circumcision and the risk of sexually transmitted infections and HIV in Rakai, Uganda. *AIDS, 18*, 2428–2430

82. Longfield, K., Glick, A., Waithaka, M. & Berman, J. (2004). Relationships between older men and younger women: Implications for STIs/HIV in Kenya. *Studies on Family Planning, 35*, 125–134

83. Kim, J., Gear, J., Hargreaves, J., et al. (2002). *Social Interventions for HIV/AIDs Intervention with Microfinance for AIDS and Gender Equity: Monograph No. 1.* (Johannesburg: Rural AIDS and Development Action Research Programme of the School of Public Health, University of Witwatersrand)

84. UNAIDS (2003). Progress report on the global response to the HIV/AIDS epidemic. (Geneva: UNAIDS)

85. Askew, I. & Berer, M. (2003). The contribution of sexual and reproductive health services to the fight against HIV/AIDS: A review. *Reproductive Health Matters, 11*, 51–73

86. USAID, UNAIDS, WHO, UNICEF and the Policy project (2003). Coverage of selected services for HIV/AIDS prevention, care and support in low and middle income countries in 2003. (Geneva: WHO)

87. Kilian, A. H., Gregson, S., Ndyanabangi, B., et al. (1999) Reductions in risk behaviour provide the most consistent explanation for declining HIV-1 prevalence in Uganda. *AIDS, 13*, 391–398

88. Asiimwe-Okiror, G., Oppio, A. A., Musinguzi, J. et al. (1997). Change in sexual behaviour and decline in HIV infection among young pregnant women in urban Uganda. *AIDS, 11*, 1757–1763

89. Jordan-Harder, B., Maboko, L., Mmbando, D., et al. (2004). Thirteen years HIV-1 sentinel surveillance and indicators for behavioural change suggest impact of programme activities in south-west Tanzania. *AIDS, 18*, 287–294

90. UNAIDS (2004). Report on the global AIDS epidemic. (Geneva: UNAIDS)

91. Aral, S. O. (2004). Sexual risk behaviour and infection: Epidemiological considerations. *Sexually Transmitted Infection, 80*(Suppl II), 8–12

92. Rugg, D., Peersman, G. & Carael, M. (2004). Global advances in HIV/AIDS monitoring and evaluation. New directions in Evaluation n. 103. (Hoboken, New Jersey: Jossey-Bass)

93. Cohen, S. (2005). Beyond slogans: Lessons from Uganda's experience with ABC and HIV/AIDS. Alan Guttmacher Institute report. Retrieved July from www.agiusa.org/pubs/journals/gr060501.pdf

94. Hayes, R., Changalucha, J., Ross, D. A., Gavyole, A., Todd, J., Obasi, A. I. N., Plummer, M. L., Wight, D., Mabey, D. C. & Grosskurth, H. (2007) The MEMA kwa Vijana Project: Design of a community-randomised trial of an innovative adolescent sexual health intervention in rural Tanzania. *Contemporary Clinical Trials*, (in press)

95. Changalucha, J., Ross, D. A., Todd, J., Everett, D., Plummer, M., Anemona, A., Obasi, A. I. N., Balira, R., Weiss, H. A., Mosha, F., Chilongani, J., Grosskurth, H., Mabey, D. C. & Hayes, R. J. (2003). MEMA kwa Vijana, a randomised controlled trial of an adolescent sexual and reproductive health intervention programme in rural Mwanza, Tanzania: 4. Results: Biomedical outcomes. Abstract No. 0699. (Ottawa, Canada: ISSTDR Congress, July 27–30, 2003). *See also* Gavyole, A., Ross, D. A., Changalucha, J., Plummer, M., Obasi, A. I. N., Todd, J., Cleophas-Mazige, B., Wight, D., Grosskurth, H., Mabey, D. C., Bukenya, D. & Hayes, R. J. (2003). MEMA kwa Vijana, a randomised controlled trial of an adolescent sexual and reproductive health intervention programme in rural Mwanza, Tanzania: 5. Summary and implications. Abstract No. 0700. (Ottawa, Canada: ISSTDR Congress, July 27–30, 2003)

96. Kamali, A., Quigley, M., Nakiyingi, J., et al. (2003). Syndromic management of sexually-transmitted infections and behavior change interventions on transmission of HIV-1 in rural Uganda: A community randomized trial. *The Lancet, 361*, 645–652

97. Victora, C. G., Habicht, J. P. & Brice, J. (2004). Evidence-based public health: Moving beyond randomized trials. *Public Health Matters, 94*, 400–405

98. Cleland, J., Boerma, T., Carael, M. & Weir, S. S. (Eds.). Measurement of sexual behaviour. *Sexually Transmitted Infection*, (Suppl II)

99. Ross, D., Changalucha, J. & Obasi, A., et al. (2007) Effects of an Innovative Adolescent Sexual Health Intervention on HIV and Other Outcomes: A Community Randomized Trial in Rural Tanzania (Accepted) AIDS

100. Speizer, I. S., Magnani, R. J. & Colvin, C. E. (2002). The Effectiveness of adolescent reproductive health interventions in developing countries: A review of the evidence. *Journal of Adolescent Health, 33*(5), 324–348

101. Merson, M. H., Dayton, J. M. & O'Reilly, K. (2000). Effectiveness of HIV prevention interventions in developing countries. *AIDS 14*(Suppl 2), S68–S84

102. Johnson, B. T., Carey, M. P., Marsh, K. L., et al. (2003). Interventions to reduce sexual risk for the human immunodeficiency virus in adolescents, 1985–2000: A research synthesis. *Archives of Pediatrics and Adolescent Medicine, 157*, 381–388

103. Bertrand, J. T. & Anhang, R. (2006). The effectiveness of mass media in changing HIV/AIDS related behavior among young people in developing countries. *World Health Organization Technical Report Series, 938*, 205–241

104. Eloundou-Enyegue, P. M., Meekers, D., Calves, A. E. (2005). From awareness to adoption: The effect of AIDS education and condom social marketing on condom use in Tanzania (1993–1996). *Journal of Biosocial Science, 37*, 257–268

105. Gallant, M. & Maticka-Tyndale, E. (2004). School-based HIV prevention programmes for African youth. *Social Science and Medicine, 58*, 1337–1351

106. Kirby, D., Obasi, A. & Laris, B. A. (2006). The Effectiveness of sex education and HIV Education interventions in schools in developing countries. *World Health Organization Technical Report Series, 938*, 103–150

107. Maticka-Tyndale, E. & Brouillard-Coyle, C. (2006) The effectiveness of community interventions targeting HIV and AIDS prevention at young people in developing countries. *World Health Organization Technical Report Series, 938*, 243–285

108. Korenromp, E. L., White, R. G., Orroth, K. K., et al. (2005) Determinants of the impact of sexually transmitted infection treatment on prevention of HIV infection: A synthesis of evidence from the Mwanza, Rakai, and Masaka intervention trials. *Journal of Infectious Diseases, 191*(Suppl 1), S168–S178

109. Laga, M., Alary, M., Nzila, N., et al. (1994). Condom promotion, sexually transmitted diseases treatment, and declining incidence of HIV-1 infection in female Zairian sex workers. *The Lancet, 344*, 246–248

110. Ghys, P. D., Diallo, M. O., Ettiegne-Traore, V., et al. (2001). Effect of interventions to control sexually transmitted disease on the incidence of HIV infection in female sex workers. *AIDS, 15*, 1421–1431

111. Cote, A. M., Sobela, F., Dzokoto, A., et al. (2004). Transactional sex is the driving force in the dynamics of HIV in Accra, Ghana. *AIDS, 18*, 917–925

112. Alary, M., Mukenge-Tshibaka, L., Bernier, F., et al. (2002). Decline in the prevalence of HIV and sexually transmitted diseases among female sex workers in Cotonou, Benin, 1993–1999. *AIDS, 16*, 463–470

113. Steen, R. & Dallabetta, G. (2003). Sexually transmitted infection control with sex workers: Regular screening and presumptive treatment augment efforts to reduce risk and vulnerability. *Reproductive Health Matters, 11*, 74–90

114. Okonofua, F. E., Coplan, P., Collins, S., Oronsaye, F., et al. (2003). Impact of an intervention to improve treatment-seeking behavior and prevent sexually transmitted diseases among Nigerian youths. *International Journal of Infectious Diseases, 7*, 61–73

115. Grosskurth, H., Mosha, F., Todd, J., et al. (1995). A community trial of the impact of improved sexually transmitted disease treatment on the HIV epidemic in rural Tanzania: 2. Baseline survey results. *AIDS, 9*, 927–934

116. Mmari, K. N. & Magnani, R. J. (2003). Does making clinic-based reproductive health services more youth-friendly increase service use by adolescents? Evidence from Lusaka, Zambia. *Journal of Adolescent Health, 33*, 259–270

117. Auvert, B., Taljaard, D., Lagarde, E., Sobngwi-Tambekou, J., Sita, R., Puren, A. (2005). Randomized, controlled intervention trial of male circumcision for reduction of HIV infection risk: The ANRS 1265 trial. *PLOS Medicine, 2*, e298

118. Scott, B. E., Weiss, H. A., Viljoen, J. I. (2005), The acceptability of male circumcision as an HIV intervention among a rural Zulu population, Kwazulu-Natal, South Africa. *AIDS Care, 17*, 304–313

119. Lagarde, E., Dirk, T., Puren, A., Reathe, R. T., Bertran, A. (2003). Acceptability of male circumcision as a tool for preventing HIV infection in a highly infected community in South Africa. *AIDS, 17*, 89–95

120. Mattson, C. L., Bailey, R. C., Muga, R., Poulussen, R., Onyango, T. (2005), Acceptability of male circumcision and predictors of circumcision preference among men and women in Nyanza Province, Kenya. *AIDS Care, 17*, 182–194

121. Kebaabetswe, P., Lockman, S., Mogwe, S., et al. (2003). Male circumcision: An acceptable strategy for HIV prevention in Botswana. *Sexually Transmitted Infection, 79*, 214–219

122. Monasch, R. & Mahy, M. (2006). Young people: The centre of the HIV epidemic. *World Health Organization Technical Report Series, 938,* 15–41

123. Stover, J., Walker, N., Garnett, G., et al. (2002). Can we reverse the HIV/AIDS pandemic with an expanded response? *The Lancet, 360,* 73–77

124. Sweat, M. D. & Denison, J. A. (1995). Reducing HIV incidence in developing countries with structural and environmental interventions. *AIDS, 9*(Suppl A), S251–S257

125. Tawil, O., Verster, A. & O'Reilly, K. (1995). Enabling approaches for HIV/AIDS prevention: Can we modify the environment and minimise the risk? *AIDS, 9,* 1299–1306

126. Sumartojo, E. (2000). Structural factors in HIV prevention: Concepts, examples, and implications for research. *AIDS, 14*(Suppl 1), S3–S10

127. Ainsworth, M. & Teokul, W. (2000). Breaking the silence: Setting realistic priorities for AIDS control in less-developed countries. *The Lancet, 356,* 55–60

128. African Union (2003). *The Abuja Declaration on HIV/AIDS and other related infectious diseases.* (At the African Summit on HIV/AIDS, TB and other related infectious diseases, Abuja 26–27 April, 2003). Retrieved from www.uneca.org/adf2000/Abuja%

129. Wellings, K., Collumbien, M., Slaymaker, E., et al. (2006). Sexual behaviour in context: A global perspective. *The Lancet, 368*(9548), 1706–1728

CHAPTER 8. SEXUAL BEHAVIOUR CHANGE, MARRIAGE AND HIV PREVALENCE IN ZAMBIA

EMMA SLAYMAKER AND BASIA ZABA
Centre for Population Studies, London School of Hygiene and Tropical Medicine, London UK

Abstract. There have been a series of nationally representative surveys in Zambia between 1996 and 2003 that contain information on sexual behaviour in the general population. These show that risky sexual behaviours have become less common. There is evidence of a decline in reported early sexual debut. In a generalized epidemic the sexual behaviour of married people, and the similarity of behaviour patterns within couples, may become an important determinant of HIV transmission. Using Demographic and Health Survey data, the behaviours of married couples were compared between 1996 and 2001/2. Over this period there was less change in the risk behaviour of married couples than in the total survey population. The risk behaviours that showed a significant decline were sex with more than one partner in the last year (men only) and sex before the age of 15. Married couples became more similar to each other with respect to sex before the age of 15. Marital status changed over this period. Monogamously married couples in 2001 were less likely to have the same history of previous marriage than those in 1996. There was an increase in the proportion of men in monogamous second marriages. The distribution of women's marital status did not change. These changes are consistent with increases in adult mortality (a consequence of increases in HIV prevalence) and suggest that marital dynamics are changing in Zambia. Marriages (either polygamous or monogamous) in which the man has been married before are becoming more common. HIV testing is uncommon: in 2001 only 3% of couples had both been tested for HIV infection. HIV prevalence has remained stable in Zambia between 1996 and 2001. If the declines in risk behaviour that have been observed in this period do not eventually lead to a decline in HIV prevalence this may indicate that the transmission patterns of HIV have changed. The data on marital history are not sufficiently detailed to fully characterize the changes that have taken place in Zambia. However the results suggest that this is an area which needs further investigation; HIV prevention and surveillance efforts may need to pay more attention to married people as behaviour change and increases in HIV associated mortality begin to change the dynamics of marriage.

M. Caraël and J.R. Glynn (eds.), HIV, Resurgent Infections and Population Change in Africa, 155–170.

Introduction

There have been five nationally representative surveys of sexual behaviour in Zambia between 1996 and 2003 [1–5]. Comprehensive rounds of ANC sentinel surveillance for HIV were carried out in 1994, 1998 and 2001. In the 2001/2 Zambia Demographic and Health Survey (ZDHS) HIV and syphilis testing were included for the first time.

The sexual behaviour data show that reported sexual risk behaviours have become less common in Zambia between 1996 and 2003. National HIV prevalence is apparently stable but there are some regional variations.

From the 1996 and 2001/2 ZDHS, cohabiting couples can be identified and their behaviours can be compared. The behavioural characteristics of cohabiting couples are assessed in the light of the changes in individual behaviour observed between 1996 and 2003.

Background

Declines in the prevalence of reported sexual risk behaviours between 1996 and 2003 have been seen among both men and women in Zambia. Most change has occurred among young people. The risk behaviours that have shown the most obvious decline among both men and women are: having had sex before age 15, having had multiple partnerships in the last year, and having had unprotected sex with non-cohabiting partners. Other changes include declines in the proportion of all men who report sex with a commercial sex worker in the last year (from 22% in 1996 to 1% in 2003). The proportion of women who have had sex in their lifetime but not in the last year has increased: and the proportion of women who report having had sex with a non-cohabiting partner in the last year has decreased [6].

It is encouraging to see decreases in the proportion of individuals who report sexual risk behaviours. However the impact of these changes on HIV prevalence may be modified by the degree to which the behaviour of each individual's partners also changes. If changes mean that couples become concordant in terms of their sexual risk behaviours this may slow HIV transmission more effectively than if couples diverged in their risk behaviours, even if the overall declines in the prevalence of risk behaviours are the same, since the infection would be confined to a smaller sub-population. It is therefore worthwhile to compare the sexual risk behaviours of married couples in 1996 and 2001.

At the national level, HIV prevalence appears to have been relatively stable since 1996 at between 17% and 18% (based on the Epidemic Projection Package (EPP) [7, 8] model fit to the ante-natal clinic (ANC) sentinel surveillance data). Among women of reproductive age (15–49) tested in the 2001/2 DHS the prevalence was 17.8%. Prevalence among men aged 15 to 49 was 12.9%, giving a national estimate of 15.6%.

We would expect declines in risk behaviour to occur before declines in prevalence, but the usual time lag between these changes is not known. However, declines in risky behaviour that are not followed by prevalence decline may point (in the absence of treatment) to changes in the patterns of transmission of HIV. As epidemics become established and HIV infection becomes more widespread the behavioural markers that are associated with exposure to HIV will change.

In a population experiencing a generalized epidemic, marriage may lose its protective value. Married people may be at lower risk of contracting infection in concentrated or low-level epidemics in which HIV infection is most often found among people who have specific sexual or drug injecting behaviours that are typically less common among married people. The Four Cities study showed that marriage was actually a risk factor for HIV infection [9]. It is therefore of interest to see whether the behaviours that have changed among married men and women in Zambia have resulted in couples having a more similar risk profile in 2001 than they did in 1996.

Methods

Data for women, men and couples from the 1996 and 2001/2 ZDHS were obtained from MEASURE DHS [1, 4]. Couples are men and women who were both interviewed in the DHS, who lived in the same household and who named each other as a spouse.[1] In each survey, the sample of women was three times larger than the sample of men. Polygamously married men were matched to all interviewed wives, and so may appear more than once in the data. Data on all current unions were used, except where stated. Preliminary analysis of these data showed that there was no difference between the results for monogamous unions only and for all unions. Data were recoded to identify individuals with specific risk behaviours and new variables were created to indicate whether the couple was concordant for specific behaviours.

Some of the currently married men and women who were interviewed do not feature in the couple data because their spouse could not be interviewed, despite being eligible. The risk behaviours that we are interested in may be different between the married people whose spouse was interviewed and those whose spouse was not interviewed. The characteristics of the currently married men and women who were in the couple sub-sample were compared with those who were not included.

The observed changes in behaviour have been most pronounced among young people. The average age of married respondents is substantially higher than that of unmarried respondents and so the behaviours of married respondents may not have altered to the same extent. Therefore the first stage of the analysis was to ascertain whether there had been changes in the reported behaviour of the currently married respondents between the 1996 and 2001 survey. The same sexual behaviour indicators were then compared with regard to the concordance between the man and woman in each couple for each risk behaviour.

---

[1] Spouse refers to a partner legally married to the respondent, or a partner who is cohabiting with the respondent as though married. It is used in this sense throughout.

All respondents were included in the denominator for each indicator.[2] The indicators of risk behaviour chosen were: the proportion who had had sex before the age of 15, the proportion who had had sex with more than one person in the year before the survey, and the proportion who had had sex with a non-cohabiting partner in the year before the survey.

Trends in the proportion of respondents who report having had sex before age 15 are vulnerable to reporting bias. Respondents, who are all aged 15 or over, cannot change their behaviour with regard to this indicator. The proportion of all respondents who reported this behaviour changed dramatically between the surveys [6] and this was due in part to a change in the propensity to report this behaviour.

Genuine change in this behaviour between 1996 and 2001 should be evident only among the most recently married respondents: those who were not yet married in 1996. The prevalence of sex before the age of 15 was compared between 1996 and 2001 surveys for two groups: all married respondents and those who had been married for five or fewer years at the time of the survey. Whilst both groups are vulnerable to changes in propensity to report this behaviour, in the group of recently married respondents there may have been real changes in behaviour between the two surveys.

The prevalences of previous marriage, and re-marriage were investigated in both the matched couples and among all respondents in the 1996 and 2001 surveys. Investigation was limited by the way in which information on previous marriage was collected. Experience of a marriage that ended was derived from current marital status (separated, divorced, widowed) for those not currently married and from a question on previous marriage for those currently married. For polygamously married men the answer to the latter question is always yes, but it is not possible to ascertain whether these men are still married to all of the wives they have ever married. Consequently people in polygamous marriages are excluded from the results concerning marital history.

Changes in marriage patterns may in part be due to changes in population structure and the availability of partners. Estimates of population size were needed to interpret trends in marital status and these were obtained by age group and sex for 1995 and 2000 from the United Nations Population Division online database [10]. These were projected forwards one year using the DHS mortality estimates.

The unit of analysis was first the married man or woman and then the couple. The prevalences of individual and couple characteristics, with 95% confidence intervals, were calculated taking into account the complex survey design. The sample weights derived for the men's sub-sample were used throughout the analysis. Chi-squared tests, adjusted for survey design, were used to test for the significance of any changes. Analysis was carried out using Stata 8 [11]. Logistic regression models, adjusted for survey design, were used to assess changes, between the two surveys, in the concordance of couples with respect to the indicators.

---

[2] Although this analysis uses data from matched couples, the men and women concerned were sampled independently and their results were later matched.

Results

Data were available for 842 couples in 1996 and 1107 couples in 2001. After sample weights were applied the effective total for analysis was 1930. The sample weights used did not average 1 because weights were based on the total sample of men. The data from 14 couples (1 from 1996 and 13 from 2001) were excluded from the analysis because, although they had been matched as cohabiting partners, the man did not report having had sex with a spouse in the last 12 months, but the woman reported recent sex with a spouse. It should be noted that in some of the remaining couples there was substantial disagreement between the reports of the two partners. For example, 21% of couples gave marital durations which differed by more than one year (this could only be calculated for the 1124 couples for whom both partners were in their first marriage).

The accuracy of a couple's reporting can also be assessed by comparing each partner's report of the time since they last had sex. In 1996 this information was available for all but two of the monogamous couples (742). In 2001 it was only possible to make this comparison in monogamous couples for whom the spouse was the most recent sexual partner for both the man and woman (923 out of 988). These data were collected as the number of days, weeks, months or years as appropriate for each respondent. The results have been given in days (transformed from the units given) because husbands and wives were not necessarily interviewed on the same day and in some cases reported in different units.

In both surveys a quarter of the couples gave identical responses (24% in 1996, 25% in 2001). The most commonly given estimates were within seven days of each other (40% in 1996 and 45% in 2001). In 1996 18% of the couples gave estimates that differed by more than 30 days: this was lower in 2001 at 12%. There was a significant change between 1996 and 2001 (p = 0.01) but this may be partly due to the changes in the way this information was collected.

The age of the female partners (mean 29, range 15 to 49) and male partners (mean 35, range 15 to 59) was similar in both surveys as was the mean age difference between spouses (mean of six years). The level of education attained by the female partners was significantly higher in the second survey (p = 0.03) but there was no change for men. Ethnic and religious backgrounds were the same in both surveys and similar proportions of couples came from urban areas. The proportions of newly married (5%) and polygamous couples (11%) were the same in both surveys.

Sexual Behaviour

Sex before age 15 declined between the surveys. In 1996 it was reported by 27% of the male partners and 25% of the female partners. In 2001 this had decreased to 16% and 18% respectively (**Table 1**). There was a significant decline in the proportion of couples who were discordant for this behaviour, from 38.5% in 1996 to 28% in 2001 (**Table 2**).

In 1996, there was little difference, in the proportion reporting sex by age 15, between all couples and those who married within the five years before the survey. By 2001,

Table 1. Percentage of the married men and women in the couple sub-sample with selected risk behaviours, by survey year.

		1996	2001	p-value
Sex by age 15	Men	27.2	15.6	**<0.0001**
	Women	24.5	18.2	**0.001**
More than one partner in last year	Men	20.0	23.0	0.2
	Women	1.6	1.2	0.5
Unprotected sex with non-cohabiting partners	Men	10.6	11.0	0.8
	Women	1.3	0.8	0.4
Previously married*	Men	27.8	32.6	**0.04**
	Women	16.4	16.6	0.9

*Restricted to monogamously married couples

the more recently married couples differed from all married couples. More recently married couples were more similar to each other in this risk behaviour because there was a greater proportion of couples for whom neither partner had had sex by age 15, due to a large decline in the proportion of couples for whom only the man had reported this behaviour (**Table 2**).

The proportion of married men who reported having had sex with more than one partner in the year preceding the survey was about 20% in both years. In contrast fewer than 2% of the married women reported this risk behaviour (**Table 1**). This difference was not due to polygyny: among monogamously married men 19% reported having more than one partner in 1996 and 18% reported this in 2001. There was no change in the proportion of couples who were discordant for this behaviour (**Table 2**).

The proportion of married men who reported having had sex with a non-cohabiting partner in the year before the survey and not using a condom the last time (11%) was much higher than the proportion of married women who reported this behaviour (1%). These proportions did not change between the surveys and nor did the proportion of couples who were discordant for this behaviour (**Table 2**).

There was no difference in any of these risk behaviours, or in the prevalence of previous marriage, between men whose wives were interviewed and those whose wives were not. For women there were no differences in sex with more than one partner, or in unprotected sex with a non-cohabiting partner, between women whose husbands were interviewed and those whose husbands were not, in either 1996 or 2001. In 1996 there was no difference in age at sexual debut between married women whose husbands were or were not interviewed, but in 2001 the proportion of currently married women who reported sex by age 15 was significantly lower in the couples who were both interviewed (18%) than in those women whose partners were not interviewed, (22%, p = 0.009). In both periods the proportion of monogamously

Table 2. Percentage of couples with different combinations of risk behaviour, by survey year.

		1996	2001	p-value
Couples married ≤ 5 years at time of survey:				
Sex by age 15	Neither	55.9	71.8	**0.0006**
	Man only	26.4	11.5	**0.0001**
	Woman only	13.2	11.4	0.6
	Both	4.5	4.2	0.9
All Couples:				
Sex by age 15	Neither	54.8	68.7	**<0.0001**
	Man only	20.3	12.1	**<0.0001**
	Woman only	18.2	15.9	0.1
	Both	6.7	3.3	**0.0008**
More than one partner in last year	Neither	79.1	76.4	0.2
	Man only	19.3	22.4	0.1
	Woman only	0.98	0.59	0.4
	Both	0.7	0.7	0.99
Unprotected sex with non-cohabiting partners	Neither	88.4	88.6	0.9
	Man only	10.4	10.6	0.9
	Woman only	1.1	0.4	0.1
	Both	0.6	0.4	0.4
Previous marriage*	Neither	68.1	61.8	**0.01**
	Man only	15.4	21.3	**0.003**
	Woman only	4.0	5.4	0.2
	Both	12.3	11.1	0.4

*Restricted to monogamously married couples

married women who had previously been married was significantly lower in the women whose spouse was interviewed (18% and 17% in 1996 and 2001 respectively) compared to women whose spouse was not interviewed (22% and 21% in 1996 and 2001 respectively) and there was no change in this between the two surveys (p = 0.02 and 0.002, 1996 and 2001 respectively).

Multivariate Analysis

Logistic regression models were used to assess whether couples in 2001 were more similar to each other than those in 1996 with respect to: 1) having had sex before the age of 15 and 2) history of previous marriage. The first analysis included only couples who had been married for less than 5 years (27% in 1996 and 25% in 2001/2).

This necessitated the exclusion of couples in which neither partner was in their first marriage (14%) because it was not possible to calculate the duration of the current marriage for those couples. The second analysis included only monogamous couples because it was not possible to ascertain whether men currently in polygamous marriages have ever been in a marriage that had ended.

In both analyses the potential confounders considered were: the age of the male partner and the age difference between the partners; the educational status of both partners; and a categorical measure of agreement for the partners' reports of when they last had sex. This latter was included to control for differences between couples that may have arisen from inaccurate reporting of the outcome behaviours. The risk status of the man for the outcome measure (had sex by age 15, was previously married) was included in each regression model to control for the change in concordance that results from changes in the prevalence of a risk behaviour. After controlling for potential confounders, the chance of a recently married couple having the same history of sex by age 15 increased significantly between 1996 and 2001 (adjusted OR 1.72) (**Table 3**).

Between 1996 and 2001 there was a decrease in the proportion of monogamous couples who had the same prior marriage history (adjusted OR 0.67). The man's age remained as a significant term in the model but did not have an important confounding effect. Men with more education were more likely to be in marriages with women who had the same previous marriage history. Women who first married at a later age were more likely to have a different marriage history to their husbands (see Table 4). The effect of a prior marriage in the male partner suggests that most previously married men choose women who have not previously been married. This is evident from Table 2 which shows that fewer than half of the previously married men were in a marriage with a woman who had been married before.

Table 3. Crude and adjusted odds ratios for concordance within couples regarding history of sex before age 15. Couples were concordant if both partners, or if neither partner had had sex by age 15. Analysis is restricted to couples who married in the five years before the survey.

Same history of sex by age 15 (N 505 couples)		Crude OR	Adjusted OR	p-value
Year	1996	1	1	
	2001	2.07 (1.37–3.13)	1.72 (1.06–2.8)	0.03
Man has higher education	No	1	1	
	Yes	1.94 (1.25–3.03)	2.01 (1.17–3.45)	0.01
Man had sex by age 15	No	1	1	
	Yes	0.04 (0.03–0.08)	0.05 (0.03–0.09)	<0.001

Table 4. Crude and adjusted odds ratios for concordant history of previous marriage, among monogamous couples.

Same history of previous marriage* (1732 couples)		Crude OR	Adjusted OR	Adj p-value
Year	1996	1	1	
	2001	0.66	0.67	
		(0.52–0.83)	(0.51–0.89)	0.005
Man's age (by year)		0.97	1.02 (1–1.04)	
		(0.96–0.98)		0.01
Woman's age at first		0.93	0.93	
marriage (by year)		(0.9–0.96)	(0.89–0.97)	<0.001
Man's education	None	1	1	
	Primary	1.38	1.89	
		(0.85–2.25)	(1.04–3.44)	0.04
	Secondary	1.56	1.74	
		(0.94–2.58)	(0.92–3.31)	0.09
	Higher	1.86	2.04	
		(1.14–3.03)	(1.13–3.68)	0.02
Man's previous	No	1	1	1
marriage	Yes	0.05	0.04	<0.001
		(0.03–0.06)	(0.03–0.06)	

*Monogamous couples only.

Marital Status in the Wider Population

In both surveys women were significantly more likely than men to report a marriage that had ended. The proportion of monogamously married or unmarried individuals who had experienced a marriage that ended was about 21% of the total for men and 23% of the total for women in both surveys (p = 0.003). The proportion of married women who were in polygynous marriages was 16% and the proportion of all women who were in polygynous marriages was 10% in both surveys. The proportion of married men who currently had more than one wife did not change between surveys. The mean number of current wives reported by all men has increased from 0.57 to 0.65 (p < 0.002); but has remained the same for all married men (1.1 wives) and polygamously married men (2.16 wives). There are no significant differences in the average number of current wives reported by all men once the different age structures of the two surveys are taken into account.

Fig. 1 shows the distribution of the entire DHS survey sample in both years, by marital status. The marital status of Zambian women did not change between 1996 and 2001 but there were significant changes in the proportion of all men who were: never married (p-value 0.0001) and who were mongamously married but had had a marriage that ended (p-value 0.002). The decrease in the proportion of men who were never married was not significant once adjusted for the different age structures

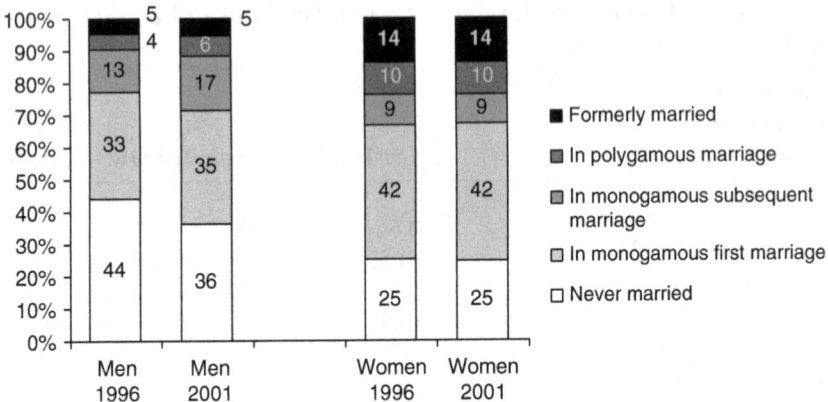

Fig. 1. Distribution of the entire DHS male and female samples, in 1996 and 2001, by marital status

of the two surveys. Men's age at first marriage did not change in this period, but the median age at first marriage increased from 18 to 19 for women.

The difference between the surveys in the proportion of monogamously married couples in which the man had previously been married arises partly from differences in the patterns of remarriage. Most previously married men remarried (85%) compared to only half of the previously married women (52%); this did not change significantly with age. Between 1996 and 2001 there was no change in the proportions of people who entered into another marriage after a marriage that ended.

Marriages in which one or both partners have previously been married are different to first marriages. Compared to monogamous couples for whom neither partner had been previously married the age difference between the spouses was greater in marriages in which only the man had been married before, smaller in marriages in which only the woman had been married before and was about the same in couples in which both partners had been previously married. **Fig. 2** shows the distribution of spousal age differences (male age–female age), comparing men who had been married before with those who had not. For ease of interpretation this is only shown for those couples in which the woman had not previously been married.

Women who remarry are more likely to be a second or subsequent ranking wife than women who are on their first marriage; after controlling for age the odds of being a second or subsequent ranking wife were 5.4 times higher in women who had experienced a previous marriage (95% CI 4.6–6.4) than for women married for the first time.

These observed changes in marriage patterns may be partially the result of differential growth rates among different age groups in the population which in turn may be related to HIV infection and HIV associated mortality. In Zambia in 2001, the age-specific HIV prevalence was very different for men and women (**Fig. 3**). HIV prevalence among women peaked at a higher level and at a younger age than HIV prevalence among men. As a result, the age-specific mortality curves [4] are also different for men and for

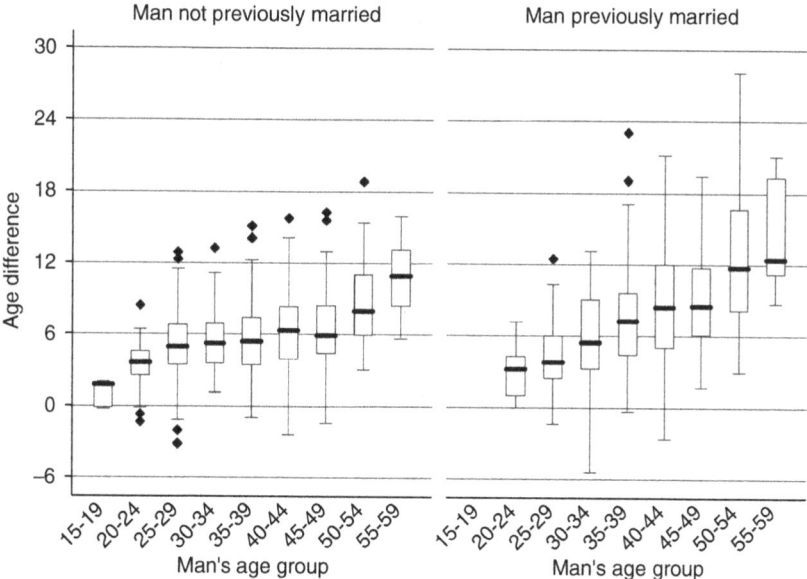

Fig. 2. Box plot of the age difference in monogamously married couples in which the woman has not been married before, by the man's age group and whether he had been married before

Note: age difference is man's age–woman's age

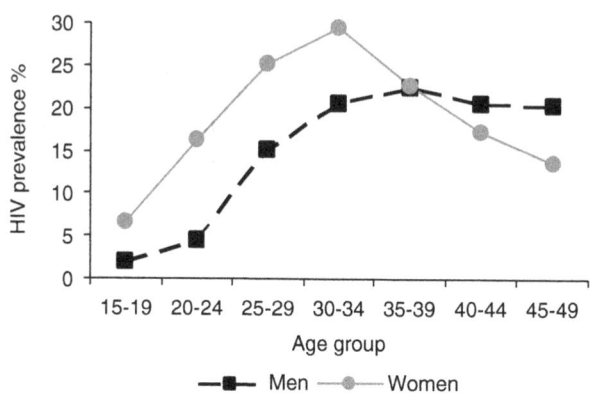

Fig. 3. National age-specific HIV prevalence among men and women in 2001. Source: ZDHS 2001 HIV test results [4]

women (**Fig. 4**). Mortality has increased between 1996 and 2001/2 (**Fig. 5** and **Fig. 6**). There were many more deaths among young women than among young men (**Fig. 7** and **Fig. 8**) and this difference was more marked in the later time period.

The marital status distributions from the DHS were applied to the 1996 and 2001 estimates of population size (projected from UN data), by five-year age group and

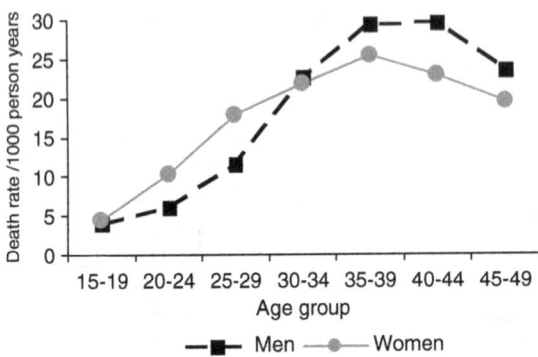

Fig. 4. National age-specific mortality rates for men and women in 2001. Redrawn from ZDHS 2001 Final Report [4]

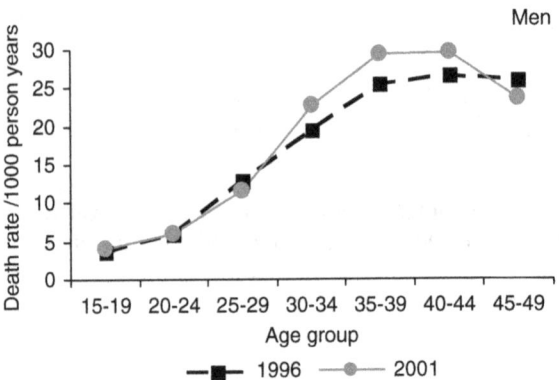

Fig. 5. National age-specific mortality rates for men in 1996 and 2001. Estimates from ZDHS 2001 Final Report [4]

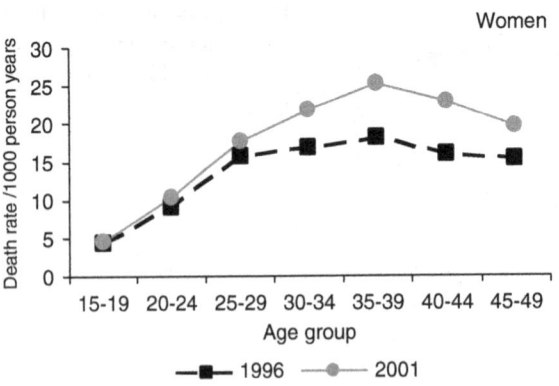

Fig. 6. National age-specific mortality rates for women in 1996 and 2001. Estimates from ZDHS 2001 Final Report [4]

sex. **Table 5** shows, for the entire Zambian population, estimates of the sex ratio within each marital status group and percentage change in the absolute size of each group between 1996 and 2001. The only group not to have increased in size between 1996 and 2001/2 was women in polygamous marriages. The groups of monogamously married men in their first marriage and monogamously married women in a subsequent marriage have not increased in size as much as would be expected given

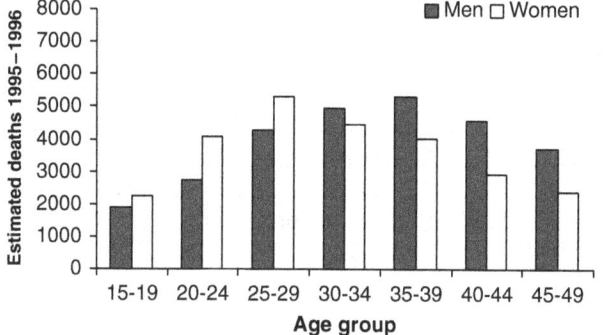

Fig. 7. Estimated annual deaths by age and sex for 1996. Based on UN Population Division population estimates for Zambia [10] and DHS mortality rates

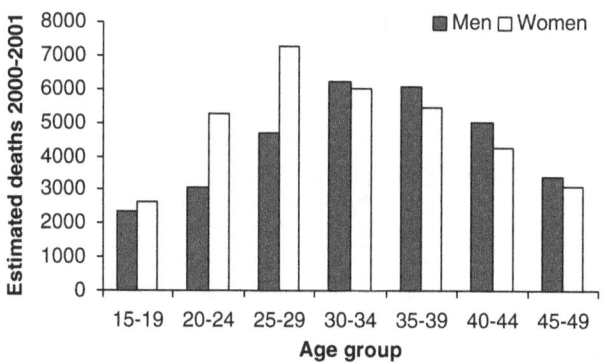

Fig. 8. Estimated annual deaths by age and sex for 2001/2. Based on UN Population Division population estimates for Zambia [10] and DHS mortality rates

Table 5. Sex ratio (men : women) in 1996 and 2001 and percentage increase in size for each marital status group status for men and women aged 15 to 49. Base: Male and female survey samples, 1996 and 2001 DHS.

Current marital status	Sex Ratio		% Increase 1996 to 2001	
	1996	2001	Men	Women
Never married	1.78	1.71	10.6	15.0
Monogamous, on first marriage	0.80	0.78	8.6	11.3
Monogamous, on subsequent marriage	1.26	1.48	19.8	2.3
Polygamously married	0.41	0.42	2.1	−1.2
Formerly married	0.35	0.36	13.9	8.3
Total	0.98	0.99	10.9	9.6

the overall population growth. A substantial increase has been seen in the number of monogamously married men who are in their second marriage and the sex ratio has also increased. The decline in the number of women in polygamous marriages could be linked to this if, in 2001 compared to 1996, a woman was more likely to marry a man whose marriage had ended, than to enter in to a polygamous union.

Discussion

Between 1996 and 2001 sexual behaviour has not changed as much among married people as it has among unmarried people in Zambia. There have been more changes in the risk behaviours of married men than married women, in part because men reported higher levels of risk behaviour at the earlier survey. Changes over time in the proportion of all men who had more than one partner in the year preceding the survey did not affect married men and did not affect the proportion of couples that were discordant for this behaviour [6].

The proportion of married men and women who reported having had sex by age 15 declined significantly between 1996 and 2001 and this resulted in greater similarity within couples. This increase in similarity between marital partners over time remained significant (adjusted OR 1.72, 95% CI 1.06–2.8) after controlling for potential confounders.

The proportion of monogamously married men who reported having been married more than once increased between 1996 and 2001. This resulted in more difference among the couples—in 1996 80% had the same past marriage history but this was 73% in 2001. This decrease in similarity within couples over time also remained significant after controlling for potential confounders (adjusted OR 0.67, 95% CI 0.51–0.89).

In the total sample, changes over time were observed in the proportions of men who were in the different categories of marital status, but no changes were observed for women. There must be some reciprocity in the marriage patterns between the sexes; the differences in the proportions are probably explained by differences in the size and growth rates of the male and female population. Some men and women marry partners outside the age range of the survey which will also cause some imbalance.

Men and women experience different age-specific mortality rates: women's mortality is greater than men's in the younger age groups but lower from the mid-thirties onwards. Mortality rates for both sexes increased between the surveys. The observed mortality patterns may affect marriage in two ways: there is likely to be a larger increase in the number of widowed men than in the number of widowed women; the widowed men may choose much younger partners when they re-marry, because of a shortage of women of a similar age.

The absolute change in the estimated size of each marital status group between the two surveys shows that marriage patterns have changed for women as well as men. If women who would have entered a polygynous relationship the first time they got married are now entering a monogamous marriage with a previously married man (perhaps because his first wife died) that would explain the differential change in monogamous marriage between the sexes.

Remarriage following the death of a spouse has long been considered as an HIV risk though data in support of this are limited. If one spouse dies of AIDS and the remaining spouse remarries there is obvious potential for the spread of infection. In Zambia there has been a tradition of levirate marriage, in which a widow marries a brother of her deceased husband, but the importance of this may have been over-played [12] and it may be declining in prevalence [13]. However marriages in which the man has been married before are becoming more common.

It has not been possible to fully explore the changes in marriage dynamics in Zambia because of limitations in the data. The analysis would have been aided by information on how marriages ended (death, divorce, separation), the duration of the current marriage (as well as the time since first marriage), dates of the end of any previous marriages and, for polygynous men, whether they remain married to all their wives.[3] It will be important to understand future marriage patterns and how these change in response to the HIV epidemic and HIV associated mortality increases.

In a generalised epidemic it is likely that much HIV infection will be acquired within marriage: either because an infected person marries someone who is uninfected or because, in a marriage where both (or all) spouses are initially uninfected, one partner gets infected outside the marriage and then infects their spouse(s). In an established epidemic, pre-marital (relationship) counselling and testing becomes an important preventive measure. In a Lusaka study of married couples discordant for HIV infection and followed after VCT (and therefore aware of their status) the incidence of HIV seroconversion was 8/100 person years [14]. 87% of these infections were acquired from the spouse [15]. This was in couples who are aware that one partner was infected. Most married people do not know their status or that of their partner. In the 2001 ZDHS 9.4% of women reported ever having been tested for HIV and this did not vary by marital status. 14% of men and 17% of married men had been tested. In the DHS, respondents were not asked why they had been tested but this information was collected in the 2003 Sexual Behaviour Survey. In that survey 4% of the women and 3% of the men who had been tested said that they had been tested before marriage. It is worth noting that the percentage of women who reported a test in this survey was similar to the DHS (9%) but the proportion of all men was much lower (9%) as was the proportion of married men (11%) though there was still a significant difference between all men and married men. It appears that pre-marital testing is still uncommon in Zambia. In most of the married couples in the 2001 DHS neither partner had been tested for HIV (78%); in 3% of couples both partners had been tested at some point in their lifetime. In 5% only the woman had been tested and in 14% only the man had been tested.

Changes in marital history, knowledge of HIV status and willingness to be tested for HIV, among married couples and among those who are about to get married, is an important area of research that may be used to identify whether patterns of transmission are changing, and to provide information to prevention programmes. More detailed information on marital history is required.

---

[3] This information is available in the 2001 survey.

References

1. Central Statistical Office Republic of Zambia, Ministry of Health (1997). Zambia Demographic and Health Survey, 1996. (Calverton, Maryland: Central Statistical Office/Macro International)

2. Central Statistical Office Republic of Zambia (1999). MEASURE evaluation. Zambia Sexual Behaviour Survey 1998 with selected findings from the quality of STD services assessment; 1999

3. Central Statistical Office Republic of Zambia, MEASURE Evaluation. Zambia Sexual Behaviour Survey 2000; 2002

4. Central Statistical Office Republic of Zambia, Central Board of Health Republic of Zambia, Macro O. (2003). Zambia demographic and health survey 2001/02. (Calverton, Maryland: Central Statistical Office/Central Board of Health/ORC Macro)

5. Central Statistics Office Republic of Zambia, Ministry of Health (2004). MEASURE Evaluation. Zambia Sexual Behaviour Survey 2003. (Chapel Hill, North Carolina: Central Statistics Office/Central Board of Health/MEASURE Evaluation Project)

6. Slaymaker, E. & Buckner, B. (2004). Monitoring trends in sexual behaviour in Zambia, 1996–2003. *STI*,*80*(Suppl II), ii85–ii90

7. Walker, N., Stanecki, K. A., Brown, T., Stover, J., Lazzari, S., Garcia Calleja, J., et al. (2003). Methods and procedures for estimating HIV/AIDS and its impact. The UNAIDS/WHO methods for end of 2001. *AIDS*, *17*(15), 2215–2225

8. The UNAIDS Reference Group on Estimates Modelling and Projections (2002). Improved methods and assumptions for estimation of the HIV/AIDS epidemic and its impact: Recommendations of the UNAIDS reference group on estimates, modelling and projections. *AIDS*, *16*(9), W1–W14

9. Auvert, B., Buve, A., Ferry, B., Carael, M., Morison, L., Lagarde, E., et al. (2001). Ecological and individual level analysis of risk factors for HIV infection in four urban populations in sub-Saharan Africa with different levels of HIV infection. *AIDS*, *15*(Suppl 4), S15–S30

10. United Nations Population Division (2002). World population prospects: The 2002 revision population database. (New York: UN)

11. StataCorp. (2003). Stata/SE 8.2 for Windows. In 8.2 edn. (College Station, USA: State Corporation)

12. Gausset, Q. (2001). AIDS and cultural practices in Africa: The case of the Tonga (Zambia). *Social Science and Medicine*, *52*(4), 509–518

13. Malungo, J .R. (2001). Sexual cleansing (Kusalazya) and levirate marriage (Kunjilila mung'anda) in the era of AIDS: Changes in perceptions and practices in Zambia. *Social Science and Medicine*, *53*(3), 371–382

14. Allen, S., Meinzen-Derr, J., Kautzman, M., Zulu, I., Trask, S., Fideli, U., et al. (2003). Sexual behavior of HIV discordant couples after HIV counseling and testing. *AIDS*, *17*(5), 733–740

15. Trask, S. A., Derdeyn, C. A., Fideli, U., Chen, Y., Meleth, S., Kasolo, F., et al. (2002). Molecular epidemiology of human immunodeficiency virus type 1 transmission in a heterosexual cohort of discordant couples in Zambia. *Journal of Virology*, *76*(1), 397–405

CHAPTER 9. MIGRATION, HIV/AIDS KNOWLEDGE, PERCEPTION OF RISK AND CONDOM USE IN THE SENEGAL RIVER VALLEY[1]

RICHARD LALOU
Institut de Recherches pour le Développement, Dakar, Sénégal

VICTOR PICHÉ
Département de Démographie, Université de Montréal, Montréal, Canada

FLORENCE WAÏTZENEGGER
Consultant in Demography

Abstract. Literature on AIDS has shown associations between migration and HIV infection. Yet the various types of mobility and different social contexts that characterize migration and non-migration are what tend to determine risk and sexual behaviour. Thus, it is important to acknowledge the diversity of migration and non-migration situations and to examine how migration affects HIV/AIDS knowledge, perception of risk and sexual behaviour. This study is based on a survey carried out in 2000 in the Senegal River valley (Sénégal). We investigated the impact of different types of migration on HIV/AIDS knowledge, perception of risk, and protective behaviour both in origin and destination areas. We explored whether migration experiences influenced HIV/AIDS awareness in various ways, either through diffusion of information and/or through contact with the epidemic. Our analysis shows that in the Senegal River valley, internal and international migrants were not better informed about HIV/AIDS than the non-migrant population in the origin area. However, international migrants were more likely to use condoms in the host countries where they engaged in risky sexual behaviour than in their home communities. Back home, the protective strategy of international migrants was fidelity rather than condom use. By these means, migrants both conformed to social norms and avoided the risk of being stigmatized. While international migrants were considered by their origin community to be a high risk-group, upon returning the international migrants themselves believed the risk of infection, which they associated with "others" and with "foreigners", to be behind them. As they were not engaged in risky sexual behaviours in their home area, they did not perceive themselves to be at risk of infection. By contrast, internal migrants, who perceived themselves at risk, were more likely to use condoms than were non-migrants. They attributed the risk of infection more to the sexual encounter than to "others". The constancy of their perception of personal risk (which stems from continuing risky sexual behaviour) could

---

[1] We wish to thank Abdoulaye Tall, Macoumba Thiam and Fara Mbodji for their collaboration in this project; IDCR-Dakar, IRD and the University of Montreal for financing this research.

M. Caraël and J.R. Glynn (eds.), HIV, Resurgent Infections and Population Change in Africa, 171–194.

explain the regular use of condoms during migration and upon their return. These findings indicate that there was no direct link between knowledge of the disease and condom use. The gap existing between knowledge and behaviour (particularly among international migrants) is largely the result of differences in the perception of the risk of infection and in socio-cultural constraints.

Introduction

Since the beginning of the HIV/AIDS epidemic, migration has been identified as a risk factor associated with acquiring and spreading HIV infection [1–9]. But the literature sheds little light on the social and cultural contexts in which migrants and non-migrants operate, nor on the diversity of migration patterns; nor on the impact of these varying contexts and patterns on AIDS knowledge, perceived risk of AIDS and sexual behaviour among migrants and non-migrants. Only a few studies, moreover, have assessed the impact of migration on the level of HIV knowledge in sub-Saharan Africa [2, 10, 11].

This paper begins by summarizing findings from the literature. We then describe the regions of Richard-Toll and Matam in the Senegal River Valley where we conducted our survey "Mobility and STI/AIDS in Senegal", and outline the data collection methods there. We examine how HIV/AIDS knowledge, perception of risk and protective behaviour among migrants and non-migrants relates to different forms of mobility in both origin and destination areas. More specifically, we investigate whether i) the level of condom use among migrants is the same in destination and return areas, and ii) migration experience promotes a different risk management strategy among returnee migrants than among non-migrating counterparts. We end with a discussion of our findings and the conclusions we draw from them.

Literature

Social science research discusses the complex dynamic between migration, knowledge and sexual behaviour. On the one hand, mobility may enhance exposure to new information networks during urban stays and international migration. Thus, migration is sometimes regarded as a factor favouring the "modernization of attitudes". In high HIV and AIDS prevalence destination areas migrants are in contact with the reality of HIV/AIDS. Back in their own communities, migrants, who as returnees have a valued social status, are likely to act as a reference group, and diffuse information on HIV/AIDS, thereby influencing their households and communities [12].

On the other hand, migrants are likely to be vulnerable in the destination area and less receptive than the local population to media messages and awareness campaigns [11, 4]. This is a common theme of analyses based on studies of labour migration in western and southern Africa where migrants are often in a situation of insecurity and vulnerability [5]. Some studies highlight the limited ability of migrants to understand HIV/AIDS messages in destination areas due to the language barrier. But even when language is not an issue, migrant populations in receiving areas are not always receptive to media messages as they do not generally feel fully integrated in the host community, and believe themselves to be protected by their culture and religion. Some studies indicate that migrants access information on HIV/AIDS both at home and in their destination areas, and that these two sets of information are sometimes conflicting. [10].

Recent findings show that migrants and mobile persons (such as truck drivers and travellers) generally have a good knowledge of HIV/AIDS and of its means of prevention [13]. Knowledge of HIV/AIDS is sometimes higher among migrant populations than among populations of the sending communities [14]. During the last ten years, awareness of HIV/AIDS has increased greatly among migrants living in developed countries. Community-level interventions, often taken over by migrant associations, help to explain this increase. Yet, notwithstanding this increase, the level of knowledge on HIV/AIDS still remains lower among migrants in developed countries than among the local host population [15, 16], due to the language barrier, higher illiteracy and a lack of concern about HIV/AIDS [11].

From the onset of the epidemic, dissemination of HIV/AIDS information has been a major strategy in the fight against the disease. The principle is simple: a wide dissemination of medical knowledge should induce individuals to adopt healthy attitudes and sexual practices [17, 18]. This approach, however, has its limitations. It implies a direct relationship between knowing and doing. As with many other health-related risks, understanding the risk of HIV/AIDS infection depends not only on understanding the mechanism of disease transmission, but also on witnessing the disease firsthand. Contact with the illness is at least as effective as radio broadcasts in affecting behaviour. Sexual behaviour, moreover, is a complex construct involving both individual and community-level factors [19]. Health-education alone cannot change risky sexual practices without taking into account the social and cultural context in which these practices occur.

Studies on protective practices reveal that mobile persons show a favourable attitude towards condoms and report using them very frequently during their moves [14, 13]. Back home, on the other hand, migrants make less use of condoms, particularly with regular partners. Some studies suggest that migrants are more often infected with HIV/AIDS than non-migrants [20], but in a study in South Africa no statistical association was found between HIV/AIDS-prevalence and the migrants' regular partners [21]. Ultimately, the personal and socio-economic characteristics of individuals, as well as their sexual and social experiences and types of relationships, help to determine their protective behaviours [22,23].

Most analyses of the relationship between HIV/AIDS and migration do not acknowledge migration as a multi-faceted phenomenon. There is little discussion of how the level of vulnerability and exposure to risk varies according to the type of mobility. Is the migrant alone or accompanied by his/her family? Is he or she looking for work, or travelling for business, study or political reasons? Is the move for a short or long period, circulatory or permanent? And do the origin and destination areas have high or low HIV/AIDS prevalence?

Different themes and assumptions emerge from the literature:
• General awareness of HIV/AIDS, or more specific knowledge regarding severity and transmission, is a necessary condition for changes in sexual behaviour. Knowledge of HIV/AIDS can evolve from scientifically-based and experience-related information.

- Migration can enhance scientifically-based and experience-related knowledge, and alter perception of the risk of AIDS.
- Migrants shape their sexual behaviours according to their knowledge and to the social and cultural context (destination and origin areas) in which they operate.
- Migrants' behaviour in destination and return areas depends on the type of migration, and the duration and destination of the move. We have distinguished three categories of spatial mobility: international migration, internal migration and temporary short-term moves. Migration and return migration can affect migrants' perceptions of risk and sexual behaviours differently [24, 25].

Context

This study was carried out in the Senegal River Valley, in the regions of Saint Louis and Matam (Senegal). Situated on the northern border of Senegal, this zone has a long-standing tradition of high mobility. As in the rest of Senegal, there are intense flows of internal migration towards the main urban centres. But in this region, the rural exodus is also the result of a strong international migration. Both international and internal migrations involve mostly men.

Senegal is an African country with a relatively low HIV/AIDS prevalence: 1.4% of the whole population [26]. Nevertheless, Senegal includes some "pockets" of high HIV/AIDS prevalence, particularly in regions with high international mobility. The region of Matam, one of our study sites, has been mentioned as a high mobility zone with a higher level of HIV/AIDS prevalence than elsewhere in Senegal. Since 2003, the region of Matam has been officially included in the sentinel HIV/AIDS surveillance sites. In 2004, the HIV/AIDS prevalence rate was 2.2% [26], similar to the 2% estimated in 1990 [3]. A study conducted in 1990 among the general population ($N = 600$) in 8 villages in the region of Matam (the Senegal River Valley) showed significant differences in HIV/AIDS infection between international migrants and other individuals [3]. Research carried out in the region of Ziguinchor in 1990 found a similar association between HIV sero-positivity and temporary rural-urban migration [27].

The economy, socio-cultural characteristics and migration patterns of the four project sites differ considerably. One of the sites belongs to the delta region (the town of Richard-Toll), while the three others are located in the Middle Valley, not far from the town of Matam.

As a result of urbanization, there is great ethnic diversity in Richard-Toll, which is composed of all the large groups of Senegal (the Haalpoular, Soninkè, Wolof, Sereer, Diola...). By contrast, the largely rural zone of Matam is mainly inhabited by the Haalpoular (77% of the population). The population of Richard Toll is better educated than that of Matam. The proportion of the population who never attended school is 1.45 times higher in Matam than in Richard Toll. The sugar industry and the derived commercial activities employ the majority of Richard-Toll's working population. Nearly a third (31.5%) of Richard-Toll's active males are employed by the *Compagnie Sucrière du Sénégal*. Agriculture and livestock farming are the primary economic activities in Matam.

Migration patterns are very different in the two zones. With the expansion of industrial and commercial activities, Richard-Toll has become an important regional attraction pole. Given that the activity of the *Compagnie Sucrière du Sénégal* is mostly seasonal, internal migration towards Richard-Toll is also mostly seasonal. In the Matam area (the middle valley), international migration is more prevalent. According to our data, nearly 22% of males in Matam (aged 15–49) reported having lived abroad at some time since 1985. Very different international migration patterns are observed in these two areas: international flows are mostly directed towards neighbouring countries (Mauritania) in Richard-Toll, whereas in Matam they are mainly headed towards Côte d'Ivoire (65%) and Central Africa (Central African Republic, Congo, Burundi, etc.), i.e. countries with higher HIV prevalence. In Mauritania, HIV prevalence is slightly lower than in Senegal.

Overall, the areas of Richard-Toll and Matam constitute two contrasting settings, within which HIV/AIDS knowledge, perceived susceptibility to AIDS and sexual behaviour should express themselves differently. Urbanization, schooling and the development of wage employment, as in Richard-Toll, probably mean better access to HIV/AIDS information, but also increased risky sexual behaviours due to the loosening of social ties. Commercial sexual services are readily available in Richard-Toll. In this context, we assume that there is relatively weak social control over sexuality. By contrast, the socio-cultural conditions in the Matam area suggest strong social control over sexuality, particularly for young girls. Migrants are often perceived to be individuals who spread disease and break sexual taboos.

Data and Methods

The survey "Mobility and STI/AIDS in Senegal" (MISS – Mobilité et IST/Sida au Sénégal) was conducted in the Senegal River valley in January and February 2000 on a representative sample of 1,872 individuals aged 15–49 [9]. Of the 1,320 respondents (one per household), 46% were males, 13.6% had experienced an international migration since 1985 and 81% had already had sexual relations. There were differences between the sample and the surveyed population. This was not the consequence of refusals, which were very low (0.4%), but of the high mobility of the surveyed population. To maximize the surveyed international migrants, the listings preceding the survey included all international migrants likely to be present (such as for a visit for Muslim holidays) at the study site at the time of the survey. A high percentage of them were still away at the time of the survey.

Both household and individual questionnaires were used in Richard-Toll and in the three sites of the Matam region. Household questionnaires focused mainly on the household's economic situation and on housing conditions. The individual questionnaire included questions on the socio-economic and demographic characteristics of the respondents and on their migration history. Data were collected on the respondents' sexual history in their actual residence, during their last internal or international migration and during their last short-term move. Finally, respondents were questioned on their knowledge and perceptions of sexually transmitted infections (STI) and HIV/AIDS.

We used ordered and binary logistic regressions to assess the effect of migration on HIV/AIDS knowledge, perception of the risk of AIDS and condom use. For the analyses of knowledge and perception of risk, data the Richard-Toll area and the Matam zone were analysed separately.

To assess AIDS-related knowledge, questions covered HIV/AIDS awareness, AIDS seriousness and routes of transmission and means of protection. We constructed a global index of knowledge, scoring 13 questions on different topics: general aware-ness on HIV/AIDS and other STI, perception of HIV/AIDS severity (its curability and the concept of asymptomatic infection), routes of transmission (sexual, mother-to-baby, blood borne), false beliefs (i.e. touching the body or sharing food with some-one with the HIV/AIDS virus, mosquito bite) and condom awareness as a means of HIV/AIDS prevention. The constructed scale for this variable ranged from zero to thirteen and three levels of knowledge were specified: 1) low score (0–7); 2) medium score (8 –10); 3) high score (11–13).

We assessed condom use both during migration and in the return area. First, we asked respondents whether they had used condoms (always, often, seldom, never) with casual partners or sex workers during their last migration. Second, we asked about use of con-doms for each reported sexual partner, other than a marital partner (fiancée, girlfriends, casual partners, commercial sex workers), in the last twelve months in the return area.

We used a logistic regression analysis to identify predictors of the likelihood of using condoms in the last twelve months. We defined the outcome as consistent condom use versus non-consistent use with all partners (apart from marital partners) in the last twelve months preceding the survey. The unit of observation was the sexual part-nership reported by respondents. Consequently, the analysis was based not on the 239 persons who declared multiple or extra-marital partners, but on the 332 sexual partnerships reported by these same respondents. We adjusted the analysis to allow for the non-independence of data within individuals.

We analyzed the third outcome, perception of risk of AIDS, as a binary variable: those who did not perceive themselves at risk compared to all the others, whatever their perceived risks.

We distinguished three types of spatial mobility according to the destination area, the duration of the migration and the reference period, using the following definitions:
• An **international migrant** is an individual born in Senegal who has left the country for a period of at least six months during the fifteen years preceding the survey, i.e. between January 1985 and January 2000. We chose the year 1985 because of its proximity to the year when the first cases of AIDS were declared in Senegal (in 1986). Since the survey was carried out in the places of origin of international migrants, nearly all the interviewed international migrants are returnee migrants. This long recall period (15 years) was necessary in order to take into account international moves which sometimes last more than 10 years; this also allowed us to interview returnee migrants when they were back in their areas of origin. Among the international migrants, more than 70% left Senegal since 1990 and more than 50% since 1992.

- An **internal migrant** is an individual who has moved within Senegal and outside the limits of his or her place of residence for a period of six months or more. The move must have occurred during the fifteen years preceding the survey, i.e. between January 1985 and January 2000.
- A **temporary short-term move** is carried out by an individual who is away from his or her place of residence for a period of at least one night and at most three months. The move must have occurred during the three months preceding the survey.

Since a single individual can have undertaken different types of migration, for the purpose of this analysis, we created four mutually exclusive categories:
- Non migrants, i.e. sedentary individuals who have not travelled during the three months preceding the survey and who have not migrated since 1985. The 556 individuals in this category represent 42.1% of the sample.
- International migrants, i.e. individuals who have migrated abroad at least once since 1985. There are 178 in this category, or 13.5% of the sample.
- Internal migrants, i.e. individuals who have not lived abroad since 1985, and who have migrated in Senegal at least once. There are 310 in this category, or 23.5% of the sample.
- Travellers, i.e. individuals who have moved for a short period and who have not migrated outside or within Senegal since 1985. There are 276 in this category, or 20.9% of the sample.

We adjusted for the following confounding variables: (1) area of residence, (2) sex, (3) age at the time of the survey, (4) marital status, (5) the respondent's educational level, (6) knowing someone with HIV/AIDS, (7) the household's economic status, and (8) level of knowledge about HIV/AIDS. The age and the marital status were specified at the beginning of the migration for migrants and at the time of the survey for non-migrant individuals or temporary travellers. The economic indicator of household wealth was created using the "score method" based on the condition of the house and the possession of goods (radio, television, a living room, cart, ...), animals and farmlands. Given the sample size, we used three categories: the poor, the moderately poor and the non-poor. We categorized AIDS knowledge according to three levels: low, medium and high. We used the area of residence as a proxy for the effect of social context on risky sexual practices.

For the analysis of condom use in the last twelve months, the model also included variables describing sexual relations: (9) type of partner: fiancée, girlfriend, casual partner, commercial sex worker, etc., (10) sexual activity and (11) other known or suspected sexual partners of the respondent's actual partner. Since there were only 79 partnerships in the data from the Matam area, we conducted the analysis for the sites together and adjusted for site, and for interaction between migration status and area of residence.

We tested all independent variables individually (Wald test). These variables entered the first model, after adjusting for migration, age and sex, if they were associated with consistent condom use below a 0.25 level of significance. The use of a backward step-wise binary logistic regression was used, taking into account the structure of the data according to sampling design (stratification and cluster sampling (svylogit in STATA®)). The final model includes only statistically significant variables ($p < 0.05$).

This analysis used the STATA program (STATA® 8.0, 2003; Stata Corporation, College station, Texas, USA).

In retrospective surveys, the temporal sequence of the perception of risk and behaviour is unknown. Individuals assess their personal risk of infection based on their awareness of HIV/AIDS and their sexual behaviour. In turn, their perceived personal risk is likely to affect their sexual and protective behaviours. Therefore, the analysis of condom use was not adjusted for perception of risk.

Results

This study addresses three key questions. First, does migration experience increase HIV/AIDS- related knowledge? Second, does migration experience lead to increased use of condoms during risky sexual practices? We define a risky sexual behaviour as any sexual encounter with an occasional partner or a commercial sex worker, regardless of the use of condoms. And third, how do migrants perceive their personal risk of infection upon their return and handle sexual risks in their area of origin?

The Experience of Migration and HIV/AIDS Related Knowledge

Awareness of HIV/AIDS and condoms is high in both Richard-Toll and Matam, as 99% of respondents reported that they knew of HIV/AIDS and 94% stated that they knew about condoms. Likewise, almost all respondents who had heard of HIV/AIDS knew about its severity. In both populations, 92% of respondents knew that HIV/AIDS is lethal and 91% of them were aware that there is no cure for the disease. However, high levels of HIV/AIDS knowledge (a knowledge index above 10) was 3.4 times more frequent in Richard-Toll than in Matam, while low knowledge levels were 3.7 times more frequent in Matam. Within each of the study sites, HIV/AIDS knowledge was higher among men. In Richard-Toll and Matam, proportions of males with good HIV/AIDS knowledge were respectively 1.5 and 4.1 times higher than that of females (Table 1).

The proportions of people who reported knowing someone with HIV/AIDS were much higher in the three Matam sites than in Richard-Toll (OR = 3.16, p < 0.001). As Figure 1 shows, there were small and non-significant variations between the Matam study sites. Overall, these results are in line with medical observations. The prevalence of HIV/AIDS reported by medical authorities (health centres, regional hospital) was higher in the department of Matam than in that of Dagana, where Richard-Toll is located. In Richard Toll, the risk of knowing someone with HIV/AIDS rose as the age of the respondents increased, for both men and women. In Matam, there were no significant trends with age.

Our previous work suggested that migration experience does not influence global HIV/AIDS-related knowledge among the populations of the Senegal River Valley. Nevertheless, migrants were more likely to be aware of asymptomatic transmission than non-migrants (OR = 1.66; p = 0.015). This advantage, however, is restricted to the

Table 1. Factors associated with knowledge on HIV/AIDS by survey area (ordered logistic regression) (MISS, 2000).

					Richard-Toll				
		N	% with good knowledge	% with medium knowledge	Crude OR	Adjusted OR*	p	95%CI	
Sex	Females	476	39.9	45.5	1	1	—		
	Males	441	60.4	31.9	2.25	1.95	<0.001	1.46 - 2.62	
Age (years)	15–19	210	40.5	39.6	1	1	—		
	20–29	245	50.8	37.0	1.62	2.15	<0.001	1.43 - 3.24	
	30–49	462	53.6	39.5	1.93	3.63	<0.001	2.18 - 6.05	
Marital status	Single	358	52.1	34.1	1	1	—		
	Married	521	48.8	41.4	0.97	0.82	0.36	0.53 - 1.26	
	Divorced/widowed	38	40.1	55.3	0.80	1.06	0.88	0.51 - 2.21	
Migration status	Non-migrants	393	49.7	36.4	1	1	—		
	International	109	54.9	35.2	1.30	1.25	0.40	0.75 - 2.08	
	Internal	211	48.4	42.3	1.05	0.95	0.79	0.68 - 1.34	
	Travellers	204	49.6	41.7	1.11	0.91	0.59	0.64 - 1.29	
Schooling	None	424	34.5	46.8	1	1	—		
	≥Primary	493	61.7	32.7	3.22	3.60	<0.001	2.65 - 4.89	
Household's economic status	Poor	457	46.2	41.0	1	1	—		
	Moderately poor	371	47.4	40.0	1.03	0.80	0.13	0.60 - 1.07	
	Non-poor	89	69.8	28.0	6.68	1.54	0.075	0.96 - 2.48	
Know someone with HIV/AIDS	Yes	139	58.5	38.2	1.65	1.81	0.003	1.22 - 2.66	
	No	778	48.3	39.0	1	1	—		

(continued)

Table 1. (continued)

				Matam				
	N	% with good knowledge	% with medium knowledge	Crude OR	Adjusted OR*	p	95%CI	
Exposure to media								
Low	192	38.4	44.4	1	1	—	—	—
Moderate	449	45.5	40.8	1.35	1.47	0.029	1.04	2.07
High	276	63.9	32.3	3.07	2.42	<0.001	1.64	3.58
Total	917							
Sex								
Females	229	6.6	48.6	1	1	—	—	
Males	158	26.5	37.2	1.99	2.85	<0.001	1.72	4.72
Age (years)								
15–19	85	10.3	44.3	1	1	—		
20–29	139	17.0	46.6	1.66	2.28	0.006	1.27	4.07
30–49	163	15.3	41.6	1.24	1.52	0.23	0.77	3.03
Marital status								
Single	142	17.1	39.4	1	1	—		
Married	227	12.7	46.9	1.08	1.44	0.23	0.79	2.62
Divorced/ widowed	18	15.2	49.1	1.00	2.49	0.11	0.81	7.63
Migration status								
Non-migrants	154	12.2	42.3	1	1	—		
International	69	15.3	41.8	1.19	0.48	0.04	0.23	0.98
Internal	97	24.7	37.8	1.63	0.80	0.43	0.46	1.39
Travellers	67	5.7	56.8	1.18	0.77	0.35	0.45	1.33
Schooling								
None	253	6.7	45.1	1	1	—		
≥Primary	134	27.7	42.4	2.88	1.99	0.004	1.25	3.16
Household's economic status								
Poor	204	10.3	43.9	1	1	—		

		n	%	%						
	Moderately poor	123	13.3	52.2	1.77	1.42	0.14	0.90	-	2.25
	Non-poor	60	31.5	28.3	1.35	1.38	0.33	0.73	-	2.61
Know someone with	Yes	135	21.0	50.3	2.28	2.00	0.002	1.30	-	3.07
HIV/AIDS	No	252	10.9	40.5	1	1	—			
Exposure to media	Low	116	9.1	31.4	1	1	—			
	Moderate	139	6.0	45.6	1.46	1.53	0.14	0.88	-	2.67
	High	132	25.8	51.1	5.27	5.13	<0.001	2.88	-	9.16
Total		387								

* Adjusted for all other variables in the table

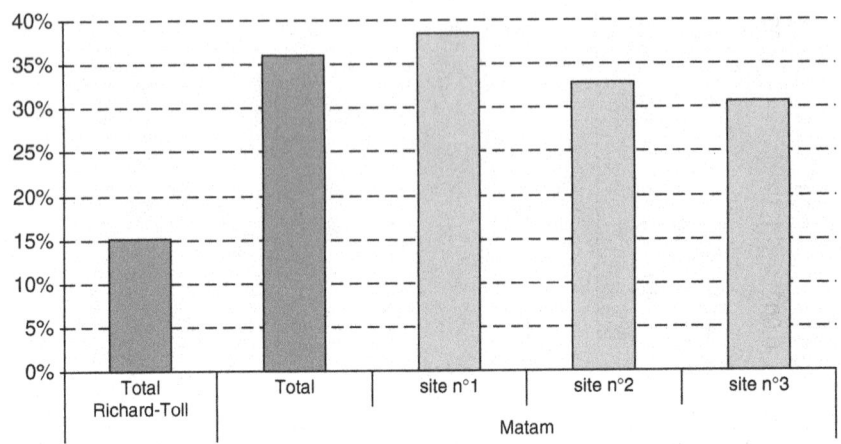

Fig. 1. Percentage of respondents who reported knowing someone with AIDS (presumed or not) by place of residence (MISS, 2000)

international migrants in Richard-Toll, i.e. individuals who have migrated mainly to Mauritania [9].

We ran the ordered logistic model for all variables shown in Table 1. It shows that the level of knowledge was associated with similar factors in Richard-Toll and Matam. There was a higher accuracy of knowledge among men and in older age groups in both areas. As expected, level of education, exposure to the media (radio and television), and knowing someone with HIV/AIDS greatly increased the level of HIV/AIDS knowledge. The multivariate analysis (Table 1) suggests that there is little association between any type of mobility experience – temporary move, internal or international migration – and HIV/AIDS knowledge, in either Richard-Toll or Matam, although international migrants in Matam were less knowledgeable about HIV/AIDS than non-migrants in the adjusted analysis (adjusted OR = 0.48; p = 0.04).

Mobility, Condom Use and Perception of Risk

We conducted the descriptive analysis of the relationship between mobility and condom use in two phases. First, we examined whether migrants change their protective behaviour in destination areas. To assess this change, we compared the sexual behaviour of migrants during migration, with that of non-migrants during the last twelve months before the survey, after adjusting for confounding factors such as age, sex, marital status and education. Second, we compared the protective behaviour of migrants in destination and return areas (survey sites).

These two comparisons attempt to assess the influence of social and cultural contexts (in origin and destination areas) on the protective behaviour of migrants. Notwithstanding the long recall period (7 years on average among international migrants), which could lead to underreporting of condom use in destination areas, or to increased HIV/AIDS knowledge and consequent behaviour changes, the results reveal a lower use of condoms in survey sites than in destination areas.

In these two analyses, we compare consistent condom use with casual partners and commercial sex workers during migration with consistent condom use in return areas in all types of relationships (including girlfriends, but excluding marital partners). Although this comparison could result in an underestimation of condom use in the survey sites, systematic condom use with a girlfriend was as frequent as with a casual partner (respectively 54% and 57%). Condoms were used less with fiancées (36%), but this situation accounted for only 9% of sexual encounters.

Protective Behaviors in Migration Areas
In Richard-Toll and Matam, international and internal migrants reported engaging in more risky sexual behaviour (i.e. sexual relations with occasional partners and commercial sex workers) in the migration areas than did non-migrants after adjustment for age, sex, education, and marital status [24].

Results in Table 2 show condom use by male migrants and non-migrants in both study sites. Nearly 80% of international migrants reported using condoms consistently during each intercourse with occasional partners and sex workers in the migration areas. While consistent condom use for internal migrants and travellers in the destination areas was 54% and 20% respectively. After adjusting for age, education, marital status and area, consistent condom use was much higher in international migrants, than in non-migrants, with no significant differences between internal migrants or travellers and non-migrants (Table 2).

Protective Behaviors in Return Areas
International migrants reported a decreased use of condoms on return (Figure 2): the prevalence of condom use fell from 79.6% during migration to 36.5% in the return areas (RR = 0.48; Fischer's p = 0.001). There was no significant trend among internal migrants or temporary travellers. Moreover, international returnee migrants were not very likely to protect themselves consistently when travelling within Senegal: only a quarter of international migrants (25%) reported using a condom at each intercourse during short-term moves.

Multiple regression results show that consistent use of condoms is associated with only a few socio-demographic and economic characteristics of the respondents and their sexual partner(s) (Table 3). The respondent's age and the frequency of sexual encounters are significantly associated with protective behaviour. Respondents aged 20–29 and 30–49 were more likely to use condoms in a consistent way than were those below age 20 (OR = 3.1 and OR = 2.7, respectively). If there was less than one sexual encounter per month, consistent protective behaviour was likely to increase (OR = 2.3; p = 0.01). However, consistent use of condoms was not significantly associated with the following variables: place of residence, marital status, respondent's level of education, household's economic status or other characteristics of the sexual relationship. HIV/AIDS knowledge was not associated with consistent use of condoms.

Table 2. Consistent condom use in destination areas for male migrants and in survey areas for non-migrant males (MISS, 2000).

		N	% consistent condom use	Crude OR	Adjusted OR*	p	95%CI		
	Non-migrants	71	40.7	1	1	—			
	International migrants	49	79.6	5.67	6.42	0.01	1.66	-	11.65
	Internal migrants	29	53.2	1.69	0.73	0.54	0.27	-	2.00
Migration Status	Travellers	16	19.6	0.35	0.70	0.72	0.094	-	5.18

N is the number of men reporting sexual relations with occasional partners or commercial sex workers
* OR adjusted for survey areas, marital status, age and education.

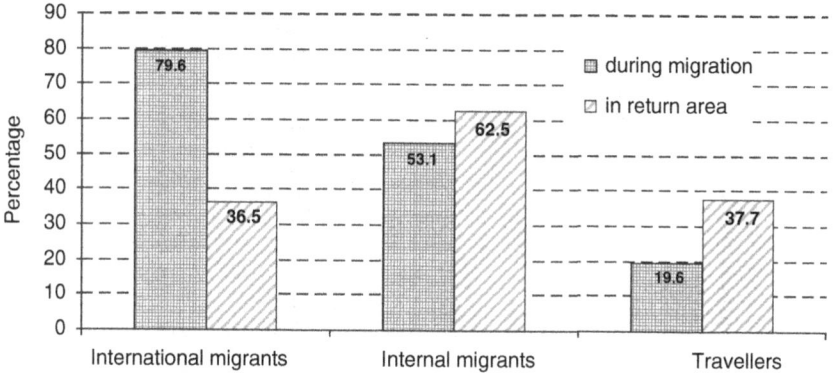

Fig. 2. Consistent condom use during migration or short-term move and in return area, by migration status (MISS, 2000)

The only association between migration status and consistent condom use on return was for internal migrants, with higher proportions of internal migrants than of non-migrants reporting consistent condom use. There was no such association for short-term travellers or international migrants (Table 3). There was no interaction between migrant status and place of residence.

Mobility and Perception of Risk in Return Areas
A binary logistic regression model was used to identify the factors associated with the perception of the risk of AIDS (low or high risk) in return areas. We adjusted the model for the following variables: sex, age, marital status, migrant status, education, household wealth, and knowing someone with HIV/AIDS. Table 4 shows that in return areas international migrants did not perceive themselves more at risk than did non-migrants. Although international migrants were aware of HIV/AIDS risks (the proportion of international migrants that knew someone living with HIV/AIDS was 1.8 times higher than among other respondents), they were not more likely to perceive themselves as being at risk than were non-migrants.. However, while internal migrants in Richard-Toll did not perceive HIV risks differently than did other individuals of this community, in Matam, internal migrants perceived themselves more at risk than non-migrants (OR = 2.21 ; p = 0.03).

Discussion

Overall in the Senegal River valley, after adjusting for other factors, internal and international migrants were not better informed about HIV/AIDS than their non-migrating counterparts. The experience of migration in contexts with broader coverage of awareness campaigns (as in urban areas), or in countries with higher HIV prevalence (Côte d'Ivoire, central and southern African countries), does not seem to have increased knowledge of the routes of transmission and the means of prevention of HIV/AIDS.

Table 3. Factors associated with consistent condom use during a sexual relationship in the twelve months preceding the survey. (Binary logistic regression) (MISS, 2000).

Variables	N	% Always use condom	Crude OR	Adjusted OR	p	95%CI	
Age (years)							
15–19	77	30.6	1	1	—		
20–29	153	61.2	3.58	3.10	0.01	1.30 -	7.40
30–49	102	56.8	2.98	2.75	0.03	1.08 -	6.97
Sex							
Female	47	30.3	1	1			
Male	285	58.0	3.17	3.34	0.01	1.27 -	8.73
>1 sexual relationship per month							
Yes	224	48.4	1	1	—		
No	108	63.9	1.89	2.25	0.01	1.21 -	4.19
Migration status							
Non-migrants	115	49.1	1	1	—		
International	73	44.5	0.83	0.61	0.38	0.20 -	1.83
Internal	84	67.8	2.18	2.49	0.02	1.16 -	5.33
Travellers	60	48.7	0.98	0.77	0.57	0.70 -	4.98
Total	332						

Other variables included in the model: Place of residence, interaction term between place of residence and migration status, marital status, level of education, knowledge of HIV/AIDS, the household's economic status, knowing someone living with HIV, sexual partner's identity and other partners of the respondent's partner, known or suspected by the respondent .

Table 4. Factors associated with perception of risk (no risk vs low, moderate or high risk) about HIV infection by survey area (binary logistic regression) (MISS, 2000).

		N	% feel at risk	Richard-Toll				
				Crude OR	Adjusted OR*	p	95%CI	
Sex	Females	452	20.1	1	1	—		
	Males	397	35.8	2.26	2.09	<0.001	1.47 -	2.97
Age (years)	15–19	194	11.9	1	1	—		
	20–29	231	32.0	3.48	3.64	<0.001	2.11 -	6.28
	30–49	424	32.5	3.57	4.37	<0.001	2.31 -	8.28
Marital status	Single	334	25.6	1	1	—		
	Married	480	30.0	1.25	0.82	0.41	0.50 -	1.32
	divorced/widowed	35	16.5	0.57	0.48	0.16	0.18 -	1.32
Migration status	Non-migrants	363	24.6	1	1	—		
	International	101	27.1	1.13	0.85	0.59	0.48 -	1.53
	Internal	198	26.7	1.11	1.06	0.80	0.70 -	1.59
	Travellers	187	34.3	1.60	1.30	0.20	0.87 -	1.94
Schooling	None	394	26.2	1	1	—		
	≥Primary	459	28.6	1.10	1.29	0.15	0.91 -	1.84
Household's economic status	Poor	428	27.9	1	1	—		
	Moderately poor	339	27.9	0.98	0.95	0.79	0.68 -	1.35
	Non-poor	82	25.4	0.86	0.75	0.29	0.45 -	1.28
Know someone with HIV/AIDS	Yes	133	39.1	1.69	1.68	0.014	1.11 -	2.54
	No	716	29.5	1	1	—		
Total		849						

(continued)

Table 4. (continued)

		N	% feel at risk	Crude OR	Matam Adjusted OR*	p	95%CI	
Sex	Females	221	11.8	1	1	—	-	
	Males	137	44.8	5.96	5.80	<0.001	3.02	11.15
Age (years)	15–19	78	18.7	1	1	—	-	
	20–29	130	28.6	1.72	1.43	0.36	0.66	3.07
	30–49	150	23.5	1.34	1.06	0.92	0.39	2.84
Marital status	Single	128	30.1	1	1	—	-	
	Married	213	20.2	0.59	1.17	0.70	0.52	2.64
	divorced/widowed	17	20.9	0.62	1.53	0.59	0.32	7.34
Migration status	Non-migrants	145	16.2	1	1	—	-	
	International	62	28.6	2.09	1.09	0.85	0.44	2.74
	Internal	86	39.6	3.43	2.20	0.027	1.09	4.42
	Travellers	65	18.3	1.14	0.98	0.95	0.45	2.13
Schooling	None	127	28.8	1	1	—	-	
	≥Primary	231	21.0	1.55	0.92	0.80	0.50	1.71
Household's economic status	Poor	186	25.5	1.24	1	—	-	
	Moderately poor	118	21.0	0.76	0.75	0.36	0.40	1.39
	Non-poor	54	25.3	0.99	0.90	0.80	0.39	2.08
Know someone with HIV/AIDS	Yes	126	30.6	1.72	1.66	0.076	0.95	2.90
	No	232	20.4	1	1	—		
Total		358						

* Adjusted for all the variables shown in the Table

As for other diseases, knowledge regarding HIV/AIDS depends not only on the information conveyed by health professionals and the mass media, but also on the experience obtained through contacts with the illness. Proximity to HIV/AIDS seems to increase sensitivity and interest for this illness and its health risks. In the Matam study sites, the populations had greater contact with the illness given the higher prevalence of HIV/AIDS in this area. HIV/AIDS was a more tangible reality in Matam than in Richard-Toll. We measured experience-related knowledge of HIV/AIDS with the variable "knowing someone with HIV/AIDS". Despite its appeal, the interpretation of this variable is limited. Respondents can report knowing someone who really has HIV/AIDS, but it can also be someone whom they believe to have HIV/AIDS. The index increases significantly if there are well-known people with HIV/AIDS in the community. Moreover, there is likely to be a cluster bias, particularly if several people are interviewed within a family, although in this survey, only one person per household was questioned.

Yet, even if migrants are not better informed about HIV/AIDS than non-migrants, they report using condoms more frequently with occasional partners or sex workers in destination areas. This protective conduct varies considerably according to the type of migration. International migrants reported almost always using condoms while abroad. Of interest, migrants in Mauritania (a low HIV prevalence country) used condoms as consistently as migrants in Central Africa and Côte d'Ivoire (higher HIV/AIDS prevalence countries), suggesting that protective behaviour was not so much in response to the level of HIV risk in African countries, but more to the risk of the relationship. Once back in Senegal, international migrants apparently gave up this means of protection. On the basis of several opinion questions, it seems that international migrants were more reluctant than non-migrants to use condoms [9]. International migrants usually rejected condom use to avoid stigmatisation. They felt under suspicion of HIV infection when they came back home, so they chose fidelity to their regular or marital partner in their home community [24].

High proportions of internal migrants used condoms consistently in destination areas; and once back home, unlike international migrants, kept on using them, even more frequently than non-migrants. Finally, short-term travellers seldom used condoms, either during the move or in their place of residence.

There is the possibility of reporting biases in the responses to queries about condom use. We cannot exclude the possibility that respondents adjusted their answers to medical norms and thus were inclined to answer "always" when they were asked whether they used condoms. Alternatively, moral prejudices or religious taboos could result in a reluctance to report condom use. We found that international migrants had a more reluctant attitude towards condom use than non-migrants. Yet, they claimed to use condoms consistently while abroad and one fourth of them declared using them during short-term moves within Senegal. Consequently, we do not feel that differences in reported condom use were due to differential reporting bias by migration status of respondents. This is detailed in the MISS survey report [9].

This study reveals that the connection between health-related knowledge and behaviours was not linear and direct. The same knowledge resulted in different protective behaviours depending on the social and cultural context in which the migrants operated. The behaviour change appeared to be determined more by crossing the national border than by other moves, perhaps because migrants perceived the risk to be higher there. However behaviour reflects constraints imposed by the social and cultural context as well as perceived risk.

For international migrants, as for many other residents of the Senegal River valley, HIV/AIDS is thought to be the disease of "others" and of "elsewhere". The home community represents a space safeguarded by Islam and its culture: a space protected from the "transgressions" which favour HIV transmission (multiple sexual partnerships and extra-marital relations). Female sexuality is still controlled, notably by early marriages and the levirate, and extra-marital sexual relations are always condemned and sometimes punished, especially for women. However the perception of the community as a protected space has changed markedly over the last few years. International migrants who wish to marry within the community may occasionally be HIV-tested, sometimes without them knowing. In these villages AIDS is not a disease that exists only in radio broadcasts. Persons with AIDS are a reality. Undoubtedly it is this tangible presence of AIDS, rather than any real or imagined change in sexual codes, that resulted in the fact that more than 70% of respondents at the time of the study perceived AIDS as a serious threat for their community.

International migrants used condoms because they were aware of HIV/AIDS, its severity and the means of protection. But because they related HIV/AIDS to foreigners and to foreign countries, international migrants were more likely to protect themselves abroad than within Senegal during sexual relations with casual partners.

Internal migrants associated the risk of infection with multiple and casual sexual partnerships. More than one-third of male internal migrants had several sexual partners other than their spouse(s) in the return area. Multiple partnerships were more frequent among internal migrants than among non-migrants. These differences from non-migrants were not observed among international migrants and short-term travellers [24]. A perpetuation of internal migrants' sexual behaviour – with its related perception of risk – helps to explain the more frequent use of condoms in the return area.

The level of condom use is in response not only to perceived risks, but also to the social context within which migrants operate. Understanding protective behaviour requires understanding the societal incentives or constraints for using condoms.

Generally, international migrants, particularly in the middle valley of the Senegal River, acquire prestige and power upon their return to their home communities. In this region of Senegal, a large part of the economic and social life of villages and towns depends on international migrants. Migrant remittances ensure every day life for families who remain in the villages, contribute to the improvement of housing and enhance community development (health centre, school). Remittances also help to modernize farm activities and develop private businesses.

Upon return to their home communities, international migrants seek to re-integrate through conformity rather than social change. In Matam, 60% of international migrants asserted having changed their behaviour since they became aware of HIV/AIDS and reported being faithful. The choice of fidelity probably explains why the personal perception of risk has changed. Sexuality is under strict regulation by the community, and behavioural changes will only last if they are accepted [28].

In the last twelve months, 9% of international migrants reported multiple casual partners compared to 20% for the rest of the population. In previous studies, we showed that the choice of fidelity among international migrants upon their return to Matam corresponded to a means of protection with a lesser social cost than condom use [24, 29]. Interestingly, 66% of respondents in Matam reported that HIV/AIDS is transmitted by sexual contact abroad, and 25% indicated that international migrants are a high-risk group. These proportions were higher in Matam than in Richard-Toll [9].

In contrast to international migrants, the return of internal migrants is not a key social issue. While internal migration is economically important for the migrant and his family, the social status of internal migrants does not change when they return home, or not as significantly as does that of international migrants. Internal migrants integrate less obtrusively back into their home communities and are not suspected of being "disease importers" as are international migrants. Their sexual behaviours do not change on return. In Matam, a large number of internal migrants had multiple sexual partners, both during migration and at home. However they reported behaviour change in response to HIV/AIDS. They perceived themselves at risk of infection and were more likely to use condoms than were other respondents [29]. The perception of risk, then, is probably linked to a personal sexual history (more frequent multiple partnerships) and to the perception that HIV/AIDS is a serious threat to the health of the community (more pronounced in Matam than in Richard-Toll) [24].

Conclusion

The survey Mobility and STI/AIDS in Senegal (MISS – Mobilité et IST/Sida au Sénégal) allowed an in-depth analysis of the relationship between mobility and HIV/AIDS. The literature on HIV often addresses these associations in a simplified way - the migrant being represented as a carrier of the infection or as a vulnerable person at risk of becoming infected – without acknowledging the variety of population movements in Africa [24].

Our study explicitly examined the link between migration, HIV/AIDS-related knowledge and protective sexual behaviour in return areas (risk of diffusion) by using a conceptual framework that considered: 1) various types of mobility; 2) different social contexts, and 3) the difference between migrants and non-migrants in AIDS-related knowledge and protective behaviours. The influence of the macro-social level was studied by using two areas of the Senegal River valley with contrasting mobility and socio-economic factors. By conducting the study in the migrants' area of origin, i.e. the area of socialization and of sexual initiation, we were able to identify the differences in knowledge and protective behaviours between migrants and non-migrants.

Overall, results of this study show that migration towards urban areas and countries with high HIV/AIDS prevalence – with probably better coverage of HIV/AIDS awareness campaigns – did not enhance the knowledge of migrants from the Senegal River valley. Still, international migrants were more likely to use condoms in the host countries where they engaged in risky sexual behaviour than in their places of origin. Back in their home communities, international migrants, no longer perceiving themselves at risk and wishing to conform to societal sexual codes, gave up the use of condoms. Unlike internal migrants who perceived themselves at risk both during migration and at home and thus adopted the use of condoms more often than non-migrants.

Findings of this research suggest that there is no direct link between knowledge and condom use. The gap which exists between knowledge and behaviour (particularly among international migrants) seems to result from differences in the perception of the risk of infection and from socio-cultural constraints. Indeed, international migrants, once they returned, did not feel more at risk than non-migrants. They considered that the risk of infection, which they related to "others" and to "foreigners", was now behind them. To conform to social norms and avoid the risk of being stigmatized, their protective strategy involved fidelity rather than condoms.. Conversely, internal migrants from Matam perceived themselves significantly more at risk than non-migrants. They associated the risk of infection more with the sexual encounter than with "others". The constancy of their perception of personal risks (which arises from continuing risky sexual behaviours) probably explains their regular use of condoms during migrations and upon return.

Behavioural change requires a minimal level of knowledge of HIV/AIDS and its risks. But, scientific knowledge on health risks does not necessarily predict health-based behaviour. Migration is an important reality of the diffusion of HIV/AIDS in sub-Saharan Africa. HIV/AIDS prevention strategies, nonetheless, must not ignore the socio-cultural context within which migration occurs. There is a need to understand risky mobility situations and how migrants manage their sexual risks in complex societal settings.

References

1. Amat-Roze J.M., Coulaud J.P. and Chamot G. (1990). La géographie de l'infection par les virus de l'immunodéficience humaine (VIH) en Afrique Noire : mise en évidence de facteurs d'épidémisation et de régionalisation. *Bulletin de la Société de Pathologie Exotique. 83*, 137–148.

2. Anarfi, J. K. (1993). Migration and AIDS. Health *Transition review 3*(Numéro supplémentaire), 45–67.

3. Kane F., Alary M., Ndoye I., Coll A.M., Mboup S., Gueye A., Kanki P.J. and Joly J.R. (1993). Temporary expatriation is related to HIV-1 infection in rural Senegal. *AIDS. 7*, 1261–1265.

4. Lalou, R. and Piché, V. (1994). *Migration et sida en Afrique de l'ouest. Un Bilan des connaissances.* (Paris: Cahiers du Ceped. Ceped)

5. Taverne, B. (1995). Sida et migrants au Burkina Faso : l'illusion d'une prévention ciblée. *Médecine d'Afrique Noire 43*, 31–35.

6. Hunt, C. (1996). Social vs Biological: Theories on the Transmission of AIDS in Africa. *Social Science and Medicine 20(9)*, 1283–1296.

7.   Decosas, J. and Adrien, A. (1997). Migration and HIV. *AIDS. 11*, 2–9.

8.   Soskolne, V. and Shtarkshall, R.A. (2002). Migration and HIV prevention programmes: linking structural factors, culture, and individual behaviour-an Israeli experience. *Social Science & Medicine. 55*, 1297–1307.

9.   Piché, V., R. Lalou, A. Tall, F. Waïtzenegger and M. Thiam (2003). *Migration, sexualité et sida dans la vallée du fleuve Sénégal.* (Paris: Marseille, IRD/Université de Montréal)

10. Fleury, F., M. Haour-Knipe and S. Ospina (1991). *Sida/Migration/Prévention: Dossier portugais, dossier espagnol.* (Lausanne: Institut universitaire de Médecine sociale et préventive)

11. Yelibi, S., P. Valenti, C. Volpe, A. Caprara, S. Deby and G. Tape (1993). Sociocultural Aspects of AIDS in an Urban Peripherical Area of Abidjan (Côte d'Ivore). *AIDS Care 5*(2), 187–197.

12. Palloni A. (1998) *Theories and Models of Diffusion in Sociology*, Center for Demography and Ecology, University of Wisconsin-Madison, CDE Working Papers, n 98–11.

13. Lydié, N., N. Robinson, B. Ferry, E. Akam, M. De Loenzien and S. Abega (2004). Mobility, Sexual Behavior and HIV in a Urban Population in Cameroon. *Journal of Acquired Deficiency Syndromes 35*(1).

14. Morris, M., M. Wawer, F. Makumbi, J. Zavisca and N. Sewankambo (1999). Condom Acceptance Is Higher Among Travellers in Uganda. *AIDS 14*(6), 733–741.

15. Haour-Knipe, M. (1993). AIDS, Prevention, Stigma and Migrant Status. *Innovation in Social Science Research 6*(1), 19–35.

16. Haour-Knipe, M., F. Fleury and F. Dubois-Arber (1999). HIV/AIDS prevention for migrants and ethnic minorities: three phases of evaluation. *Social Science and Medicine 49*(10), 1357–1372.

17. Ajzen, T. (1991). The Theory of Planned behavior. *Organizational Behavior and Human Decision Processes 50*, 179–211.

18. Becker, M. H. (1974). The health belief model and personal health behavior. *Health Education Monographs*, 220–243.

19. Fraisse, P. (1963). *Manuel pratique de psychologie expérimentale.* (Paris: Presses Universitaires de France)

20. White, R.G. (2003). What can we make of an association between human immunodeficiency virus prevalence and population mobility? *International Journal of Epidemiology*, (32), 753–754.

21. Lurie, M., B. Williams, M. Khangelani Zuma, D. Mkaya-Mwamburi, D. Garnett, A. Sturm, M. Sweat, J. Gittelsohn and S. Abdool Karim (2003). The Impact of Migration on HIV-1 Transmission in South Africa: A Study of Migrant and Nonmigrant Men and their Partners. *Sexually Transmitted Diseases, 30*(2), 149–156.

22. Van Campenhoudt, L. (1999). The relational rationality of risk and uncertainty reducing processes explaining HIV risk-related sexual behaviour. *Culture, Health and Sexuality 1*(2), 181–191.

23. Bajos, N., M. Bozon, A. Ferrand, A Giami, A. Spira et Le Groupe ACSF (1998). *La sexualité au temps du sida.* (Paris: Presses Universitaires de France.

24. Lalou, R. and Piché V. (2004). Les migrants face au sida. Entre gestion des risques et contrôle social. L'exemple de la vallée du fleuve Sénégal. Population-E 59(2), pp. 195–228.

25. Thiam, M. (2004). Sexualité et sida au Sénégal. Thèse soutenue à l'Université de Montréal, département de démographie, Octobre 2004.

26. Comité National de Prévention du Sida du Sénégal (2004). Bulletin séro-épidémiologique n°11 de surveillance du VIH, République du Sénégal, 45 pages + annexes.

27.   Pison G., Le Guenno B., Lagarde E., Enel C. and Seck C. (1993). Seasonal Migration: A Risk Factor for HIV Infection in Rural Senegal. *Journal of Acquired Immune Deficiency Syndromes.* 6, 196–200.

28.   Balandier, G. (1984). Le sexuel et le social, lecture anthropologique. *Cahiers Internationaux de Sociologie LXXVI,* 5–19.

29.   Lalou, R. & Msellati, P. (2007). Le risque et le stigmate. Les comportements sexuels des migrants de retour et des séropositifs, deux exemples ouest-africains. (In P. Vimard, A. Adjamagbo & P. Msellati (Eds.), *Santé de la reproduction et fécondité dans les pays du Sud. Nouveaux contextes et nouveaux comportements* (pp. 360–399). Louvain-la-Neuve, Academia-Bruylant.)

OWEN MUGURUNGI
AIDS and TB Unit, Ministry of Health and Child Welfare, Zimbabwe

SIMON GREGSON
*Department of Infectious Disease Epidemiology, Imperial College
London, London, UK*

A. D. McNAGHTEN
*CDC Zimbabwe and Centers for Disease Control & Prevention,
Atlanta, USA*

SABADA DUBE AND NICHOLAS C. GRASSLY
*Department of Infectious Disease Epidemiology, Imperial College
London, London, UK*

Abstract. HIV spread rapidly in Zimbabwe in the mid-late 1980s. By the mid-1990s, one-quarter of adults in the country were infected with HIV. HIV-1 subtype C is believed to be the predominant sub-type within the country and its spread has been mediated overwhelmingly by heterosexual sex. Sexual networks shaped by cultural and colonial influences, and the combination of a relatively high level of development and marked socio-economic inequalities, have facilitated the spread of HIV infection into the majority rural population, and have thereby fueled the large national epidemic. Classic sexually transmitted infections such as syphilis, gonorrhoea and Chlamydia have been controlled during the epidemic through a pioneering syndromic management programme, but *Herpes simplex* virus type 2 is extremely common. Male circumcision is only practised in minority groups. Blood transfusions were screened for HIV from an early stage in the epidemic and there is little evidence that contaminated needles have made more than a modest contribution to HIV transmission. The socio-demographic effects of the epidemic have been devastating and include sustained, crisis-level adult mortality, particularly in the most economically-active age-groups, a reversal of previous gains in early childhood survival, a rapid decline in population growth, and an inexorable rise in orphanhood. Since the late 1990s there have been signs of a leveling out in the HIV epidemic and of a decline in HIV incidence. There is evidence of reductions in rates of sexual partner change and of a decline in HIV prevalence in young people. These encouraging trends may reflect saturation of the epidemic within high risk groups, heightened mortality due to ageing of HIV

M. Caraël and J.R. Glynn (eds.), HIV, Resurgent Infections and Population Change in Africa, 195–213.
© Springer Science + Business Media B.V. 2008

infections, and changes in behaviour adopted in the face of the extreme adult mortality. Zimbabwe's well-educated population and extensive primary health care network are conducive to a relatively rapid response to the HIV epidemic and the Government's intensified efforts to control HIV transmission supported by those of its partners are also likely to have played a part in placing a brake on the national epidemic.

Introduction

Zimbabwe is a land-locked country of some 11.6 million people in southern Africa lying to the west of Mozambique, to the east of Botswana, to the north of South Africa and to the south of Zambia and Malawi. The country gained independence in 1980, since when the Government has greatly expanded access to education and primary health care services, even in rural areas far from the main urban centres. Despite recent economic difficulties, Zimbabwe remains one of the more developed countries in sub-Saharan Africa [1] with a GNI of US$2,120 per capita, an educated population and a well-developed transport and communications infrastructure. Mortality rates were amongst the lowest in the region prior to HIV/AIDS and fertility rates were already in decline in the 1980s.

The HIV epidemic in Zimbabwe appears to have taken hold in the mid-1980s [2] and the country has been one of the most severely affected in sub-Saharan Africa [3]. In this article, we provide an overview of the current understanding of the course of the HIV epidemic in Zimbabwe, of the epidemiology of HIV infection within the country and factors that may have contributed to the size of the local epidemic, of the demographic effects of the HIV epidemic and of its current status, as well as summarising the national response to the epidemic.

Levels and Trends in HIV Prevalence

Current Estimates

HIV-1 subtype C is understood to be the predominant strain of HIV infection in Zimbabwe [4]. In accordance with WHO/UNAIDS recommendations for countries with widely disseminated HIV epidemics, routine data for sentinel surveillance purposes are collected from pregnant women attending for check-ups at antenatal clinics (ANCs) [5]. The unadjusted ANC data for 2002 yielded an estimate of HIV prevalence among women attending antenatal clinics in Zimbabwe as a whole of 25.7% (1,784/6,938).

However, experience has shown that ANC surveillance data can provide biased estimates of HIV prevalence amongst adults in the general population due to problems such as non-representative selection of clinics included in the national surveillance system, over-representation of more sexually-active individuals, sub-fertility in HIV-infected women, and differences in HIV prevalence between men and women [6]. Furthermore, the effects of these biases can differ between countries. UNAIDS and their partners have therefore developed the Epidemic Projection Package (EPP) and the Spectrum package to adjust for the effects of these biases in different settings and to provide improved estimates of levels of HIV prevalence in individual countries that are informed by past as well as the most recent data [5]. When these methods were applied to meet United Nations requirements for a national estimate for HIV prevalence among men and women aged 15–49 years as at the end of 2003 [7], a figure of 24.6% (UNAIDS plausible range: 20%–28%) was obtained.

The 24.6% national HIV prevalence estimate for 2003 [7] was substantially lower than the previous estimate for 2001 (33.7%) [3]. However, this was mostly due to improvements in the methods of estimation resulting from devolution of the estimation process to the country level and the availability of new demographic data, rather than to a real reduction in HIV prevalence occurring over time. Indeed, a downward revision of the 2001 estimate to 24.9% was released at the same time as the estimate for 2003 [7].

Perhaps the most important of the innovations made in 2003 was the identification of a separate "other" population stratum which covered centres of formal sector employment such as rural administrative centres, mining areas and large-scale farming estates. For the 2001 and earlier rounds of national estimates, ANC surveillance sites were categorised as either urban or rural (with "other" areas being included in the rural category), HIV prevalence for all rural sites was reduced by 20% to take account of a peri-urban bias in the selection of these sites, EPP was used to generate separate HIV prevalence estimates for the urban and rural populations, and these estimates were combined using weights for the respective populations obtained from Census data to yield an overall national estimate. However, the Zimbabwe National HIV/AIDS Estimates Working Group 2003, comprised of Ministry of Health, National AIDS Council, Central Statistics Office, and other locally-based epidemiologists and demographers, established that the 20% adjustment for over-representation of peri-urban sites within the rural ANC sites was inadequate and the HIV prevalence estimate for 2001 had been overstated.

Newly available Census data for 2002 showed that the "rural" population constituted 68% of the total and that one-seventh of this population lived in "other" areas [8]. However, more than one-third of the ANC sentinel surveillance sites categorised as "rural" in 2001 were located in "other" areas and local studies indicated that HIV prevalence was much higher in these areas than in truly rural locations. For example, HIV prevalence in small towns and estates in Manicaland province between 2001 and 2003 were 33% and 21%, respectively, whilst HIV prevalence in rural business centres and villages was 16%. In a national population-based survey (the ZiChiRe Study) of 16–29 year-olds in growth points (administrative centres designated by the Government as foci for rural development) conducted in 2001, HIV prevalence was found to be 26% (15% and 34% in males and females, respectively) [9]. It was therefore decided to fit EPP separately to the ANC data from urban, other and the remaining rural sites in the 2003 exercise and this contributed to the downward revision in the 2001 estimate. In addition, one sixth of the remaining rural ANC surveillance sites were identified as lying in growth points and trading centres located along major roads where HIV prevalence is also higher than in the subsistence farming villages in which the great majority of Zimbabwe's rural population live. Detailed analysis of the ANC data and data from population-based studies indicated that HIV prevalence estimates derived from these sites should be reduced by 30% to adjust for this bias.

Other modifications made in the 2003 round of national HIV/AIDS estimates included minor changes to the standard UNAIDS assumptions on the relationship between HIV prevalence in women attending antenatal clinics and women in the general population and on the ratio of HIV prevalence in women to HIV prevalence in men in the three population strata. The female-male sex ratio of HIV prevalence in each population stratum is currently of the order of 1.35:1 [7, 10–12]. Comparisons of HIV prevalence in pregnant women and women of reproductive age made in localised population-based surveys [13] suggested that ANC estimates in urban areas are close to HIV prevalence in women rather than the adult population as a whole as is usually assumed. This may be because age at first sex is delayed and contraceptives are widely used in urban areas of Zimbabwe. This modification also slightly reduces the HIV prevalence estimates for current and past years.

Other factors that contributed to the revision in HIV/AIDS estimates for previous years included inclusion of newly available ANC surveillance data and omission of duplicate sites and data points from two sites (Chiredzi, data points prior to 2001; and Musume, data for 2000) that the National HIV/AIDS Estimates Working Group considered to be inconsistent and implausibly high. The resulting ANC-based national estimates for 2003 indicated that HIV prevalence in adults aged 15–49 years in 2003 was 28%, 35% and 21% in urban, other and rural areas, respectively.

Some independent corroboration for the resulting 2003 round of ANC-based estimates is provided by data from the Zimbabwe Young Adult Survey, a nationally representative, population-based survey of HIV risk behaviours and prevalence among young adults aged 15–29 years [12]. These data indicate that HIV prevalence was 10% and 22% among men and women aged 15–29 years, respectively, in 2001. Extrapolating from these data using the ratios of HIV prevalence in 15–49 year-olds to HIV prevalence in 15–29 year olds for males and females in Manicaland yielded a combined national estimate for both sexes of 22% which lies within the range for the ANC-based estimate (20%–28%) [7].

Trends in HIV Prevalence

Early data from the Zimbabwe Blood Transfusion Service indicate that HIV prevalence was still low (2–3%) even in predominantly urban areas in the mid-1980s [14]. Routine antenatal clinic (ANC) surveillance for HIV was established in 1990 by which time adult HIV prevalence was estimated to have reached approximately 9% [15]. Fig. 1 shows the trend in HIV prevalence estimated in the Zimbabwe National HIV and AIDS Estimates 2003 Report [7]. Fig. 2 also shows the same trend in HIV prevalence together with trends in crude prevalence from the individual ANC sites included in the national sentinel surveillance system. The best estimate of the national trend suggests that HIV prevalence stabilised in the mid-to-late 1990s and declined very slowly in the five years to 2003. According to these ANC data- and model-based estimates, HIV prevalence remained stable between 2001 (24.9%) and 2003 (24.6%). In the pooled ANC data, there is evidence of a small but statistically significant reduction in HIV prevalence among pregnant women attending antenatal clinics nationally from 32% in 2000 to 30% in 2002 (χ^2 test, p < 0.01) with the

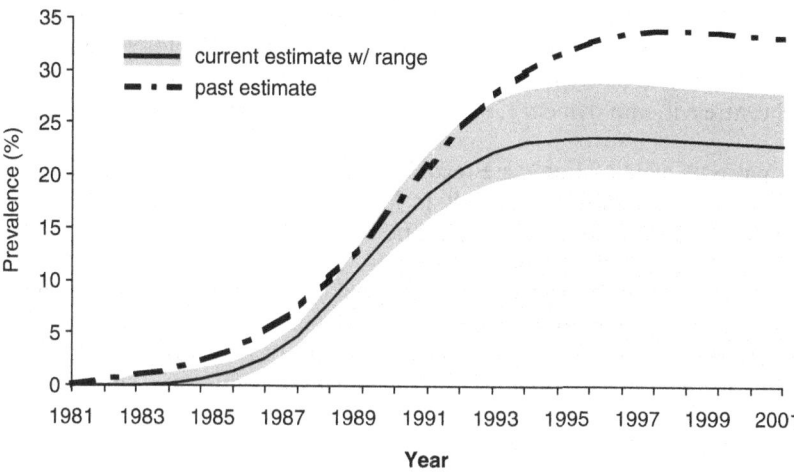

Fig. 1. Trend in best estimate of HIV prevalence in adults aged 15–49 years and range around estimates allowing for possible errors in surveillance data as projected in EPP using data from Zimbabwe's national antenatal clinic surveillance system [7]. The previous estimate is shown for comparison

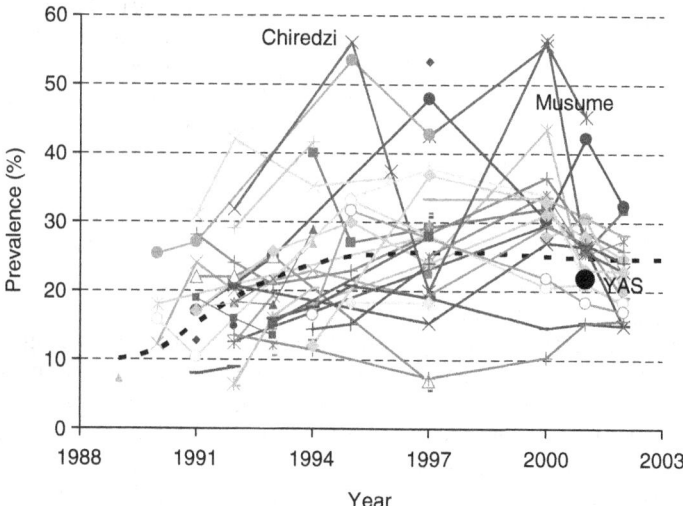

Fig. 2. Trends in crude HIV prevalence in adults aged 15–49 years for individual sites included in Zimbabwe's national antenatal clinic surveillance system, and national estimate from the Zimbabwe Young Adult Survey (YAS) 2001. EPP fit (dotted line) is shown for comparison

reduction being most pronounced in 15–24 year-olds (29% to 25%, p < 0.01) [16]. Significant reductions in the HIV prevalence in 15–49 year-olds were recorded in urban areas (35% to 30%; p < 0.01) and rural areas (30% to 26%; p < 0.01) but not in rural centres of employment (36% in both years, p = 0.9).

Similar patterns of reduction were recorded between the 1998–2000 and 2001–2003 rounds of the population-based study in Manicaland. Overall, HIV prevalence fell from 19.5% to 18% (age- and socio-economic location-adjusted odds ratio (OR), 0.84; [95% CI, 0.74–0.96]) in men aged 17–54 years and from 26% to 22% (adjusted OR, 0.88; [95% CI, 0.79–0.98]) in women aged 15–44 years [17]. Again the reduction was greatest in men and women aged under 25 years (sex-adjusted OR, 0.52; [95% CI, 0.45–0.62]. There were statistically significant reductions (p < 0.05) in HIV prevalence for men living in estates, roadside business centres and subsistence farming areas but not for those living in the two small towns (p = 0.8). Among women, there were statistically significant reductions in all socio-economic strata.

HIV Incidence and Age Patterns of Prevalence

Very few longitudinal studies have been conducted in Zimbabwe in which HIV incidence has been measured directly. Between 1993 and March 1995, HIV incidence in male factory workers in Harare was found to be 2.93% (95% CI, 2.18–3.86) [18,19]. More recently, HIV incidence has been measured in a cohort of men and women in four socio-economic strata in Manicaland (**Table 1**). Overall, HIV incidence was estimated at 1.88% per annum for men (aged 17–54 years at baseline) and 1.74% per annum for women (15–44). The results suggest that, within the rural areas, HIV is still spreading most extensively in centres of employment such as small towns and large-scale commercial farming estates. HIV incidence was highest at young ages for women (2.14% among those under 25 years of age versus 1.43% in those aged 25 years and above; p = 0.03) but was similar in younger and older men (p = 0.8).

Direct estimates of changes in the incidence of infection require at least three rounds of follow-up in a longitudinal survey. However, the age-profile of the prevalence of HIV can reveal something about past trends in HIV incidence, although this profile is also affected by age-specific patterns of new infections and the impact of AIDS and other cause mortality. The median reported age at first sex in Zimbabwe is 19 years for men and women and the distribution is well fitted by a log-logistic function. If we assume that once sexually active, the risk of becoming HIV infected is independent of age, then, accounting for HIV-related and other cause mortality, we can estimate past levels of HIV incidence from the age distribution of prevalence. We use an estimate of the median survival time after HIV infection of 11–12 years depending on the age at infection (those infected at age 15 survive for longer) [20,21].

In general the shape of the distribution of HIV prevalence by single years of age for 15 to 24 year-olds tends to be linear if incidence has been unchanged, convex if increasing and concave if decreasing (**Fig. 3a**). We estimate the linear rate of change in incidence from the nationally representative YAS and the Manicaland Study. The YAS data are consistent with a declining incidence for men (**Fig. 3d**) but for women

Table 1. HIV incidence by socio-economic stratum, Manicaland, Zimbabwe, 1998–2003.

Socio-economic stratum	Men				Women			
	HIV seroincidence per 100 PY	Seroconversions	Person years	N	HIV seroincidence per 100 PY	Seroconversions	Person years	N
Small towns	2.92	21	719.9	247	2.64	15	568.7	194
Commercial farming estates	1.95	44	2258.4	764	2.44	46	1881.6	647
Roadside business centres	1.74	10	573.1	192	0.91	14	1537.9	512
Subsistence farming areas	1.32	20	1511.1	504	1.56	48	3068.6	1031
Total	1.88	95	5062.5	1707	1.74	123	7056.8	2384

Men aged 17–54 years; women aged 15–44 years.

a scenario of no change cannot be excluded (**Fig. 3e**). In the second round of the Manicaland survey, there is evidence for a significant decline in incidence for both men (**Fig. 3c**) and women (**Fig. 3b**). Of course, these estimates will be confounded by changes with age in the risk of becoming infected. For instance, if those individuals who become sexually active early in life are at greater risk of becoming infected, then the age distribution of prevalence would tend to be convex and any declines in incidence would be underestimated. The impact of mortality on this pattern is limited since few of those infected in this age group will still be under 25 years of age when they develop AIDS.

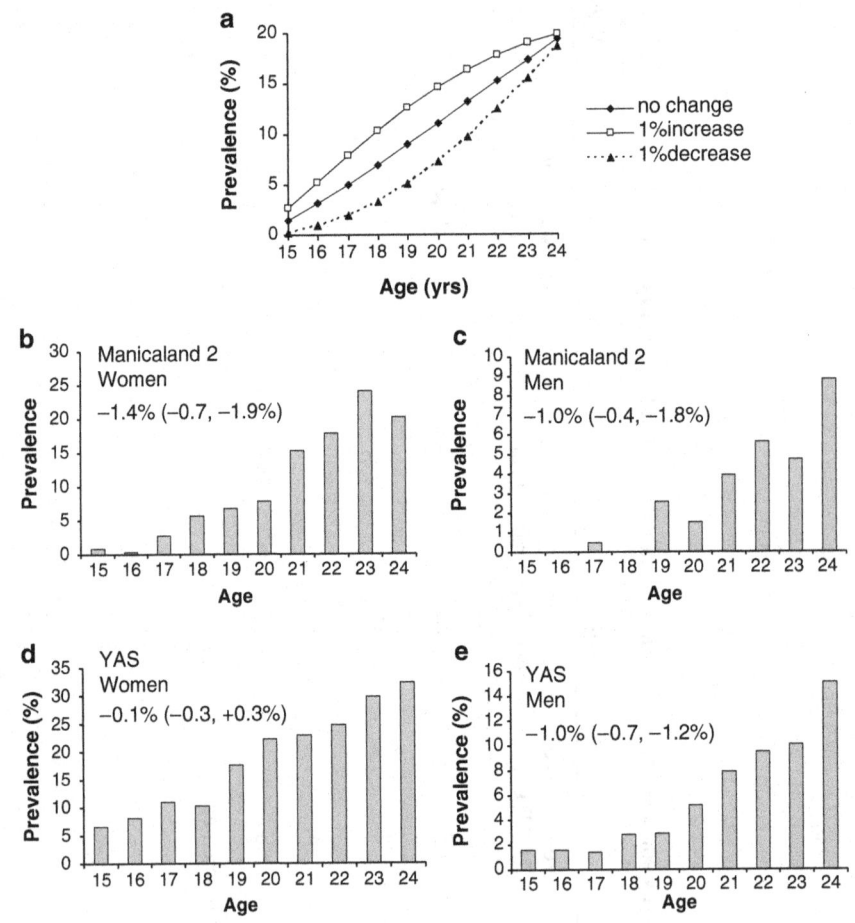

Fig. 3. Graph (a): expected age-profile of HIV prevalence where incidence has shown a linear increase of 1% per year, a 1% annual decrease or no change over the preceding 10 years. The risk of becoming infected is assumed to be the same for all ages once individuals have become sexually active. Maximum likelihood estimates (and 95% CI) of the linear annual rate of change in incidence under the same assumption for prevalence data from Manicaland for (b) women and (c) men, and from the YAS for (d) women and (e) men

Estimates of a decline in HIV incidence are what would be expected in a maturing epidemic as HIV infection becomes saturated among groups with high-risk behaviour [22]. The national estimates generated using ANC data and the EPP [6] and SPECTRUM [23] software suggest that HIV incidence peaked in 1993, fell during the mid-late 1990s, and remained constant since 2000.

Population and Individual Level Determinants of HIV Infection

Population Level Determinants

The recent downward revision of the national HIV prevalence estimates notwithstanding, Zimbabwe still has one of the largest HIV epidemics in sub-Saharan Africa. Despite its recent troubles, it is also one of the more developed countries in sub-Saharan Africa. In common with other southern African countries such as Botswana, South Africa and Namibia, Zimbabwe's large HIV epidemic may be due, in part, to its level and pattern of development [24–26]. In particular, the high level of HIV prevalence found in rural areas—relative to those in many other countries in the region—probably reflects the extensive labour-related circular migration made possible by the good quality transport infrastructure as well as the presence of employment opportunities within the rural areas themselves [27]. Circular migration is particularly common due to the colonial practice of not providing family accommodation for labour migrants [28] and the local culture which places emphasis on maintaining a rural home [29].

The emphasis that was placed on developing the primary health care system in the years following Independence in 1980, together with the early introduction of syndromic management procedures, has resulted in relatively low levels of most other sexually transmitted infections in Zimbabwe [9, 11, 15, 30]. However, *Herpes simplex* virus type-2 is very common [11, 31] and has been found to be an important determinant of the scale of HIV epidemics at the population level [32] in Africa. The widespread use of medical injections within the primary healthcare system opens up the possibility that use of contaminated needles may have contributed to the spread of HIV within Zimbabwe [33]. However, very few infections appear to occur in persons who have not started sex but who report a history of medical injections [34]. Male circumcision has been found to have a protective effect at the population level [35] and is practised by only a small minority of Zimbabwe's population. Ritual scarification is relatively rare in Zimbabwe but dry sex is widely practiced in some communities and has been suggested as a possible cofactor in HIV transmission [36–38].

Sexual behaviour is frequently found to be associated with enhanced risk of HIV infection at the individual level (see below). In univariate analyses conducted in an ecological study of 122 developing countries, later age at first sexual intercourse was associated with smaller HIV epidemics and greater frequency of non-regular sexual partnerships was associated with larger HIV epidemics. However, these effects ceased to be statistically significant as an explanation for population level differences in HIV prevalence in multivariate regression analyses [26] and did not explain the widely divergent HIV prevalence levels observed in a study conducted in four sub-Saharan African cities [35]. Age at first sex is high in Zimbabwe by African standards (median age for females 18.7 years [39]). Multiple pre-marital and extra-marital sexual partnerships were common—particularly amongst men—during the 1990s [40]. In an ecological comparison of risk factors with those found in Kisesa in rural north-west Tanzania where HIV prevalence is considerably lower, high-risk sexual behaviours were not found to be more common in Manicaland [41]. High-risk sexual behaviour is becoming less common in rural Zimbabwe [17] but appears to have been relatively constant in Kisesa [42]. Thus, it is likely that high risk sexual behaviour was considerably more common in Zimbabwe in the late 1980s and early 1990s when the HIV epidemic became established in the country. Differences in reporting bias and higher AIDS-associated mortality in persons with high-risk behaviour may also conceal underlying differences in sexual behaviour between the two populations. To the extent that rates of sexual partner change and condom use are indeed similar, it may be that patterns of sexual mixing are different. More extensive contacts with higher HIV-prevalence urban- or commercial centre-based populations could have contributed to the larger rural epidemic in Manicaland [43].

Individual Level Determinants

The primary nationally-representative source of data on individual level determinants of HIV infection is the Zimbabwe Young Adult Survey 2001/2002 [12]. Data are limited to men and women aged 15–29 years. Within this age range, HIV infection is associated with age, female sex, urban residence, and experience of marital breakdown due to divorce or widowhood. Young women with secondary school education or enhanced socio-economic status are at reduced risk of HIV infection compared to their less educated and less well-off peers but there were no equivalent differences for men. Young men and women who report higher numbers of sexual partners in their lifetimes are at increased risk of HIV infection but no association was found with reported age at first sex [44].

In a detailed study of a cohort of 2,691 male factory workers interviewed in Harare between 1993 and 1995, independent individual level risk factors for prevalent HIV infection included being aged 25–44 years compared to both younger and older ages, not being a home-owner, having a history of genital warts, genital ulcer, or urethral discharge in the past year ($p < 0.05$ in each case), multiple sexual partners in the past year (OR, 1.58; [95% CI, 1.21–2.05]), having paid for sex in the past year (OR, 2.55; [95% CI, 1.64–3.96]), and having visited a beer hall in the past week (OR, 1.62; [95% CI, 1.30–2.02]). Married and divorced men were at significantly higher risk than those who had remained single, but widowers were the most likely to be infected with HIV [45]. Between 1993 and 1995, the incidence of new HIV infections was independently associated with non-co-resident marriage (adjusted hazard ratio (HR) versus co-resident marriage, 2.21; [95% CI, 1.00–4.89]), recent genital ulcer (HR, 3.55; [95% CI, 1.52–8.29]), and number of sex partners in year preceding enrolment (HR, 1.10; [95% CI, 1.01–1.21]) [18].

In Manicaland, 1998–2000, over the wider age-range 17–44 years, older persons and women were also found to be at greater risk of HIV infection [10, 11]. After taking age and sex into account, residence in a more urban area was associated with increased risk. Married persons were at significantly greater risk of HIV infection than single people, and divorcees and widows were at significantly greater risk than married persons. Secondary school education showed a statistically significant protective effect for women up to the age of 24 years but had no effect in older women or among men [27]. A greater number of sexual partners in their lifetime was associated with increased risk of currently being infected with HIV for men and women ($p < 0.001$) [46]. Among men, a greater number of sexual partners in the last year ($p = 0.05$) and in the past month ($p = 0.05$) showed weaker but independent effects on the chances of currently being infected with HIV. For women, reporting a greater number of current sexual relationships was independently associated with current HIV infection. Amongst young people, earlier age at first sex and having an older sexual partner were associated with heightened risk of HIV infection [47].

In the same study, the lifetime experience of sexually transmitted infections was found to be associated with increased risk of HIV infection after controlling for behavioural risk factors—genital ulcers (adjusted OR, 4.49; [1.96–10.31]) and urethral/vaginal discharge (adjusted OR, 1.80; [1.13–2.88]). HSV-2 appears to be the most common cause of genital ulcers and *Trichomonas vaginalis* the most prevalent source of genital discharge in the study populations [11, 48]. Recent injections and needle-stick injuries were not found to be associated with increased risk of incident HIV infection either in men (adjusted RR, 0.33; [95% CI, 0.07–1.46]) or women (adjusted RR, 1.04; [95% CI, 0.59–1.85]) [49]. Furthermore, injections were no more common among men (RR = 1.07, $p = 0.8$) or women (RR = 1.13, $p = 0.3$) who were HIV positive at baseline than amongst those who were uninfected [49].

With one or two exceptions (e.g. the effect of earlier age at first sex), the individual-level risk factors identified in these studies done in different locations and at slightly different times in the course of the HIV epidemic in Zimbabwe are internally consistent. The risk factors also appear to be broadly consistent with findings from studies done in other countries. However, the identity and strength of individual-level risk factors can change over the course of an HIV epidemic due, for example, to the temporal spread of HIV infection through sexual networks [50] and selective patterns of behaviour change [27, 51]. Thus, one would expect some variation in findings from different studies.

Demographic Impact

Mortality

Early mathematical model projections predicted substantial rises in mortality due to HIV/AIDS during the late 1980s and early 1990s [2, 52]. For example, Robinson and Marindo [53] estimated that the adult mortality rate per 1000 person years increased from 9.8 in 1987 to between 20.6 and 24.4 in 1995. By the year 2000, they projected that between 66% and 73% of all adult deaths would be attributable to HIV infection.

Current estimates based on the EPP and SPECTRUM models indicate that 135,000 (range 110,000–154,000) adult AIDS deaths and 36,000 (29,000–41,000) child AIDS deaths occurred during 2003 in a total population of 11.9 million[7].

Despite limitations in coverage, vital registration records show clear evidence of a rise in death rates in urban areas [54] and in rural areas [55] from the late 1980s and early 1990s, respectively. Indirect estimates calculated from nationally-representative data on orphanhood and sibling survival show very substantial increases in adult mortality [56, 57].

In rural areas in Manicaland province, the increase in adult death rates was initially concentrated in men in the most sexually-active age-groups and most of the increase was accounted for by a rise in deaths from illnesses commonly associated with HIV infection [55]. Preliminary estimates indicate that death rates in a cohort of 2,645 men aged 17–54 and 3,849 women aged 15–44 years in 1998–2000 were 22.8 per 1000 person years and 18.4 per 1000 person years, respectively, over the three-year period to 2001–2003. The percentages of deaths attributable to HIV infection were consistent with the projections by Robinson and Marindo—71.5% (113/158) of male deaths and 74.3% (124/167) of female deaths occurred amongst individuals who were HIV-positive at baseline—a slightly different measure [58].

Demographic and Health Survey data indicate that the infant mortality rate in Zimbabwe increased from 49.1 per thousand in 1988 to 52.8 in 1994 and 65.0 in 1999. Over the same period, under-5 mortality rose from 70.6 per thousand in 1988 to 77.1 in 1994 and 102.1 in 1999 [39]. These increases are likely to be to be largely due to HIV [59], although severe economic recession, reductions in vaccination coverage and drought are also likely to have contributed. The increases are underestimated since the deaths of children of women who themselves died of HIV/AIDS are excluded because of the way the data are collected.

Fertility

Zimbabwe Demographic and Health Survey data indicate that the total fertility rate has declined steadily from 6.67 live births per woman in the early 1980s to 5.50 in the mid 1980s and 3.96 in the late 1990s [39]. Using data on HIV-infected and uninfected women from Manicaland, we have shown in an earlier publication that HIV-associated sub-fertility could account for as much as a quarter of the decline since the mid-1980s [60]. Likely mechanisms include more frequent widowhood and divorce, reduced coital frequency, and direct effects of HIV infection including amenorrhoea.

HIV epidemics can also affect fertility through their effects on behaviour within the wider population and on the composition of the population [61–65]. For example, women may attempt to avoid HIV infection by delaying onset of sexual activity, through condom use, and through abstinence following divorce or widowhood. At the same time, shorter periods of post-partum abstinence (to avoid partners having extra-marital relationships) and breastfeeding—as well as more effective treatment of sexually transmitted infections and selective mortality among sub-fertile women—can place upward pressures on fertility at the population level. These effects are difficult to measure but the studies in Manicaland suggest that changes in behaviour made in response to the HIV/AIDS epidemic may have contributed to fertility decline in Zimbabwe [62].

Population Growth, Population Structure and Orphanhood

Zimbabwe's population grew from 10.4 million to 11.6 million between 1992 and 2002 [8]. The average rate of growth during this period (1.1%) was considerably lower than in the previous 10 year inter-census period (3.1%) and the current growth rate is thought to be close to zero [2, 52, 66]. The fall in the growth rate reflects the long-term decline in fertility [62], international migration, and the effects of economic hardships and major droughts (particularly in 1992–1993) as well as those of the HIV/AIDS epidemic. However, there can be little doubt that the latter has been the largest single factor through its effects on mortality and fertility.

HIV epidemics can have severe effects on the dependency ratio (i.e. the ratio of the number of children and elderly to the number of adults of economically-active age in the population) at the local level [67] and there is some evidence of this in localised studies in Zimbabwe [55]. However, even very large HIV epidemics generally have little effect on the dependency ratio at the national population level due to the counter-balancing effects of higher adult mortality, lower fertility and heightened early childhood mortality [68]. HIV-associated mortality can have the effect of reducing the mean age of the working age population [69] and thereby of eroding the skills- and experience-base of a country. Detailed analysis of data from the 2002 Census should show whether this has been the case in Zimbabwe.

In the Children on the Brink report for 2002, UNICEF, UNAIDS and USAID estimate that there were over 1 million (17.6%) orphaned children less than 15 years of age in Zimbabwe in 2001. Of these 782,000 (76.8%) were orphaned by HIV/AIDS [70]. By 2010, the total number of orphans is projected to have reached 1.3 million, 88.9% of whom will have lost at least one parent due to AIDS. Using EPP and SPECTRUM and locally available data, the Zimbabwe Ministry of Health and Child Welfare obtained a similar estimate of 761,000 (range 620,000–800,000) HIV/AIDS orphans aged 0–14 years for the year 2003. However, data from the Zimbabwe Demographic and Health Survey 1999 and from the studies in Manicaland [71] support the wider view that a smaller proportion of orphans have lost their mothers (i.e. are double or maternal orphans) at this stage in the epidemic than is indicated by the Children on the Brink report. This may be because the level of background non-AIDS mortality was over-estimated in the Children on the Brink report [72].

The National Response to the HIV/AIDS Epidemic

As in most other countries, it took some time before the national response to HIV/AIDS in Zimbabwe gained momentum. And, as elsewhere, the Government's initial response to HIV/AIDS was bio-medically orientated and based primarily on a variety of individual level information dissemination approaches [14]. However, the country has taken a pioneering role in a number of respects [73]. It was one of the first countries to recognize the potential value of, and to develop and implement, the syndromic management approach to control the sexually transmitted infections that act as cofactors in HIV transmission [74, 75]. It has played a major role in the development of more participatory and contextualized interventions especially in regard to the control of HIV transmission within core groups and potential bridge populations [76, 77]. Local Non-Governmental Organisations and AIDS Service Organisations in Zimbabwe have played a pioneering role in the development of sustainable and culturally-appropriate, community-based support programmes for people living with AIDS and for orphans [78]. Similar programmes are now being scaled-up throughout the country.

In the late 1990s, a number of professionally run and widely promoted "New Start" voluntary counselling and testing centres were established by Population Services International in urban centres with support from USAID and the National AIDS Coordination Programme [15]. To date, uptake is understood to be relatively low (e.g. in comparison to utilization of similar services in Uganda) but is gradually increasing. Population Services International have also been running an active programme of social marketing of male ("Protector+") and female ("CARE") condoms throughout Zimbabwe [79, 80] together with televised debates with young people on reproductive health issues and a television serial drama ("Studio 263") which highlights circumstances that can lead to exposure to HIV infection and models strategies for dealing with these situations.

A National AIDS Council was established in 2000 to coordinate a multi-sectoral response to the HIV epidemic. The Zimbabwe Government introduced an "AIDS Levy", effectively an extra 3% on income tax, as a means of financing a National AIDS Trust Fund [81]. This highly innovative fund is being channelled through District AIDS Action Committees for disbursement at Ward and Village level to support grassroots HIV/AIDS initiatives. A prevention of parent-to-child transmission service based on single doses of Nevirapine to mother and baby around the time of delivery is being extended to all districts within the country [82, 83]. Programmes for comprehensive, holistic and integrated prevention and care services including preparations for implementation of Highly Active Anti-Retroviral Therapy (HAART) are currently under development in rural as well as urban settings.

Conclusions

In this chapter, we have provided an overview of current understanding of the pattern of spread and impact of the local HIV epidemic from an epidemiological and demographic perspective. Past estimates may have exaggerated the scale of the HIV epidemic in Zimbabwe but it remains one of the most seriously affected countries in the world with almost one-quarter of its adult population currently thought to be infected with HIV and subject to extreme levels of mortality.

Zimbabwe may have been vulnerable to a large HIV epidemic because of its particular pattern of development. The country is now struggling with serious economic difficulties caused in part by the effects of the HIV epidemic. However, its relatively strong underlying level of development may be enabling it to mobilise a faster and more effective response than has been possible in other settings [27]. HIV surveillance data from a variety of national and local sources indicate that HIV prevalence is beginning to come down, with substantial falls being seen in young age-groups UNAIDS, 2005. Furthermore, there is some evidence that this reflects major changes in behaviour rather than purely the natural dynamics of HIV epidemics [17]. Such changes could be in response to the sustained period of crisis-level adult mortality but must also reflect the high level of knowledge and awareness of HIV that exists within the country and the intensity of HIV-prevention activity that has been underway in many parts of the country for the past few years.

The challenge now is to make effective treatment and care services widely available in a systematic and locally-integrated manner whilst sustaining the reductions in behaviours that enhance exposure to HIV infection. Hopefully, the international community will continue to assist Zimbabwe in attaining this vital humanitarian goal.

Acknowledgements

The authors thank the Ministry of Health and Child Welfare for access to data from recent national HIV-related surveys.

References

1. World Bank (2002). *World Development Report.* (Washington, DC: World Bank)

2. Blair Research Institute, Oxford University (1996). *The early socio-demographic impact of the HIV-1 epidemic in rural Zimbabwe.* (Port Blair: Blair Research Institute)

3. UNAIDS (2002). *Report on the global HIV/AIDS epidemic.* (Geneva: UNAIDS)

4. Chandiwana, S. K. (2001). Why has HIV spread so rapidly in southern Africa? *Zimbabwe Science News*, *35*(1 & 2), 11–17

5. Chin, J. & Mann, J. (1989). Global surveillance and forecasting of AIDS. *Bulletin of the World Health Organization*, *67*(1), 1–7

6. Projections URGoEMa (2002). Improved methods and assumptions for estimation of the HIV/AIDS epidemic and its impact: Recommendations of the UNAIDS reference group on estimates, modelling and projections. *AIDS*, *16*, W1–W14

7. Zimbabwe Ministry of Health and Child Welfare (2003). *Zimbabwe National HIV and AIDS Estimates.* (Harare: Zimbabwe Ministry of Health and Child Welfare)

8. Zimbabwe Central Statistical Office (2002). *Census 2002: Zimbabwe Preliminary Report.* (Harare, Zimbabwe: CSO)

9. Woelk, G., Kasprzyk, D., Montano, D. E. & Mutsindiri, R. (2002). *National survey of STDs and HIV prevalence among residents in rural growth point villages in Zimbabwe.* (Barcelona: XIV International AIDS Conference 2002)

10. Gregson, S. & Chandiwana, S. K. (2001). The Manicaland HIV/STD prevention project: Studies on HIV transmission, impact and control in rural Zimbabwe. *Zimbabwe Science News*, *35*(1), 27–42

11. Gregson, S., Mason, P. R., Garnett, G. P., et al. (2001). A rural epidemic in Zimbabwe? Findings from a population-based survey. *International Journal of STD and AIDS, 12,* 189–196

12. Zimbabwe Ministry of Health and Child Welfare, Zimbabwe National Family Planning Council, National AIDS Council Zimbabwe, Centers for Disease Control and Prevention Zimbabwe (2004). *The Zimbabwe Young Adult Survey (YAS) 2001–2002:* (Harare: Zimbabwe Ministry of Health and Child Welfare and Centers for Disease Control and Prevention Zimbabwe).

13. Gregson, S., Terceira, N., Kakowa, M., et al. (2002). Study of bias in antenatal clinic HIV-1 surveillance data in a high contraceptive prevalence population in sub-Saharan Africa. *AIDS, 16*(4), 643–652

14. Jackson, H. (1992). *AIDS: Action now.* 2nd edn. (Harare, Zimbabwe: AIDS Counselling Trust)

15. Decosas, J. & Padian, N. S. (2002). The profile and context of the epidemics of sexually transmitted infections including HIV in Zimbabwe. *Sexually Transmitted Infections, 78*(Suppl 1), 40–46

16. Nesara, P., Lee, L. M., Zisengwe, L. M., Magure, T. & McNaghten, A. D. (2003). *Trends in HIV prevalence in antenatal attendees in Zimbabwe, 2000–2002.* (Nairobi: International Conference on AIDS in Sub-Saharan Africa 2003)

17. Gregson, S., Garnett, G. P., Nyamukapa, C. A., et al. (2006). HIV decline associated with behaviour change in eastern Zimbabwe. *Science, 311,* 664–666

18. Mbizvo, M., Machekano, R., McFarland, W., et al. (1996). HIV seroincidence and correlates of seroconversion in a cohort of male factory workers in Harare, Zimbabwe. *AIDS, 10*(8), 895–902

19. Ray, S., Latif, A., Machekano, R. & Katzenstein, D. (1998). Sexual behaviour and risk assessment of HIV seroconvertors among urban male factory workers in Zimbabwe. *Social Science and Medicine, 47*(10), 1431–1443

20. Morgan, D., Mahe, C., Mayanja, B., Okongo, J. M., Lubega, R. & Whitworth, J. A. G. (2002). HIV-1 infection in rural Africa: Is there a difference in median time to AIDS and survival compared with that in industrial countries? *AIDS, 16*(4), 597–603

21. Collaborative Group on AIDS Incubation and Survival including the CASCADE EU Concerted Action (2000). Time from HIV-1 seroconversion to AIDS and death before widespread use of highly-active antiretroviral therapy: A collaborative re-analysis. *The Lancet, 355,* 1131–1137

22. Anderson, R. M. & May, R. M. (1991). *Infectious diseases of humans: dynamics and control.* (Oxford: Oxford University Press)

23. Stover, J. & Kirmeyer, S. (2001). DEMPROJ (Version 4): *A computer program for making population projections.* (Washington, DC: Futures Group International, Policy Project)

24. Over, M. & Piot, P. (1993). HIV infection and sexually transmitted diseases. (In D. T. Jamison, W. H. Mosley, A. R. Measham, J. L. Bobadilla (Eds.), *Disease Control Priorities in Developing Countries* (pp. 455–528). New York: Oxford University)

25. Dyson, T. (2003). HIV/AIDS and urbanization. *Population and Development Review, 29*(3), 427–442

26. Drain, P. K., Smith, J. S., Hughes, J. P., Halperin, D. T. & Holmes, K. K. (2004). Correlates of national HIV seroprevalence: an ecological analysis of 122 developing countries. *Journal of Acquired Immune Deficiency Syndromes, 35*(4), 407–420

27. Gregson, S., Waddell, H. & Chandiwana, S. K. (2001). School education and HIV control in sub-Saharan Africa: from discord to harmony? *Journal of International Development, 13,* 467–485

28. Bassett, M. T. & Mhloyi, M. (1991). Women and AIDS in Zimbabwe: the making of an epidemic. *International Journal of Health Services, 21*(1), 143–156

29. Potts, D. H. & Mutambirwa, C. C. (1990). Rural-urban linkages in contemporary Harare: why migrants need their land. *Journal of Southern African Studies, 16*(4), 177–198

30. Montano, D. E., Kasprzyk, D., Woelk, G. & St. Lawrence, J. (2002). *National survey of behavioural risk for STDs and HIV among residents of rural growth point villages in Zimbabwe.* (Barcelona: XIV International AIDS Conference 2002)

31. Gwanzura, L., McFarland, W., Alexander, D., Burke, R., Katzenstein, D. (1998). Association between HIV and HSV-2 seropositivity among male factory workers in Zimbabwe. *Journal of Infectious Diseases, 177*, 481–484

32. Weiss, H. A., Buve, A., Robinson, N. J., et al. (2001). The epidemiology of HSV-2 infection and its association with HIV infection in four urban African populations. *AIDS, 15*(Suppl 4), S97–S108

33. Gisselquist, D., Rothenberg, R., Potterat, J. & Drucker, E. (2002). HIV infections in sub-Saharan Africa not explained by sexual or vertical transmission. *International Journal of STD and AIDS, 13*(10), 657–666

34. Gregson, S., Nyamukapa, C. A., Garnett, G. P., et al. (2005). HIV infection and reproductive health in teenage women orphaned and made vulnerable by AIDS in eastern Zimbabwe. *AIDS Care, 17*, 785–794

35. Buve, A., Carael, M., Hayes, R. J., et al. (2001). Multicentre study on factors determining differences in rate of spread of HIV in sub-Saharan Africa: Methods and prevalence of HIV infection. *AIDS, 15*(Suppl 4), S5–S14

36. Civic, D. & Wilson, D. (1996). Dry sex in Zimbabwe and implications for condom use. *Social Science and Medicine, 42*(1), 91–98

37. Ray, S., Gumbo, N. & Mbizvo, M. (1996). Local voices: what some Harare men say about preparation for sex. *Reproductive Health Matters, *(7), 34–45

38. Dallabetta, G., Miotti, P., Chiphangwi, J., Liomba, G. & Saah, A. (1990). *Vaginal tightening agents as risk factors for acquisition of HIV.* (San Francisco: Sixth International Conference on AIDS 1990)

39. Machirovi, L. M. (2000). *Zimbabwe Demographic and Health Survey, 1999.* (Harare: Zimbabwe Central Statistical Office/Macro International)

40. Zimbabwe National AIDS Council MoHaCW, The MEASURE Project, (CDC/Zimbabwe) CfDCaP (2002). *AIDS in Africa During the Nineties: A review and analysis of survey and research results.* (Chapel Hill: Carolina Population Center, University of North Carolina)

41. Boerma, J. T, Gregson, S., Nyamupaka, C. A. & Urassa, M. (2003). Understanding the uneven spread of HIV within Africa: comparative study of biological, behavioral and contextual factors in rural populations in Tanzania and Zimbabwe. *Sexually Transmitted Diseases, 30*, 779–787

42. Mwaluko, G., Urassa, M., Isingo, R., Zaba, B. & Boerma, J. T. (2003). Trends in HIV and sexual behaviour in a longitudinal study in a rural population in Tanzania, 1994–2000. *AIDS, 17*(18), 2645–2651

43. Garnett, G. P. & Anderson, R. M. Factors controlling the spread of HIV in heterosexual communities in developing countries: patterns of mixing between different age and sexual activity classes. *Philosophical Transactions of the Royal Society of London, Series B*, (342), 137–159

44. Zimbabwe Ministry of Health and Child Welfare (2004). *Monitoring the HIV/AIDS epidemic and the national response: The Zimbabwe young adult survey (YAS) 2001–2002.* (Harare: Zimbabwe Ministry of Health and Child Welfare)

45. Bassett, M. T., McFarland, W. C., Ray, S., et al. (1996). Risk factors for HIV infection at enrollment in an urban male factory cohort in Harare, Zimbabwe. *Journal of Acquired Immune Deficiency Syndromes and Human Retrovirology, 13*(3), 287–293

46. Lewis, J. J. C., Chandiwana, S. K., Nyamukapa, C. A., Garnett, G. P., Donnelly, C. A. & Gregson, S. (2002). *Patterns of sexual behaviour and the risk of HIV infection in rural Zimbabwe.* Abstract ThPeC7450. (Barcelona: XIV International AIDS Conference 2002)

47. Gregson, S., Nyamukapa, C., Garnett, G. P., et al. (2002). Sexual mixing patterns and sex-differentials in teenage exposure to HIV infection in rural Zimbabwe. *The Lancet, 359*(June), 1896–1903

48. Mason, P. R., Fiori, P. L., Cappuccinelli, P., Rapelli, P. & Gregson, S. (2005). Seroepidemiology of *Trichomonas vaginalis* and patterns of association with HIV infection in young women in rural Zimbabwe. *Epidemiology and Infection* 2001; 2005;133:315–323

49. Lopman, B., Garnett, G. P., Mason, P. R. & Gregson, S. (2005) Evidence of absence: Injection history and HIV incidence in rural Zimbabwe. *Public Library of Science Medicine*, 2005; 2(2):142–146

50. Gregson, S. & Garnett, G. P. (2000). Contrasting gender differentials in HIV-1 prevalence and associated mortality increase in eastern and southern Africa: artefact of data or natural course of epidemics? *AIDS, 14*(Suppl 3), S85–S99

51. Hargreaves, J. R. & Glynn, J. R. (2002). Educational attainment and HIV infection in developing countries: a review of the published literature. *Tropical Medicine and International Health, 7*, 489–498

52. US Bureau of the Census (1997). *The demographic impact of HIV/AIDS: Perspectives from the world population profile, 1996.* (Washington, DC: US Bureau of the Census)

53. Robinson, N. J. & Marindo, R. (1999). Current estimates of and future projections for adult deaths attributed to HIV infection in Zimbabwe. *Journal of Acquired Immune Deficiency Syndromes, 20*(2), 187–194

54. Murimwa-Moyo, I. M. (1991). Mortality levels, patterns and trends in the city of Harare, Zimbabwe. MSc. in Medical Demography. (London: London School of Hygiene and Tropical Medicine)

55. Gregson, S., Anderson, R. M., Ndlovu, J., Zhuwau, T. & Chandiwana, S. K. (1997). Recent upturn in mortality in rural Zimbabwe: evidence for an early demographic impact of HIV-1 infections? *AIDS, 11*(10), 1269–1280

56. Timaeus, I. (1998). Impact of the HIV epidemic on mortality in sub-Saharan Africa: evidence from national surveys and censuses. *AIDS, 12*(Suppl), S15–S27

57. Feeney, G. (2001). The impact of HIV/AIDS on adult mortality in Zimbabwe. *Population and Development Review, 27*(4), 771–780

58. Gregson, S., Mushati, P., Nyamupaka, C. A. (2007). Adult mortality and erosion of household viability in AIDS-afflicted towns, estates and villages in eastern Zimbabwe. *Journal of Acquired Immune Deficiency Syndromes, 44*, 188–195

59. Aiken, C. G. A. (1992). HIV-1 infection and perinatal mortality in Zimbabwe. *Archives of Disease in Childhood, 67*, 595–599

60. Terceira, N., Gregson, S., Zaba, B. & Mason, P. R. (2003). The contribution of HIV to fertility decline in rural Zimbabwe. *Population Studies, 57*(2), 149–164

61. Gregson, S. (1994). Will HIV become a major determinant of fertility in sub-Saharan Africa? *Journal of Development Studies, 30*(3), 650–679

62. Gregson, S., Zhuwau, T., Anderson, R. M. & Chandiwana, S. K. (1997). HIV-1 and fertility change in rural Zimbabwe. *Health Transition Review, 7*(Suppl 2), 89–112

63. Zaba, B. & Gregson, S. (1998). Measuring the impact of HIV on fertility in Africa. *AIDS, 12*(Suppl), S41–S50

64. Grieser, M., Gittelsohn, J., Shankar, A. V., et al. (2001). Reproductive decision making and the HIV/AIDS epidemic in Zimbabwe. *Journal of Southern African Studies, 27*(2), 225–243

65. Guilkey, D. K. & Jayne, S. (1997). Fertility transition in Zimbabwe: Determinants of contraceptive use and method choice. *Population Studies, 51*(2), 173–190

66. Zimbabwe National AIDS Co-ordination Programme (1998). *HIV/AIDS in Zimbabwe: Background, projections, impact and interventions*. (Harare: Zimbabwe Ministry of Health and Child Welfare)

67. Low-Beer, D., Stoneburner, R. L. & Mukulu, A. (1997). Empirical evidence for the severe but localized impact of AIDS on population structure. *Nature Medicine, 3*(5), 553–557

68. Anderson, R. M., May, R. M. & McLean, A. (1987). Possible demographic consequences of AIDS in developing countries. *Nature, 332*, 228–234

69. Gregson, S., Garnett, G. P. & Anderson, R. M. (1994). Assessing the potential impact of the HIV-1 epidemic on orphanhood and the demographic structure of populations in sub-Saharan Africa. *Population Studies, 48*, 435–458

70   UNAIDS (2005). *Evidence for HIV decline in Zimbabwe: A comprehensive review of the epidemiological data*. (Geneva: UNAIDS)

71. UNAIDS, UNICEF, USAID (2002). Children on the brink 2002. (Washington, DC: TvT Associates)

72. Nyamukapa, C. A. & Gregson, S. (2005). Extended family' and women's roles in safeguarding orphans' education in AIDS-afflicted rural Zimbabwe. *Social Science and Medicine, 60*, 2155–2167

73. Grassly, N. C., Lewis, J. J. C., Mahy, M., Walker, N. & Timaeus, I. M. (2004). Comparison of survey estimates with UNAIDS/WHO projections of mortality and orphan numbers in sub-Saharan Africa. *Population Studies, 58*, 207–217

74. Gomo, E. & Chandiwana, S. K. (2001). A review of the HIV/AIDS situation in Zimbabwe. *Zimbabwe Science News, 35*(1 & 2), 4–10

75. Latif, A. S., Katzenstein, D. A., Bassett, M. T., Houston, S., Emmanuel, J. C. & Marowa, E. (1989). Genital ulcers and transmission of HIV among couples in Zimbabwe. *AIDS, 3*, 519–523

76. Grosskurth, H., Mosha, F., Todd, J., et al. (1995). Impact of improved treatment of sexually transmitted diseases on HIV infection in rural Tanzania: Randomised controlled trial. *The Lancet, 346*, 530–536

77. Dube, N. & Wilson, D. Peer education programs among HIV-vulnerable communities in Southern Africa. (In B. Williams, C. Campbell (Eds.), *HIV/AIDS management in southern Africa: Priorities for the mining industry* (pp. 107–110). Johannesburg: Epidemiology Research Unit)

78. Morris, M., Podhisita, C. & Wawer, M. J., (1996). Handcock MS. Bridge populations in the spread of HIV/AIDS in Thailand. *AIDS, 10*(11), 1265–1272

79. Foster, G., Makufa, C., Drew, R., Kambeu, S. & Saurombe, K. (1996). Supporting children in need through a community-based orphan visiting programme. *AIDS Care, 8*(4), 389–403

80. Meekers, D. (1999). *Patterns of use of the female condom in urban Zimbabwe*. (Washington, DC: Population Services International)

81. Meekers, D. (2001). The role of social marketing in STD/HIV protection in 4600 sexual contacts in urban Zimbabwe. *AIDS, 15*(2), 285–286

82. Parirenyatwa, D. (2002). *Social Aspects of HIV/AIDS in sub-Saharan Africa 2002*. (Pretoria: Zimbabwe National AIDS Trust Fund).

83. Guay, L. A., Musoke, P., Fleming, T., et al. (1999). Intrapartum and neonatal single-dose nevirapine compared with zidovudine for prevention of mother-to-child transmission of HIV-1 in Kampala, Uganda: HIVNET 012 randomised trial. *The Lancet, 354*, 795–802

84. Zimbabwe Ministry of Health and Child Welfare (2002). *Strategic framework for introducing Nevirapine based prevention of mother-to-child transmission of HIV in Zimbabwe*. (Harare: Zimbabwe Ministry of Health and Child Welfare)

CHAPTER 11. THE IMPACT OF HIV INFECTION ON TUBERCULOSIS IN AFRICA

JUDITH R. GLYNN
Department of Epidemiology and Population Health,
London School of Hygiene and Tropical Medicine, London, UK

Abstract. Tuberculosis (TB) notification rates in Africa have doubled since the early 1980s, with the largest rises in countries most affected by the HIV epidemic. HIV increases the risk of TB in those latently infected with *M tuberculosis* and increases the risk of active disease soon after new infection or re-infection with *M tuberculosis*. Overall, the risk of TB in those with HIV infection is about four to ten times that in those without HIV infection. The risk starts to rise soon after infection with HIV, and continues to increase with progressive immunosuppression. At a population level, the relative risk for the association of HIV and TB increases as the HIV epidemic progresses, and will continue to increase for some time after a fall in HIV incidence due to the long latent period of HIV. The proportion of TB currently directly attributable to HIV in Africa has been estimated at 31%, but the true impact of HIV on TB will be even greater because of onward transmission from the extra TB cases. Antiretroviral treatment for advanced HIV-disease can decrease the risk of TB, but would have to be used early and extensively to have a large effect at the population level.

Introduction

There are about 1.8 million deaths from TB each year worldwide, about half a million in Africa [1]. Tuberculosis is increasing in many countries. In Africa notified case rates have doubled since the mid 1980s, just after the start of the HIV epidemic. There is considerable variation in the completeness of reporting systems, as well as in the effectiveness of case detection, but in general those countries with the largest HIV epidemics show the largest increase in TB [1]. **Fig. 1** shows the trends for selected countries with different HIV epidemics. In Botswana, Zimbabwe and Zambia, where the HIV prevalence in antenatal clinic attenders is over 30%, and in Kenya, Malawi and Tanzania where HIV prevalence is 15–20%, TB case rates have risen two to seven-fold. In Benin, Senegal and Cameroon, with an HIV prevalence of less than 10%, little increase is recorded.

M tuberculosis infections can occur at any age. Disease may occur soon after infection or later in life. Disease some years after the initial infection may be due

M. Caraël and J.R. Glynn (eds.), HIV, Resurgent Infections and Population Change in Africa, 215–228.

TB notification rates

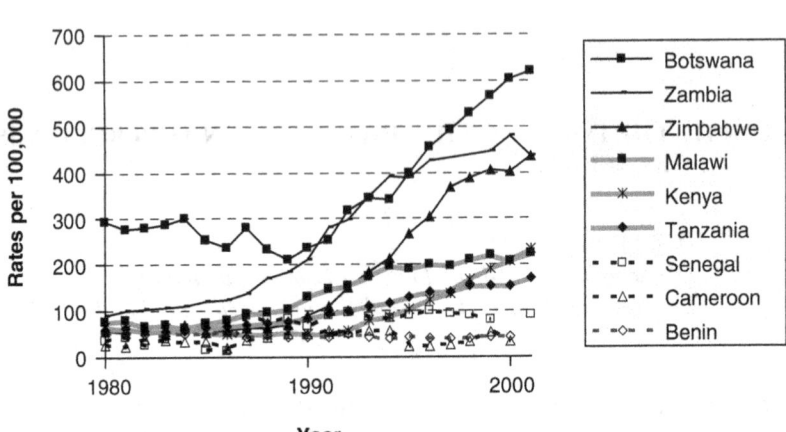

Fig. 1. TB notification rates in African countries with HIV epidemics of different levels. Botswana, Zimbabwe and Zambia: HIV prevalence in adults > 30%. Kenya, Malawi and Tanzania: HIV prevalence in adults = 15–20%. Benin, Burkina Faso and Cameroon: HIV prevalence in adults < 10%

to reactivation of the initial infection, or to exogenous re-infection. HIV infection increases the reactivation of latent tuberculosis in those infected some time in the past, and also increases the likelihood of progressing to active tuberculous disease soon after infection or re-infection. Whether it also increases the risk of infection or re-infection with *M tuberculosis* is unknown. Mortality rates in HIV infected TB patients are high and some studies have found high recurrence rates, perhaps due to higher rates of disease due to re-infection. In this chapter I review the evidence for the interaction of HIV and TB in Africa.

The Influence of HIV Infection on TB Incidence

The incidence of TB in individuals infected with HIV has been measured directly in several studies. Although TB incidence in the population depends on infection rates with *M tuberculosis*, incidence in those already infected with *M tuberculosis* (as measured by the tuberculin test) can be compared in different studies. Studies that have recorded incidence of TB in dually infected individuals are summarised in **Table 1**. Since there are few studies in Africa, studies in other places are also shown [2–18]. Some variation is expected, depending on: the exclusion criteria used in the studies; the rates of re-infection with *M tuberculosis*; the extent to which the tuberculin test accurately reflects *M tuberculosis* infection (which varies from setting to setting) [19]; and the stage of the HIV epidemic. Despite this, studies show a remarkably consistent TB incidence rate of 5–10% per year in HIV infected individuals in most settings, which contrasts with an estimated lifetime risk of developing TB following infection of about 10% in the absence of HIV [20].

Table 1. Incidence of tuberculosis (TB) in HIV-positive individuals with tuberculin reactions of at least 5 mm who had not received isoniazid.

Ref	Place	Year	Patient group	Exclusion criteria	Follow-up (years)	Risk n/N	Rate/100 pyar (95 % CI)
[2]	Port-au-Prince, Haiti	86–92	Symptom-free, newly diagnosed	Previous TB, abnormal chest X-ray, abnormal LFTs	2.4	6/25	10.0 (3.6–21.4)
[3]	New York, USA	85–88	IVDUs in methadone maintenance programme	? none	1.8	7/36	10.8 (4.3–22.2)
[4]	New York, USA	88–90	IVDUs in methadone maintenance programme	Documented previous TB	1.7	4/25	9.7 (2.6–24.7)
[5]	Hartford, USA	84–92	IVDUs seen as in or outpatients	? none	3.8	2/18	2.9 (0.4–10.6)
[6]	6 cities, USA	88–94	Mixed. 23% IVDUs. No or < 6 months isoniazid	TB in last 12 months, acute pulmonary disease, AIDS	?3.8	?/34	4.5 (1.6–9.7)
[7, 8]	Madrid, Spain	85–94	Referred patients, 90% IVDUs	Previous or active TB	2.8	24/84	10.4 (6.7–15.5)
[9]	Madrid, Barcelona, Spain	89–92	Newly diagnosed, refused or discontinued isoniazid	Previous or active TB	4.9 / 1.7	43/92 / 7/26	9.4 (6.8–12.7) / 16.2 (6.5–33.5)
[10, 11]	Italy	90–93	In and outpatients, 73% IVDUs	TB in last 18 months	1.4	15/197	5.4 (3.0–9.0)
[12]	Nairobi, Kenya	89–92	Commercial sex workers	Previous TB	2.4	11/69	6.7 (3.3–11.9)
[13]	Nairobi, Kenya	92–94	Commercial sex workers and clinic attenders	Previous TB, possible current TB, abnormal LFTs, pregnant, life-threatening intercurrent illness	1.8	10/69	8.0 (3.9–14.8)

(continued)

Table 1. (continued)

Ref	Place	Year	Patient group	Exclusion criteria	Follow-up (years)	Risk n/N	Rate/100 pyar (95 % CI)
[14, 15]	Kampala, Uganda	92–95	Clinic attenders	Previous TB, active TB, white cell count < 3000/mm³, Hb < 80 g/L, abnormal LFTs, pregnancy, advanced HIV disease, major underlying illness	1.3 2.2	21/464 42/464	3.4 (2.1–5.2) 4.2 (3.0–5.6)
[16]	Lusaka, Zambia	92–96	Clinic attenders, referrals from blood bank and voluntary testing centres	Previous TB, possible current TB, abnormal LFTs, pregnancy, life threatening illness	1.6	9/60	9.2 (4.2–17.4)
[17]	Rio de Janeiro, Brazil	91–98	Clinic attenders (some receiving antiretroviral therapy)	Previous TB, AIDS, combination antiretroviral therapy	3.6	35/169	4.8 (3.5–6.6)
[18]	Chennai, India	89–98	STD clinic attenders	? none	2.6	14/88	7.1 (3.4–10.8)

IVDU = intravenous drug user, LFT = liver function test, Hb = haemoglobin, CI = confidence interval, n/N = number with TB/total number, pyar = person years at risk

The 5–10% annual risk is likely to be an underestimate. Some included individuals will not actually be infected with *M tuberculosis* since the tuberculin test can be "positive" for other reasons [19]. Furthermore, HIV infected individuals with advanced disease become anergic, so the tuberculin test becomes negative. These anergic individuals are not included in the studies, but they probably have the highest risk of TB if infected [7]. A fuller picture of the influence of HIV on TB can be obtained by studying cohorts of HIV infected and non-infected individuals.

The Association Between HIV Infection and TB

Many studies have examined the relative risk of TB in those with and without HIV infection. Cohort studies that have been conducted in Africa are summarised in **Table 2** [12, 21–30]. All studies have shown an increase in risk in those with HIV infection compared to those without, but the relative risk has varied from less than four to more than 20. Some of the variation in the relative risk may be due to study design. The relative risk may be underestimated if some of the HIV negative cohort become infected during follow-up, or if sick people are excluded; or overestimated if HIV positive individuals are identified because they are already ill.

Case control studies have given similar results. Case control studies are often difficult to interpret because of the problems in choosing controls [31]. TB cases are usually identified in hospital, but hospital controls would be likely to have a much higher HIV prevalence than the general population. Blood donors are sometimes used as controls, but they are unlikely to be representative of the population HIV prevalence, especially if they are pre-screened or paid. Population based controls are preferred, though this assumes that the population has good access to hospital services. Population based case-control studies in Africa have found age, sex and area adjusted odds ratios for the association of HIV infection and TB between four and 12 [32–36].

Most studies are consistent with a relative risk for the association of HIV and TB of about seven, but the true relative risk will vary. The relative risk should increase as the HIV epidemic progresses, as a higher proportion of HIV infected individuals become immunosuppressed. In an established and stable HIV epidemic this proportion will become constant. If the HIV incidence starts to go down, the proportion of HIV infected individuals who are immunosuppressed will rise even further. The predicted rise in the relative risk over time has been seen in Karonga District, Malawi. Population based case-control studies in the late 1980s and early 1990s found relative risks of 7.4 (95% CI 4.4–12.4) for all TB, and 6.3 (3.6–11.0) for smear positive TB [35]. By the late 1990s the relative risks in the same population had risen to 12.0 (9.0–16.1) for all TB and 9.9 (7.3–13.4) for smear positive TB [36]. Studies on the South African goldmines also found an increase in the relative risk, from 2.8 (1.5–5.0) in 1991–1994, and 5.9 (4.2–8.2) in 1995–1997, to 14.8 (8.7–25.2) in 1998–1999, though the earlier risks may have been underestimated by the inclusion of (unknown) seroconverters during the long follow-up period in that study [26, 27].

Table 2. Cohort studies in Africa comparing TB incidence in HIV positive and negative individuals.

Ref	Place	Study population	Year enrolled	Follow-up (months)	HIV+ Risk (%)	HIV+ Rate/100 pyar (95% CI)	HIV− Risk (%)	HIV− Rate/100 pyar (95% CI)	Rate ratio	Comments
[21]	Rwanda	Antenatal women	1988	48	17/215 (7.9%)	2.9 (1.8–4.6)	1/216 (0.5%)	0.16 (0.02–1.1)	18.2 (2.4–137.0)	Excluded seroconverters
[22]	Rwanda	Antenatal women	1988	24	20/460 (4.3%)	2.4 (1.6–3.7)	2/998 (0.2%)	0.1 (0.03–0.40)	21.8 (5.1–92.9)	35 HIV+, 3 HIV− subjects, lost to follow-up excluded
[23]	Zaire	Antenatal women	1986	36	19/249 (7.6%)	3.1 (2.0–4.9)	1/310 (0.3%)	0.12 (0.02–0.85)	25.8 (5–125)	
[24]	DR Congo	Employees and wives	1987	36	16/330 (4.8%)	2.4 (1.4–3.9)	81/11278 (0.72%)	0.38 (0.30–0.48)	6.3 (3.4–10.8)	Calculated from data in the paper
[12]	Kenya	Female sex workers	1989	36	49/587 (8.3%)	3.5 (2.6–4.6)	0/132 (0%)	0		
[25]	Malawi	Community	1987	120	7/182 (3.9%)		62/11059 (0.56%)		7.4 (OR) (3.3–16.6)	Retrospective cohort study. Pyar not available. Adjusted OR 6.3 (2.7–14.5)

Ref	Country	Population	Year	pyar						Notes
[26]	South Africa	Miners	1991	60	135/1374 (9.8%)	4.9 (4.1–5.7)	78/2648 (2.9%)	1.1 (0.8–1.3)	4.5 (3.4–6.1)	
[27]	South Africa	Miners	1998	12	128/1792 (7.1%)	8.5 (7.2–10.1)	15/2970 (0.5%)	0.58 (0.32–0.95)	14.8 (8.7–25.2)	
[28]	South Africa	Miners	1991	72	451/6108 (7.4%)	2.7 (2.4–2.9)	289/20503 (1.4%)	0.80 (0.71–0.90)	3.6 (3.1–4.2)	Pulmonary only. 45% were new seroconverters
[29]	Uganda	Community	1990	120	24/275 (8.7%)	2.1 (1.4–3.2)	1/246 (0.41)	0.075 (0.002–0.42)	28.6 (3.9–212)	Pulmonary only. 61% were new seroconverters
[30]	Ethiopia	Factory workers	1997	53	10/95 (10.5%)	4.5 (2.2–8.1)	14/709 (2.0%)	0.68 (0.37–1.1)	6.6 (2.6–16.0)	

pyar = person years at risk

Changes in the relative risk for the association of HIV and TB following a decrease in HIV incidence have not been reported in Africa but have been seen dramatically in Thailand. In Chiang Rai the HIV incidence rose rapidly and then fell sharply. This is shown in surveys in 21 year-old male military conscripts: the HIV prevalence peaked at 17% in 1992, but dropped to 7% by 1994 and 3% by 1997. The relative risk for the association with TB estimated in later years, comparing hospital TB cases to controls from the same time period, rose very high. This reflected the earlier high HIV prevalence in the population, resulting in a high proportion of HIV infected individuals being immunosuppressed [37].

These examples illustrate how the risk can change over time at a population level. At an individual level it is known that TB tends to occur earlier than the other HIV-related opportunistic infections, and the risk of TB has been correlated with CD4 count [38, 39]. Although the risk increases with duration of HIV infection, it was found in a study on the South African goldmines that the risk of TB doubled even in the first year after seroconversion [40].

Since the risk of TB increases with duration of HIV infection, and since most young people have recently acquired HIV infection, the relative risk for the association of HIV infection and TB should be lower in younger individuals. This is however not found, and instead several studies have found slightly higher relative risks for the association of TB and HIV in younger adults than in older adults [32, 36, 37, 41–44]. A possible explanation is that HIV infection has a greater impact on first or recent *M tuberculosis* infections than on latent infections. Young people are more often meeting *M tuberculosis* for the first time, and in many populations are probably also at greater risk of re-infection due to increased population mixing at younger ages.

A further indication that HIV may have different influences on latent and recent infection comes from studies of recurrent TB. Recurrence of active TB following treatment and apparent cure is more common in HIV infected individuals [45]. Recurrence can arise either from reactivation of the same infection or following a new (re-)infection. These scenarios can be differentiated by examining the DNA finger-prints of the "strains" of *M tuberculosis* from the two episodes: identical (or closely related) fingerprints suggesting a relapse, and unrelated fingerprints suggesting a new infection. Studies have confirmed that both mechanisms occur but the proportion of recurrent disease due to new infections varies considerably [46]. Among HIV infected individuals re-infection may be much more important than in HIV negative individuals. Re-infection accounted for 13/21 recurrences in HIV positive individuals compared to 1/18 recurrences in HIV negative individuals in South Africa [47].

The Impact of HIV on TB in the Population

The traditional method of estimating the impact of HIV on TB at the population level is to calculate the population attributable fraction (PAF). **Fig. 2** shows the PAF that would be seen for relative risks between four and ten as the HIV prevalence increases. For example, with a relative risk of seven, the proportion of TB attributable to HIV reaches 50% when the HIV prevalence is 17%. As we have already

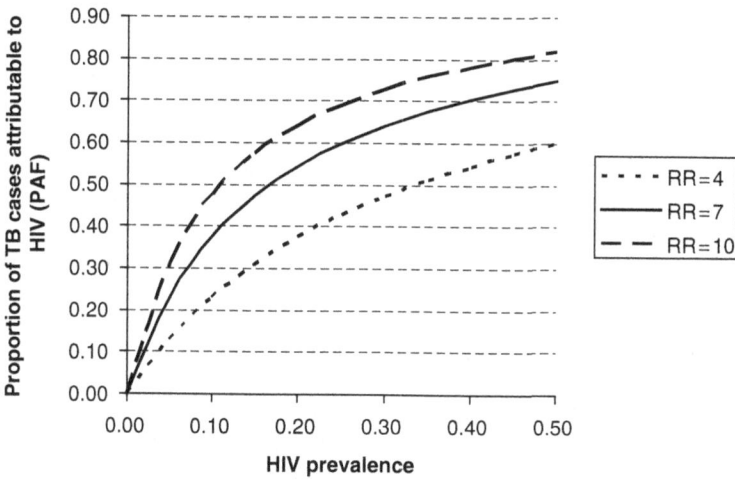

Fig. 2. Proportion of TB directly attributable to HIV for different rate ratios (RR) for the association of HIV and TB, by HIV prevalence

seen, this is an oversimplification since the relative risk varies with stage of the HIV epidemic and perhaps also depending on the population group and the background incidence of *M tuberculosis* infection.

These estimates underestimate the true impact of HIV, because they ignore the fact that TB is infectious. The PAF measures the direct impact of HIV infection on the first generation of TB cases. These extra cases will add to the transmission of *M tuberculosis* in the population and generate more cases [48]. The extent of this indirect impact is difficult both to estimate and to measure.

The annual risk of *M tuberculosis* infection (ARI) is monitored using tuberculin tests in children. This method has several problems [19], but allows broad trends to be assessed. Using this technique it was found that the ARI was decreasing in many countries before the arrival of HIV. There is evidence from Kenya that this trend has been reversed in areas where the HIV prevalence is particularly high [49]. However in Tanzania the ARI has continued to fall, perhaps due to strengthening of the control programme over the same period [50].

Further evidence of the indirect impact comes from monitoring trends in TB incidence in HIV negative individuals. In South Africa a doubling in TB incidence in HIV negative gold miners was found in one study, suggesting considerable ongoing transmission of *M tuberculosis* [28]. However another study, also in gold miners, found no such increase [51].

Although some indirect effect is likely, the actual extent is debated. HIV infected individuals with TB are more likely to have (non-infectious) extra-pulmonary disease than are HIV negative TB patients, and among those with pulmonary disease, a higher proportion are sputum smear negative (and therefore less infectious)

[52]. In several household studies HIV positive patients have been shown to give rise to fewer infections in their contacts, even after adjusting for sputum smear status and HIV status of the contacts [53–55], but other studies have shown no such difference [56–58]. HIV infected TB patients may be infectious for a shorter time than HIV uninfected patients: untreated patients with TB die more quickly if they are co-infected with HIV, and HIV positive TB patients may become sick enough to seek health care more quickly than those who are HIV negative, and thus get treated sooner for TB [1]. If the average duration of infectiousness is appreciably reduced the indirect effect on onward transmission will be less important than it might have been otherwise.

The indirect impact of HIV on TB may be increased by the clustering of HIV and TB in the same groups of the population, both socio-economic and occupational groups, and families. Outbreaks of TB with attack rates of over 30% in AIDS care facilities highlight the issue [59], but published data may overestimate the problem since small outbreaks with low attack rates are not reported. Spouses of TB patients are likely to be a high risk group. With an HIV prevalence in smear positive TB cases of over 60%, as found in southern and eastern Africa [36], about 40% of the spouses are likely to be HIV infected as well, so are at high risk of developing active TB.

The HIV epidemic also has an impact on TB through its effects on the TB programme, by overloading the health services and reducing the number of trained health care workers. Some countries have responded by a shift from hospital-based to home-based care [60].

Because HIV-infected TB cases have a lower survival rate than HIV-uninfected cases, the effect of HIV on mortality from TB is even larger than the effect on TB incidence. It has been estimated that 12% of TB deaths worldwide, and 39% of TB deaths in Africa are attributable to HIV [1].

The Future

Reversing the upward trend in TB rates requires continued efforts in both HIV and TB control. Reducing transmission of HIV, and finding and treating TB patients are both crucial. Isoniazid and other prophylactic regimens in HIV infected individuals have reduced TB incidence in the short [14, 16, 61] and medium term [15, 62], but outside intervention trials, uptake has been poor and there are concerns that improperly implemented prophylaxis may increase drug resistance [63, 64].

Antiretroviral drugs have been shown to reduce TB incidence in HIV infected individuals [38]. As usage increases they may become an important contributor to TB control, but it has been estimated that unless therapy started early and was widespread with good compliance the population-level impact on TB will be limited [65]. On the other hand TB patients provide a useful entry point for HIV testing, counselling and treatment, and TB control programmes may offer a model for antiretroviral use: collaboration in the control of HIV and TB is imperative [66, 67].

References

1. Corbett, E. L., Watt, C. J., Walker, N., Maher, D., Williams, B. G., Raviglione, M. C. & Dye, C. (2003). The growing burden of tuberculosis: global trends and interactions with the HIV epidemic. *Archives of Internal Medicine, 163,* 1009–1021

2. Pape, J., Jean, S. S., Ho, J. L., Hafner, A. & Johnson, W. D. (1999). Effect of isoniazid prophylaxis on incidence of active tuberculosis and progression of HIV infection. *The Lancet, 342,* 268–272

3. Selwyn, P. A., Hartel, D., Lewis, V. A., Schoenbaum, E. E., Vermund, S. H., Klein, R. S., et al. (1989). A prospective study of the risk of tuberculosis among intravenous drug users with human immunodeficiency virus infection. *New England Journal of Medicine, 320,* 545–550

4. Selwyn, P. A., Sckell, B., Alcabes, P., Friedland, G. H., Klein, R. S. & Schoenbaum, E. E. (1992). High risk of active tuberculosis in HIV-infected drug users with cutaneous anergy. *JAMA, 268,* 504–509

5. Rubinstien, E. M., Madden, G. M. & Lyons, R. W. (1996). Active tuberculosis in HIV-infected injecting drug users from a low-rate tuberculosis area. *Journal of Acquired Immune Deficiency Syndromes Human Retrovirology, 11,* 448–454

6. Markowitz, N., Hansen, N. I., Hopewell, P. C., Glassroth, J., Kvale, P. A., Mangura, B. T, et al. (1997). Incidence of tuberculosis in the United States among HIV-infected persons. *Annals of Internal Medicine, 126,* 123–132

7. Moreno, S., Baraia-Etxaburu, J., Bouza, E., Parras, F., Perez-Tascon, M., Miralles, P., et al. (1993). Risk for developing tuberculosis among anergic patients infected with HIV. *Annals of Internal Medicine, 119,* 194–198

8. Moreno, S., Miralles, P., Diaz, M. D., Baraia, J., Padilla, B., Berenguer, J. & Alberdi, J. C. Isoniazid preventive therapy in human immunodeficiency virus-infected persons. Long term effect on development of tuberculosis and survival. *Archives of Internal Medicine, 157,* 1729–1734

9. Guelar, A., Gatell, J. M., Verdejo, J., Podzamczer, D., Lozano, L., Aznar, E., et al. (1993). A prospective study of the risk of tuberculosis among HIV-infected patients. *AIDS, 7,* 1345–1349

10. Antonucci, G., Girardi, E., Raviglione, M. C. & Ippolito, G. (1995). Risk factors for tuberculosis in HIV-infected persons. A prospective cohort study. The Gruppo Italiano di Studio Tubercolosi e AIDS (GISTA). *JAMA, 274,* 143–148

11. Girardi, E., Antonucci, G., Ippolito, G., Raviglione, M. C., Rapiti, E., Di Perri, G. & Babudieri, S. (1997). Association of tuberculosis risk with the degree of tuberculin reaction in HIV-infected patients. The Gruppo Italiano di Studio Tubercolosi e AIDS. *Archives of Internal Medicine, 157,* 797–800

12. Gilks, C. F., Godfrey-Faussett, P., Batchelor, B. I. F., Ojoo, J. C., Ojoo, S. J., Brindle, R. J., et al. (1997). Recent transmission of tuberculosis in a cohort of HIV-1-infected female sex workers in Nairobi, Kenya. *AIDS, 11,* 911–918

13. Hawken, M. P., Meme, H. K., Elliott, L. C., Chakaya, J. M., Morris, J. S., Githui, W. A., et al. (1997). Isoniazid preventive therapy for tuberculosis in HIV-1-infected adults: results of a randomized controlled trial. *AIDS, 11,* 875–882

14. Whalen, C. C, Johnson, J. L., Okwera, A., Hom, D. L., Huebner, R. & Mugyenyi, P., et al. (1997). A trial of three regimens to prevent tuberculosis in Ugandan adults infected with the human immunodeficiency virus. *New England Journal of Medicine, 337,* 801–808

15. Johnson, J. L., Okwera, A., Hom, D. L., Mayanja, H., Mutuluuza Kityo, C., Nsubuga, P., et al. (2001). Duration of efficacy of treatment of latent tuberculosis infection in HIV-infected adults. *AIDS, 15,* 2137–2147

16. Mwinga, A., Hosp, M., Godfrey-Faussett, P., Quigley, M., Mwaba, P., Mugala, B. N., et al. (1998). Twice weekly tuberculosis preventive therapy in HIV infection in Zambia. *AIDS, 12,* 2447–2457

17. de Pinho, A. M., Santoro-Lopes, G., Harrison, L. H. & Schechter, M. (2001). Chemoprophylaxis for tuberculosis and survival of HIV-infected patients in Brazil. *AIDS*, *15*, 2129–2135

18. Swaminathan, S., Ramachandran, R., Baskaran, G., Paramasivan, C. N., Ramanathan, U., Venkatesan, P., et al. (2000). Risk of development of tuberculosis in HIV-infected patients. *International Journal of Tuberculosis and Lung Disease*, *4*, 839–844

19. Rieder, H. L. (1995). Methodological issues in the estimation of the tuberculosis problem from tuberculin surveys. *Tubercle and Lung Disease*, *76*, 114–121

20. Vynnycky, E. & Fine, P. E. M. (1997). The natural history of tuberculosis: the implications of age-dependent risks of disease and the role of reinfection. *Epidemiology Infection*, *119*, 183–201

21. Leroy, V., Msellati, P., Lepage, P., Batungwanayo, J., Hitimana, D. G., Taelman, H., et al. (1995). Four years of natural history of HIV-1 infection in african women: a prospective cohort study in Kigali (Rwanda), 1988–1993. *Journal of Acquired Immune Deficiency Syndromes, Human Retrovirology*, *9*, 415–421

22. Allen, S., Batungwanayo, J., Kerlikowske, K., Lifson, A. R., Wolf, W., Granich, R., et al. (1992).Two-year incidence of tuberculosis in cohorts of HIV-infected and uninfected urban Rwandan women. *American Review of Respiratory Diseases*, *146*, 1439–1444

23. Braun, M. M., Badi, N., Ryder, R. W., Baende, E., Mukadi, Y., Nsuami, M., et al. (1991). A retrospective cohort study of the risk of TB among women of childbearing age with HIV infection in Zaire. *American Review of Respiratory Diseases*, *143*, 501–504

24. Ryder, R. W., Batter, V., Kaseka, N., Behets, F., Sequeira, D., M'Boly, E., et al. (2000). Effect of HIV-1 infection on tuberculosis and fertility in a large workforce in Kinshasa, Democratic Republic of the Congo. *AIDS Patient Care and STDs*, *14*, 297–304

25. Glynn, J. R., Warndorff, D. K., Malema, S. S., Mwinuka, V., Ponnighaus, J. M., Crampin, A. C. & Fine, P. E. (2000). Tuberculosis: associations with HIV and socioeconomic status in rural Malawi. *Transactions of the Royal Society of Tropical Medicine and Hygiene*, *94*, 500–503

26. Corbett, E. L., Churchyard, G. J., Clayton, T. C., Williams, B. G., Mulder, D., Hayes, R. J. & De Cock, K. M. (2000). HIV infection and silicosis: the impact of two potent risk factors on the incidence of mycobacterial disease in South African miners. *AIDS*, *14*, 2759–2768

27. Corbett, E. L., Churchyard, G. J., Charalambos, S., Samb, B., Moloi, V., Clayton, T. C., et al. (2002). Morbidity and mortality in South African gold miners: impact of untreated disease due to human immunodeficiency virus. *Clinical Infectious Diseases*, *34*, 1251–1258

28. Sonnenberg, P., Glynn, J. R., Fielding, K., Murray, J., Godfrey Fausett, P. & Shearer, S. (2004). HIV and pulmonary tuberculosis: the impact goes beyond those infected with HIV. *AIDS*, *18*, 657–662

29. Morgan, D., Mahe, C., Mayanja, B. & Whitworth, J. A. (2002). Progression to symptomatic disease in people infected with HIV-1 in rural Uganda: Prospective cohort study. *BMJ*, *324*, 193–196

30. Wolday, D., Hailu, B., Girma, M., Hailu, E., Sanders, E. & Fontanet, A. L. (2003). Low CD4+ T-cell count and high HIV viral load precede the development of tuberculosis disease in a cohort of HIV-positive Ethiopians. *International Journal of Tuberculosis and Lung Disease*, *7*, 110–116

31. Glynn, J. R. (1998). Resurgence of tuberculosis and the impact of HIV infection. *British Medical Bulletin*, *54*, 579–593

32. Van den Broek, J., Borgdorff, M. W., Pakker, N. G., Chum, H. J., Klokke, A. H., Senkoro, K. P. & Newell, J. N. (1993). HIV-1 infection as a risk factor for the development of tuberculosis: A case-control study in Tanzania. *International Journal of Epidemiology*, *22*, 1159–1165

33. Orege, P. A., Fine, P. E. M., Lucas, S. B., Obura, M., Okelo, C., Okuku, P. & Were, M. (1993).A case control study on human immunodeficiency virus-1 (HIV-1) infection as a risk factor for tuberculosis and leprosy in Western Kenya. *Tubercle and Lung Disease*, *74*, 377–381

34. Ponnighaus, J. M., Mwanjasi, L. J., Fine, P. E. M., Shaw, M. A., Turner, A. C., Oxborrow, S. M., et al. (1991). Is HIV infection a risk factor for leprosy? *International Journal of Leprology*, *59*, 221–228

35. Glynn, J. R., Warndorff, D. K., Fine, P. E. M., Msiska, G. K., Munthali, M. M. & Ponnighaus, J. M. (1997). The impact of HIV on morbidity and mortality from tuberculosis in sub-Saharan Africa: A study in rural Malawi and review of the literature. *Health Transition Review*, *7*(Suppl 2), 75–87

36. Crampin, A. C., Glynn, J. R., Floyd, S., Malema, S. S., Mwinuka, V. M., Ngwira, B., et al. (2004). Tuberculosis and gender: Exploring the patterns in a case control study in Malawi. *International Journal of Tuberculosis and Lung Disease*, *8*, 194–203

37. Siriarayapon, P., Yanai, H., Glynn, J. R., Yanpaisarn, S. & Uthaivoravit, W. (2002). The evolving epidemiology of HIV infection and tuberculosis in northern Thailand. *Journal of Acquired Immune Deficiency Syndromes*, *31*, 80–89

38. Badri, M., Wilson, D. & Wood, R. (2002). Effect of highly active antiretroviral therapy on incidence of tuberculosis in South Africa: A cohort study. *The Lancet*, *359*, 2059–2064

39. van der Sande, M. A., Schim van der Loeff, M. F., Bennett, R. C., Dowling, M., Aveika, A. A., Togun, T. O., et al. (2004). Incidence of tuberculosis and survival after its diagnosis in patients infected with HIV-1 and HIV-2. *AIDS*, *18*, 1933–1941

40. Sonnenberg, P., Glynn, J. R., Fielding, K., Murray, J., Godfrey Fausett, P. & Shearer, S. (2002). *How soon after HIV infection does the risk of tuberculosis start to increase?* A retrospective cohort study in South African gold miners. J Infect D.; 2005: 191: 150–158

41. Van Cleef, M. R. A. & Chum, H. J. (1995). The proportion of tuberculosis cases in Tanzania attributable to human immunodeficiency virus. *International Journal of Epidemiology*, *24*, 637–642

42. Chum, H. J., O'Brien, R. J., Chonde, T. M., Graf, P. & Rieder, H. L. (1996). An epidemiological study of tuberculosis and HIV infection in Tanzania, 1991–1993. *AIDS*, *10*, 299–309

43. Long, R., Scalcini, M., Manfreda, J., Carre, G., Philippe, E., Hershfield, E., et al. (1991). Impact of HIV type I on tuberculosis in rural Haiti. *American Review of Respiratory Disease*, *143*, 69–73

44. Houston, S., Ray, S., Mahari, M., Neill, P., Legg, W., Latif, A. S., et al. (1994). The association of tuberculosis and HIV infection in Harare, Zimbabwe. *Tubercle and Lung Disease*, *75*, 220–226

45. Korenromp, E. L., Scano, F., Williams, B. G., Dye, C. & Nunn, P. (2003). Effects of human immunodeficiency virus infection on recurrence of tuberculosis after rifampin-based treatment: an analytical review. *Clinical Infectious Diseases*, *37*, 101–112

46. Lambert, M. L., Hasker, E., Van Deun, A., Roberfroid, D., Boelaert, M. & Van der Stuyft, P. (2003). Recurrence in tuberculosis: relapse or reinfection? *The Lancet Infectious Diseases*, *3*, 282–287

47. Sonnenberg, P., Murray, J., Glynn, J. R., Shearer, S., Kambashi, B. & Godfrey-Faussett, P. (2001). HIV-1 and recurrence, relapse, and reinfection of tuberculosis after cure: A cohort study in South African mineworkers. *The Lancet*, *358*, 1687–1693

48. Lienhardt, C. & Rodrigues, L. C. (1997). The estimation of the impact of HIV infection on tuberculosis: tuberculosis risks re-visited? *International Journal of Tuberculosis and Lung Disease*, *1*, 196–204

49. Odhiambo, J. A., Borgdorff, M. W., Kiambih, F. M., Kibuga, D. K., Kwamanga, D. O., Ng'ang'a L., et al. (1999). Tuberculosis and the HIV epidemic: increasing annual risk of tuberculous infection in Kenya, 1986–1996. *American Journal of Public Health*, *89*, 1078–1082

50. Tanzanian- Tuberculin-Survey-Collaboration (2001). Tuberculosis control in the era of the HIV epidemic: risk of tuberculosis infection in Tanzania, 1983–1998. *International Journal of Tuberculosis and Lung Disease*, *5*, 103–112

51. Corbett, E. L., Charalambos, S., Fielding, K., Clayton, T., Hayes, R. J., De Cock, K. M. & Churchyard, G. J. (2003). Stable incidence rates of tuberculosis (TB) among Human Immunodeficiency

Virus (HIV)-negative South African gold miners during a decade of epidemic HIV-associated TB. *Journal of Infectious Diseases, 188*, 1156–1163

52. Elliott, A. M., Halwiindi, B., Hayes, R. J., Luo, N., Tembo, G., Machiels, L., et al. (1993). The impact of human immunodeficiency virus on presentation and diagnosis of tuberculosis in a cohort study in Zambia. *Journal of Tropical Medicine and Hygiene, 96*, 1–11

53. Cauthen, G. M., Dooley, S. W., Onorato, I. M., Ihle, W. W., Burr, J. M., Bigler, W. J., et al. (1996). Transmission of *Mycobacterium tuberculosis* from tuberculosis patients with HIV infection or AIDS. *American Journal of Epidemiology, 144*, 69–77

54. Elliott, A. M., Hayes, R. J., Halwiindi, B., Luo, N., Tembo, G., Pobee, J. O. M., et al. (1993). The impact of HIV on infectiousness of pulmonary tuberculosis: A community study in Zambia. *AIDS, 7*, 981–987

55. Espinal, M. A., Perez, E. N., Baez, J., Henriquez, L., Fernandez, K., Lopez, M., et al. (2000). Infectiousness of *Mycobacterium tuberculosis* in HIV-1-infected patients with tuberculosis: a prospective study. *The Lancet, 355*, 275–280

56. Nunn, P., Mungai, M., Nyamwaya, J., Gicheha, C., Brindle, R. J., Dunn, D. T., et al. (1994). The effect of human immunodeficiency virus type-1 on the infectiousness of tuberculosis. *Tubercle and Lung Disease, 75*, 25–32

57. Klausner, J. D., Ryder, R. W., Baende, E., Lelo, U., Williame, J. C., Ngamboli, K., et al. (1993). *Mycobacterium tuberculosis* in household contacts of human immunodeficiency virus type 1-seropositive patients with active pulmonary tuberculosis in Kinshasa, Zaire. *Journal of Infectious Diseases, 168*, 106–111

58. Cruciani, M., Malena, M., Bosco, O., Gatti, G. & Serpelloni, G. (2001). The impact of human immunodeficiency virus type 1 on infectiousness of tuberculosis: a meta-analysis. *Clinical Infectious Diseases, 33*, 1922–1930

59. Girardi, E., Raviglione, M. C., Antonucci, G., Godfrey-Faussett, P. & Ippolito, G. (2000). Impact of the HIV epidemic on the spread of other diseases: the case of tuberculosis. *AIDS, 14*(Suppl 3), S47–S56

60. Salaniponi, F. M., Gausi, F., Mphasa, N., Nyirenda, T. E., Kwanjana, J. H. & Harries, A. D. (2003). Decentralisation of treatment for patients with tuberculosis in Malawi: Moving from research to policy and practice. *International Journal of Tuberculosis and Lung Disease, 7*, S38–S47

61. Bucher, H. C., Griffith, L. E., Guyatt, G. H., Sudre, P., Naef, M., Sendi, P. & Battegay, M. (1999). Isoniazid prophylaxis for tuberculosis in HIV infection: a meta-analysis of randomized controlled trials. *AIDS, 13*, 501–507

62. Quigley, M. A., Mwinga, A., Hosp, M., Lisse, I., Fuchs, D., Porter, J. D. H. & Godfrey-Faussett, P. (2001). Long-term effect of preventive therapy for tuberculosis in a cohort of HIV-infected Zambian adults. *AIDS, 15*, 215–222

63. Lugada, E. S., Watera, C., Nakiyingi, J., Elliott, A., Brink, A., Nanyunja, M., et al. (2006). Operational assessment of isoniazid prophylaxis in a community AIDS service organisation in Uganda. *International Journal of Tuberculosis and Lung Disease, 6*, 326–331

64. Bakari, M., Moshi, A., Aris, E. A., Chale, S., Josiah, R., Magao, P., et al. (2000). Isoniazid prophylaxis for tuberculosis prevention among HIV infected police officers in Dar es Salaam. *East African Medical Journal, 77*, 494–497

65. Williams, B. G. & Dye, C. (2003) Antiretroviral drugs for tuberculosis control in the era of HIV/AIDS. *Science, 301*, 1535–1537

66. Harries, A. D., Hargreaves, N. J., Chimzizi, R. & Salaniponi, F. M. (2002). Highly active antiretroviral therapy and tuberculosis control in Africa: synergies and potential. *Bulletin of the World Health Organization, 80*, 464–469

67. Harries, A. D., Nyangulu, D. S., Hargreaves, N. J., Kaluwa, O. & Salaniponi, F. M. (2001). Preventing antiretroviral anarchy in sub-Saharan Africa. *The Lancet, 358*, 410–414

CHAPTER 12. IMPACT OF HIV ON MORTALITY IN SOUTHERN AFRICA: EVIDENCE FROM DEMOGRAPHIC SURVEILLANCE

IAN M. TIMÆUS

Centre for Population Studies, London School of Hygiene and Tropical Medicine, London, UK

Abstract. This analysis examines recent increases in adult mortality resulting from HIV/AIDS in several Southern Africa populations. It assesses whether the populations share a common age pattern of mortality increase and compares their experience with an existing model age pattern of AIDS mortality in Africa. The data come from civil registration of deaths in South Africa and Zimbabwe, from two localised demographic surveillance systems based in South Africa, and from parish registers maintained by the Evangelical Lutheran Church in north-western Namibia. Principal components analysis is used to represent the variation in age-specific mortality across the schedules in terms of a few variables. Two components account for most of the variation. The first of these appears to represent background mortality and the second AIDS mortality. The age pattern of AIDS mortality is similar in all these Southern African populations. Mortality has risen between ages 25 and 65 for adult men, with the greatest rises occurring at ages 35–44 years. For women, mortality increase generally extends from about 20 to 60 years, peaking among women in their thirties. In Namibia, however, slightly older women are affected. The typical age pattern of mortality increase in Southern Africa is rather like that in the INDEPTH Pattern 5 model life tables, which are derived largely from data on Tanzania. The similarities between the left-hand sides of the resulting "humps" in the mortality schedules is particularly close. However, AIDS mortality among middle-aged men and women may be higher in Southern Africa than in the INDEPTH models. Although the age pattern of AIDS mortality differs across Africa, these differences may be small enough to permit development of a simple one-parameter model of the resulting bulge in age-specific mortality schedules that is adequate for modelling and projections.

Introduction

Sub-Saharan Africa is almost entirely without reliable routinely-collected vital statistics. The lack of such data has helped to foster the enduring scepticism of some scientists, policy-makers and commentators as to the severity of the HIV/AIDS epidemic in the continent. The most radical of these sceptics deny that AIDS is a new disease

M. Caraël and J.R. Glynn (eds.), HIV, Resurgent Infections and Population Change in Africa, 229–243.

caused by HIV. Others accept that HIV causes AIDS but believe that the severity of the epidemic has been overestimated, sometimes accusing scientists and activists working on AIDS of exaggerating the scale of the HIV epidemic to further their own careers [1]. Some of these sceptics question whether mortality has risen greatly in Africa in recent years; others believe that mortality increase is due mainly to worsening poverty or the spread of drug-resistant strains of existing infectious diseases.

In the West, it was mortality statistics that provided the first reliable quantitative data on the spread of HIV. Considerable ingenuity has gone into developing methods for back-projecting HIV infections from AIDS deaths [2, 3]. In Africa, in the absence of functioning vital statistics systems, it has been necessary to work in the opposite direction [4]. Estimates of the severity of the HIV/AIDS epidemic are based on epidemiological surveillance data and, in particular, data obtained by anonymous testing of blood samples taken from women attending antenatal clinics. Unfortunately, in most African countries these antenatal clinic surveillance data are not statistically representative of all pregnant women or even of those pregnant women who attend public-sector antenatal clinics [5]. In addition, moving from an estimate of HIV prevalence among pregnant women to one of HIV prevalence among all women and among men, and then from these estimates to estimates of the incidence of HIV infection, AIDS mortality and AIDS orphans, involves a long series of assumptions about the epidemiology and natural history of HIV. While both the sophistication of the modelling process and knowledge of the key epidemiological parameters involved in it have improved in recent years, estimates obtained in this way inevitably remain approximate [6]. Thus, they remain open to attack by sceptical critics claiming that the numbers are either baseless or systematically and grossly exaggerated.

Previous Research

The only countries in mainland sub-Saharan Africa in which the civil registration system has so far yielded useful mortality statistics at the national level are Zimbabwe and South Africa [7, 8]. Even in these countries, registration of deaths is incomplete and the data require adjustment. In addition, the civil register of deaths can be used to measure AIDS mortality in a few cities [9]. In the absence of routine vital statistics for most of Africa, attempts have been made to estimate mortality trends since the onset of the HIV/AIDS epidemic using data collected in national censuses and Demographic and Health Surveys [10, 11, 12]. Such data have their own limitations [13, 14]. In particular, they are subject to biases arising from errors in the retrospective reporting of events and provide no information on causes of death.

One further source of statistics on mortality in sub-Saharan Africa exists: demographic surveillance of the entire population of geographically defined local areas. Such demographic surveillance systems (DSS) now exist in many African countries. Many, but not all, of them collaborate in the INDEPTH network [15]. While some African DSS are long established [16], many were set up during the last decade or so. A number of these sites have a specific remit to study the HIV/AIDS epidemic and several of them have introduced population-based HIV surveillance. Most use verbal autopsies to collect information on causes of death.

An early review of the data on AIDS mortality being collected by DSS in Africa clearly documented their value [17]. It found that adult mortality had risen two- to three-fold in populations with only moderate HIV epidemics (<10 per cent). Thus, AIDS accounted for about half of all adult deaths in such populations. By combining DSS data on mortality with information on individual's serostatus, Nunn et al. [18] showed that mortality in the Masaka District of Uganda was eleven times higher in HIV positive adults than in HIV negative adults. Furthermore, a comparison of the DSS-based mortality estimates for the study area with retrospective estimates demonstrated that mortality among HIV negative adults remained similar to that in the population as a whole before HIV became prevalent [19]. Thus, the increase in adult mortality in the study area could be accounted for fully by the spread of HIV infection.

More recent studies based on DSS data have tended to confirm the conclusions of the initial reports. For example, a study in a rural area in north-western Tanzania with seven per cent HIV prevalence among adults aged 15–44, found that mortality was 15 times higher among HIV positive adults than in the HIV negative and that AIDS accounted for nearly half the deaths at ages 15–44 [20]. Moreover, in Rakai District of Uganda, with a prevalence of HIV infection of 16 per cent at ages 15–59, AIDS accounts for 73.5 per cent of adult deaths and the risk of dying among HIV positive adults is 20 times that of the uninfected [21]. Synthesizing the results of these studies and those from other DSS sites in Eastern Africa that have collected data on serostatus, Todd et al. [22] estimate that the relative risk of dying among HIV positive, compared with HIV negative, adults is approximately 15 in African populations with moderate background mortality. Recent research has also confirmed the suggestion [17] that the survival times of adults following infection with HIV in Africa differ is only slightly lower than in Western populations prior to the introduction of antiretroviral therapy. Data from the natural history cohort linked to the Masaka District DSS suggest that the median time from seroconversion to death among adults is about 10 years [23].

In a comparative study of the mortality data collected by 19 INDEPTH sites, Sam Clark identifies clusters of mortality schedules with similar age patterns of mortality and develops model life tables that embody the distinctive characteristics of each of these patterns [15]. The analysis identifies seven such patterns in the set of 140 mortality schedules. (As most sites provided data for several time periods, there are 70 mortality schedules for each sex). One of these patterns is based largely on data from Bangladesh, however, and in two more it is only the mortality schedules for women that are distinctive. One of the four remaining patterns (Pattern 5) is shaped largely by data from three large Tanzanian sites that form part of the Adult Mortality and Morbidity Project (AMMP)—Hai, Morogoro and, for men, Dar es Salaam. From these data, Clark isolates a distinctive pattern of mortality increase due to AIDS. Finally, by adding this "AIDS hump" in the age pattern of mortality to the Pattern 1 models, which are based on the largest cluster of empirical schedules, he produces models of all-cause mortality for use in African populations in which AIDS deaths are exerting a marked downward pressure on life expectancy.

These models of the impact of AIDS are potentially of great value for forecasting future mortality and projecting the population in Africa. Empirically-based evidence as to the age-specific impact on mortality of AIDS could also help to calibrate the parameters of epidemiological models of the HIV epidemic. Thereby, it could contribute to improving understanding of age patterns of HIV incidence and survival times. In particular, mortality data may provide a far firmer basis than exists at present for assessing the severity of the epidemic among men as well as women. However, one important limitation of the INDEPTH models of the impact of AIDS is that they are based very largely on data from Tanzania. The age-specific impact on mortality of the HIV/AIDS epidemic is a function of the ages at which people become infected and of their subsequent survival times. As these characteristics of the HIV epidemic are likely to vary across Africa, variation in age patterns of mortality increase is also to be expected. Indeed, the INDEPTH data also yield a second cluster of mortality schedules that, while affected less than those in Pattern 5, include significant AIDS mortality (Pattern 3, based on data from the Agincourt study in South Africa, Bandim in Guinea-Bissau and, for women, Dar es Salaam). Thus, such variation certainly occurs. It unclear either whether the pattern of AIDS mortality revealed by the AMMP data is typical of Africa or by how much age patterns of mortality increase in other parts of the African region might differ from those in Tanzania.

Scope of the Analysis

This analysis examines the increase in adult mortality associated with the spread of HIV/AIDS in Southern Africa. It has two specific objectives. The first is to examine the extent to which recent age patterns of mortality increase in several Southern African populations share common features. In particular, it examines the extent to which patterns identified in the civil registration data for South Africa and Zimbabwe are confirmed by the results of active demographic surveillance. The second objective of the paper is to compare the impact of AIDS on mortality by age in Southern Africa with the model pattern derived from the AMMP data for Tanzania.

Death registration statistics for three years are analysed for South Africa—1990, 1996 and mid-1999 to mid-2000. For Zimbabwe, registration statistics for 1986, 1992 and 1995 are used. These years are selected from among those for which data are available to span the period of rising mortality due to HIV/AIDS. Registration of deaths is incomplete in both countries and the mortality rates have been adjusted upward to correct for this [8, 24]. As AIDS is seldom reported as a cause of death, AIDS mortality in both countries is inferred from the rise in mortality over time by making the assumption that mortality from other causes remained unchanged over the decade of interest. It seems likely that other causes of death that might have increased among adults at this time, for example drug-resistant malaria or the non-communicable diseases, would have affected older people as well as young and middle-aged adults. Thus, partial empirical support for the assumption that AIDS is the sole quantitatively important condition involved in these rises in mortality is provided by the lack of trend in mortality in old age in the adjusted statistics. Indeed, in South Africa it is more likely that the rise in HIV/AIDS mortality among young men has been offset by falling mortality from violence since the first multi-racial elections in 1994 [25, 26, 27]. However, this trend is unlikely to effect estimates of AIDS mortality greatly as the drop in injury deaths is concentrated among men aged 15 to 29 and AIDS mainly kills men aged 30 or more [26].

Data obtained through demographic surveillance of two sites in South Africa are included in the analysis. The first study is the Wellcome Africa Centre for Health and Population Studies Demographic Information System (ACDIS) that covers part of Umkhanyakude district in northern KwaZulu-Natal [28]. This study uses verbal autopsies to identify causes of death. Using these diagnoses, one can calculate mortality rates for both all-cause and non-AIDS adult mortality [29]. At present, cause-specific data are available only for the first year of the study—2000. The second study is the Agincourt Health and Demographic Surveillance System in the Bushbuckridge Municipality on the borders of Limpopo and Mpumalanga provinces [30]. The mortality schedule used here is for 1995–1999 [15]. The published data on the Agincourt study are not detailed enough to allow one to distinguish AIDS and non-AIDS mortality by age and sex from either cause-specific data or the evidence of mortality trends.

The final set of mortality data analysed here is based on neither civil registration nor demographic surveillance but on the church registers maintained by the Evangelical Lutheran Church in Namibia (ELCIN) in several parishes in the North-Western part of the country [31]. About 80 per cent of the population of this part of Namibia belong to ELCIN. The congregations of the parishes studied do not represent a representative random sample of the population. Nevertheless, although the parishes are situated in diverse locations, mortality differentials between them are small. Thus, it seems unlikely that the mortality of the study population differs markedly from that of the general population of this part of Namibia. The dataset analysed here covers the years 1980–2000. Information on causes of death is not available. However, the mortality rates for the period up to 1993 show no evidence of being affected by AIDS deaths. Moreover, adult mortality was stagnating prior to the onset of the HIV epidemic [32]. Thus, once again, the rise in adult mortality between 1980–1993 and 1994–2000 can be assumed to be due to AIDS.

Results

Fig. 1 presents age-specific death rates from AIDS in Umkhanyakude and the three populations in which death rates from AIDS can be estimated from the rise in all-cause mortality. Clearly, Umkhanyakude district in 2000 had the most severe epidemic, followed by Zimbabwe in 1995. In all the populations, AIDS mortality occurs at slightly older ages for adult men than for adult women. The absolute rises in mortality are somewhat larger for men than women. However, as the increase occurs at older ages for men than for women, this does not necessarily translate into a greater number of AIDS deaths among men than among women.

The shape of the age pattern of mortality increase for women is very similar in all four populations. However the distribution is shifted four to five years upwards in North-Western Namibia, and perhaps slightly downwards in the national data for South Africa, compared with the other populations. For men, both the shape and the location

a) Men

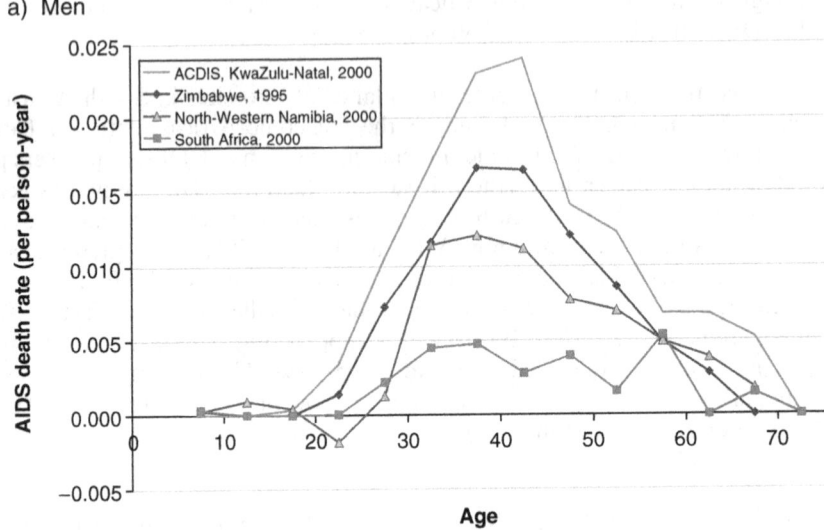

b) Women

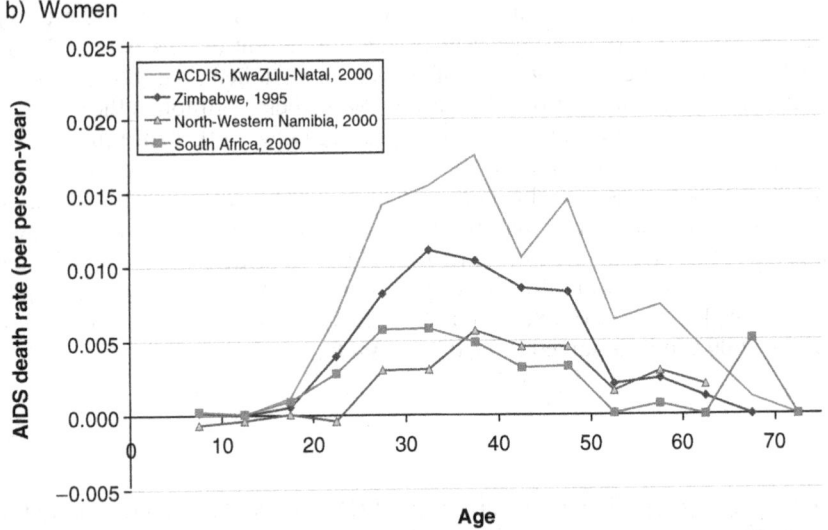

Fig. 1. Estimated age-specific AIDS death rates in four Southern African populations in which HIV has become prevalent
Sources: **ACDIS, KwaZulu-Natal [29]; Zimbabwe [8]; North-Western Namibia [32]; South Africa [24]**

on the age scale of all four distributions are very similar except that the distribution for men in Namibia is shifted a year or two towards older ages compared with the other populations.

Human mortality schedules vary by age in broadly the same way in all populations and their particularities are influenced by the severity of mortality and structure of causes of death. As with Clark's analysis of the INDEPTH data [15], one can use principal components analysis to attempt to represent the variation in age-specific mortality across these 11 populations in terms of a smaller number of variables. The technique aims to produce a parsimonious description of the age-specific mortality rates in terms of a limited number of orthogonal variables. The first of these components is calculated from the covariance matrix so as to account for as much of the variance in the rates as possible, the second component accounts for as much of the remaining variation as possible, and so on. Using the full set of 11 components, one could reproduce the observations exactly.

In this application, the mortality schedules for three of the four populations include both ones that are substantially affected by AIDS deaths and ones that are little affected (the exception being the Agincourt study). Thus, it should be possible to distinguish the component of variation in mortality by age that is associated with AIDS from the pattern of variation in background mortality by age that is common to all the life tables. Separate analyses are undertaken for men and women. The analyses are conducted on the logit probabilities of dying in each five-year age group ($_5q_x$) of women from 5–9 to 60–64 and of men from 5–9 to 65–69:

$$0.5 \cdot \text{logit}\left(_5q_x \right) = \frac{_5q_x}{1 - {_5q_x}}$$

The set of 11 observations on age group is weighted by the sum, across the populations, of the proportions of deaths in each population occurring in that age group.

The results of this analysis are shown in **Table 1**. Just two principal components for men and three components for women account for 98 per cent of the variation in the 11 mortality schedules for each sex. Examination of the component scores for the different age groups reveals that the first component, which accounts for most of the variation in the data, represents the common pattern in mortality by age shared by all 11 mortality schedules (**Fig. 2a**). As one would expect, men's mortality rises more steeply with age than that of women. The second component accounts for variation between the schedules in the relative severity of adult mortality compared with mortality in adolescence and old age. For both sexes the plot of the component scores against age is n-shaped (**Fig. 2b**). Thus, populations with a positive coefficient (usually termed loading) on this second component have relatively high mortality in the central adult ages. The component for men is shifted toward older ages than the component for women and is also somewhat broader. For both sexes, the third principal component (not shown) appears largely to capture distinctive features of the mortality schedules for North-Western Namibia. For women, it has most effect on the mortality of those in their twenties and aged above age 55 (both of which are

Table 1. Loading coefficients of 11 Southern African mortality schedules on the principal components that explain 98 per cent of the variance in the logit probability of dying by five-year age group.

Population and year	Women (5–64 years)			Men (5–69 years)	
	1	2	3	1	2
Zimbabwe, 1985	0.3272	−0.2042	−0.2478	0.3511	−0.4002
Zimbabwe, 1992	0.2954	0.1876	0.0397	0.3194	0.0762
Zimbabwe, 1995	0.2957	0.4327	0.3315	0.3113	0.4369
South Africa, 1990	0.3773	−0.2484	−0.2972	0.2978	−0.2366
South Africa, 1996	0.3430	0.0215	−0.2363	0.2968	−0.2302
South Africa, 1999–2000	0.3011	0.2988	0.0026	0.2948	−0.0023
ACDIS, KwaZulu-Natal, 2000, AIDS free	0.3313	−0.2237	−0.2583	0.3246	−0.2434
ACDIS, KwaZulu-Natal, 2000, all-cause	0.3044	0.4268	0.2427	0.3010	0.3359
North-Western Namibia, 1980–1993	0.1393	−0.0278	0.0332	0.2275	−0.0900
North-Western Namibia, 1994–2000	0.2478	−0.5855	0.7444	0.2463	0.5892
Agincourt, Limpopo, 1995–1999	0.2904	−0.0928	−0.0471	0.3253	−0.0833
Percentage of variance explained	87.2	6.1	4.3	93.4	4.6

relatively low in Namibia). For men, this component is less important and largely affects the relative severity of mortality in the age group 20–24 years.

Returning to **Table 1**, the loading coefficients of the different populations on the first component of mortality vary little across the 11 populations for either men or women. In contrast, the loadings on the second mortality component for both men and women are related largely to the importance of AIDS mortality in the all-cause mortality schedule. The component loadings rise sharply over time in the mortality schedules of both sexes in Zimbabwe and South Africa and in the men's schedules in North-Western Namibia. The loadings are also much higher in the all-cause mortality schedules based on ACDIS data than in the AIDS-free mortality schedules for this population. For women, the third mortality component also rises with time in the three populations with repeated observations and is higher in the all-cause ACDIS data. This suggests that it is picking up secondary features of the variation between the schedules in the importance of AIDS mortality. The decline over time in the loading on the second component in North-Western Namibia is matched by a particularly large rise in the loading on the third component. Finally, the mortality of the population of the Agincourt site in the second half of the 1990s appears to have been intermediate in most respects to the national schedules for South Africa for 1996 and 1999–2000.

a) First component

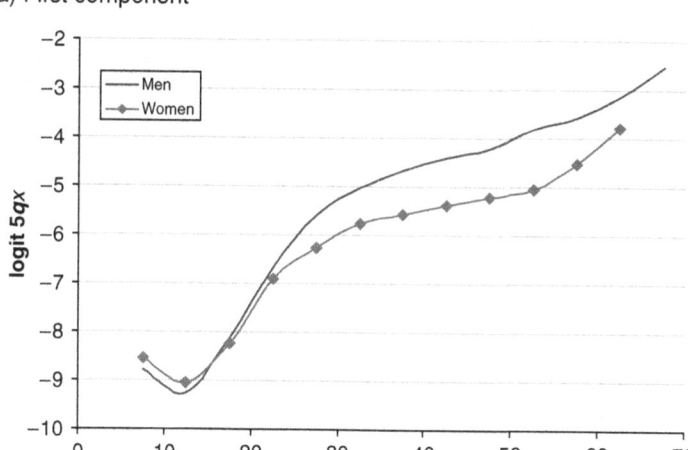

b) Second component

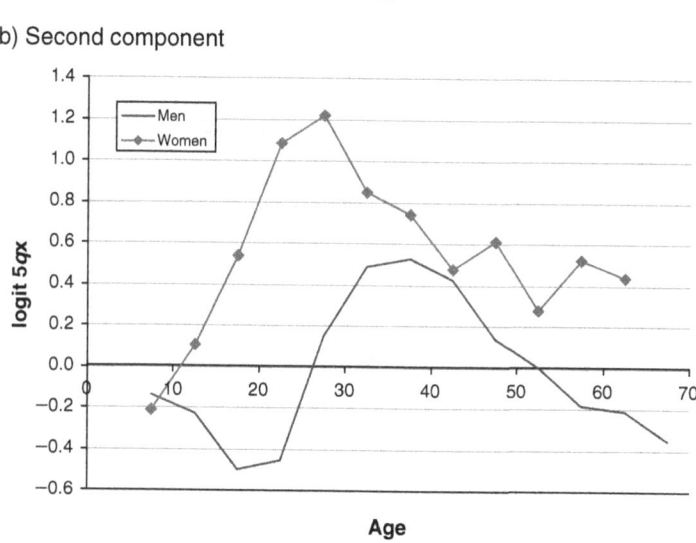

Fig. 2. a,b Logit probability of dying by five-year age group and sex in the first two principal components of 11 Southern African mortality schedules

Inspection of **Table 1** allows one to identify typical component loadings for, firstly, the mortality schedules that precede the onset of significant AIDS mortality in these populations and, secondly, the most recent data from them. The loadings on the first component average about 0.3. Treating North-Western Namibia as somewhat of an outlier, the loadings on the second component range from about −0.4 to 0.5 for men and from about −0.415 to 0.425 for women. For women the loadings on the third component rise from about −0.3 to 0.25.

Using the loadings just listed for the most important components, one can produce model age patterns of mortality in Southern Africa, as represented by these data, for both before the onset of the AIDS epidemic and according to the most recent data available (**Fig. 3**). These mortality schedules in no sense estimate the level of adult mortality in Southern Africa at any date. Nevertheless, it is indicative of the importance of the rise in adult mortality associated with AIDS that the probability of dying between ages 15 and 60 ($_{45}q_{15}$) rises from 26 per cent for women and 38 per

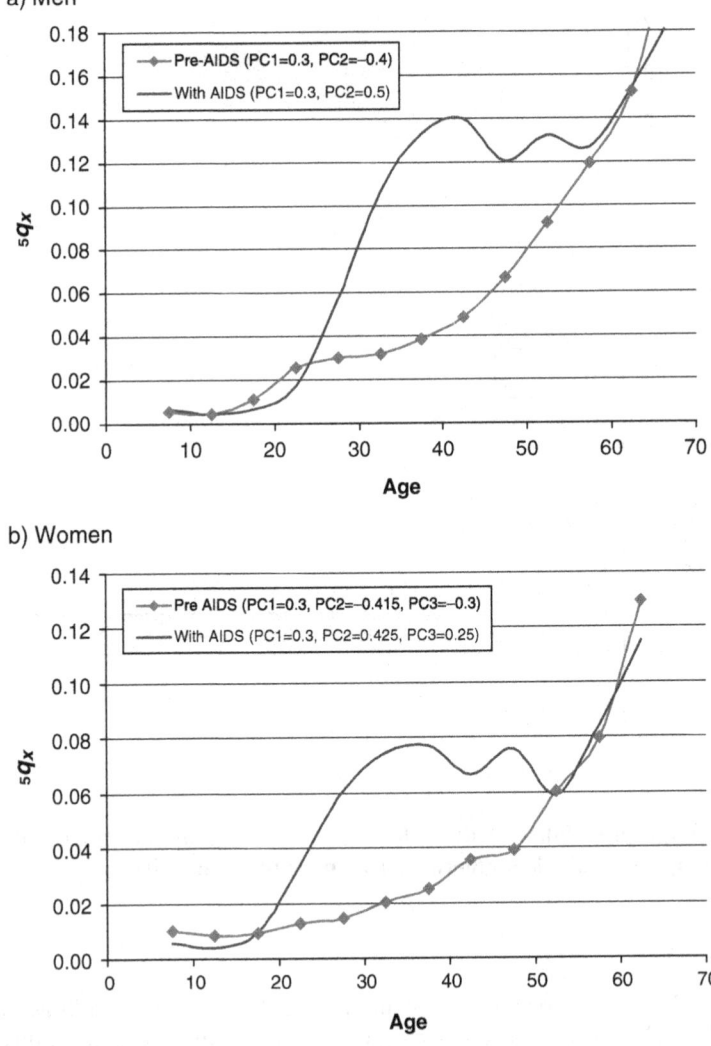

Fig. 3. Typical probabilities of dying by age ($_5q_x$) pre-AIDS and with AIDS mortality, principal component (PC) models fitted to 11 Southern African populations

cent for men in the pre-AIDS schedules to 43 per cent and 59 per cent respectively in the schedules that include AIDS mortality. With regard to their shape, a distinct injuries "hump" exists in the pre-AIDS mortality schedule for men at ages 20–29. As in the original data, the range of ages over which mortality has risen in the schedules that include AIDS and the modal age of that increase is about five years older for men than for women. The distribution for men also appears to be somewhat skewed towards older ages. Some of the erratic fluctuations in mortality between adjacent age groups in the upper part of the age range considered persist in the second component of mortality.

Fig. 4 superimposes the age pattern of mortality without and with AIDS in appropriate INDEPTH model mortality schedules on to the age patterns of mortality in these Southern African models. Non-AIDS mortality in Southern Africa rises much more sharply with age for both men and women than in the INDEPTH Pattern 1 models. This feature of Southern African life tables predates the HIV/AIDS epidemic and may be accounted for by low communicable disease mortality among young adults and relatively high non-communicable disease mortality compared with the poorer tropical countries to the north [33]. Setting aside these differences in background mortality, the location, spread and shape of the age patterns of mortality increase associated with AIDS in the two models is clearly rather similar for both men and women. However, it appears that there has been somewhat more increase in mortality in middle age in Southern Africa than in the AMMP data from Tanzania.

Discussion

The first conclusion to be drawn from this analysis is that age patterns of AIDS mortality are rather similar in the different Southern African populations considered. The patterns of mortality increase in Zimbabwe between the mid-1980s and mid-1990s and in South Africa during the 1990s closely resemble each other. In neither case are the elderly affected. No major discrepancies exist between the age patterns of AIDS mortality by sex estimated directly from the verbal autopsies conducted as part of ACDIS and those inferred from the rise in mortality revealed by the national statistics for South Africa. The AIDS epidemic in northern KwaZulu-Natal in 2000 was clearly more severe than that in the country as a whole and AIDS deaths may be somewhat more common at ages 55–69 than is suggested by the rise in mortality nationally. Overall though, it is the similarity of the age patterns of mortality increase in the two sets of data that is most striking for both men and women.

The rise in mortality due to HIV/AIDS occurs between ages 25 and 65 for adult men, with the greatest rises occurring at ages 35–44 years. The age pattern of mortality increase for adult women is offset downwards by about five years from that of men: it extends from about age 20 to about age 60, with a peak among women in their thirties. The increase in women's mortality occurs at somewhat older ages in North-Western Namibia than in Zimbabwe or South Africa. This is consistent with the median age at first sexual intercourse of women in North-Western Namibia reported in the 2000 Demographic and Health Survey which, at nearly 21 years, is markedly higher than elsewhere in the region [34]. However, the increase in men's mortality

a) Men

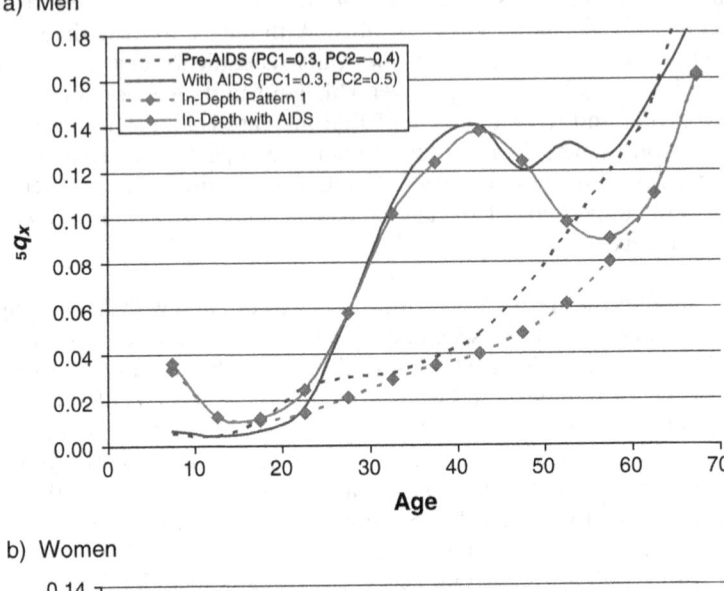

b) Women

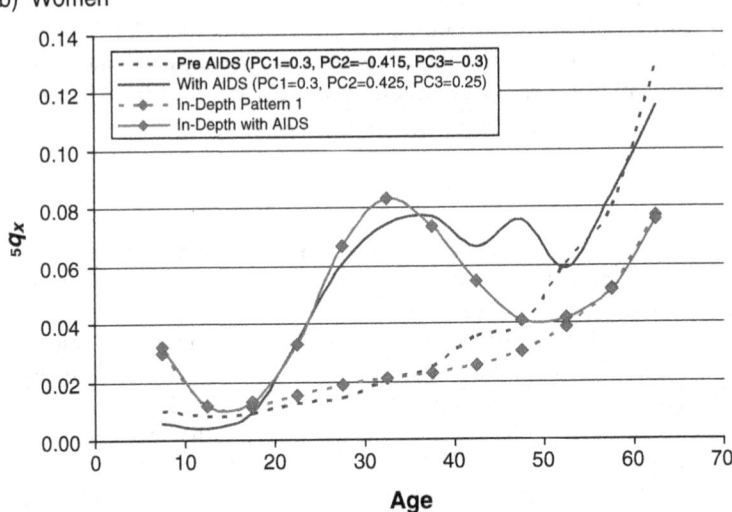

Fig. 4. Comparison of the Southern African principal component (PC) and INDEPTH models of the probability of dying by age ($_5q_x$) in populations with and without AIDS mortality

Source: author's analysis and INDEPTH models [15]

revealed by the Namibian data occurs at only slightly later ages than in the other populations.

The principal components analysis suggests that the AIDS component of adult mortality in Southern Africa has an age pattern that is rather like that in the INDEPTH Pattern 5 model life tables based on AMMP data from Tanzania. The similarities between the left-hand sides of the "humps" in the mortality schedules produced by AIDS is particularly close. However, the death rates from AIDS among women aged 40 or more and men aged 50 or more may be higher in Southern Africa than in Tanzania. This might reflect differences in patterns of sexual activity between these two regions of Africa. For example, it would be consistent with higher levels of extramarital sexual intercourse in Southern Africa. Alternatively, it might just reflect the relatively recent onset of the HIV/AIDS epidemic in Southern Africa (together with the time since the data were collected in Zimbabwe). For example, infection of older adults with HIV may be a feature of the early years of the epidemic. As the epidemic matures, HIV infections may become concentrated among new cohorts of young people commencing sexual activity, with those prone to high-risk behaviour being selected out of the population at risk too quickly to give rise to many infections at older ages.

In summary, although their coverage is very limited, the preliminary impression to be gained from this analysis is that age patterns of mortality increase due to AIDS are similar across Southern and Eastern Africa. The differences in the importance of AIDS as a cause of death in middle age between the Southern African and Tanzanian populations emphasize that some variation in the age pattern of mortality from AIDS is to be expected. Nevertheless, it may be possible to develop a simple one-parameter model of the bulge in age-specific mortality schedules produced by AIDS which, while not entirely applicable throughout Africa, is adequate for modelling and projection purposes. This should be based on a broader set of empirical data than those generated by the AMMP site in Tanzania. Nevertheless, it seems unlikely that the final models would differ greatly from those published in the INDEPTH volume or presented here.

References

1. Malan, R. (2003). Africa isn't dying of AIDS. *The Spectator*. 13 December, 2003

2. Downs, A., Heisterkamp, S., Brunet, J. & Hamers, F. (1997). Reconstruction and prediction of the HIV/AIDS epidemic among adults in the European Union and in the low prevalence countries of central and eastern Europe. *AIDS*, *11*(5), 649–662

3. Karon, J., Rosenberg, P., McQuillan, G., Khare, M., Gwinn, M. & Petersen, L. (1996). Prevalence of HIV infection in the United States, 1984 to 1992. *Journal of the American Medical Association*, *276*(2), 126–131

4. UNAIDS (2004). *Report on the global HIV/AIDS epidemic: 4th global report.* (Geneva: Joint United Nations Programme on HIV/AIDS)

5. Grassly, N. C., Morgan, M., Walker, N., Garnett, G., Stanecki, K. A., Stover, J., Brown, T. & Ghys, P. D. (2004). Uncertainty in estimates of HIV/AIDS: the estimation and application of plausibility bounds. *Sexually Transmitted Infections*, *80*(Suppl 1), i31–i38

6. Walker, N., Grassly, N. C., Garnett, G. P., Stanecki, K. A. & Ghys, P. D. Estimating the global burden of HIV/AIDS: what do we really know about the HIV pandemic? *The Lancet, 363*(9427), 2180–2185

7. Dorrington, R., Bourne, D., Bradshaw, D., Laubscher, R. & Timæus, I. M. (2001). *The impact of HIV/ AIDS on adult mortality in South Africa.* (Tygerberg: South African Medical Research Council)

8. Feeney, G. (2001). The impact of HIV/AIDS on adult mortality in Zimbabwe. *Population and Development Review, 27*(4), 771–780

9. Garenne, M., Madison, M., Tarantola, D., Zanou, B., Aka, J. & Dogore, R. (1996). Mortality impact of AIDS in Abidjan, 1986–1992. *AIDS, 10*(11), 1279–1286

10. Timæus, I. M. (1998). Impact of the HIV epidemic on mortality in sub-Saharan Africa: evidence from national surveys and censuses. *AIDS, 12*(Suppl 1), S15–S27

11. Timæus, I. M. (1999). Adult mortality in Africa in the era of AIDS. In *The African population in the 21st century: Third African population conference, Durban South Africa, December 6–10, 1999.* Volume 2 (pp. 377–395). (Dakar, Senegal: Union for African Population Studies and South Africa, Department of Welfare)

12. Timæus, I. M. & Jasseh, M. (2004). Adult mortality in Sub-Saharan Africa: evidence from Demographic and Health Surveys. *Demography, 41*(4), 757–772

13. United Nations (2002). *Methods for estimating adult mortality.* ESA/P/WP.175. (New York: Department of Economic and Social Affairs)

14. Timæus, I. M. (1991). Measurement of adult mortality in less developed countries: A comparative review. *Population Index, 57*(4), 552–568

15. INDEPTH Network (2002). *Population and health in developing countries. Volume 1: Population, health and survival at INDEPTH sites.* (Ottawa: International Development Research Centre)

16. Feachem, R. G. & Jamison, D. T. (Eds.) (1991). *Disease and mortality in sub-Saharan Africa.* (Oxford: Oxford University Press)

17. Boerma, J., Nunn, A. & Whitworth, J.(1998). Mortality impact of the AIDS epidemic: evidence from community studies in less developed countries. *AIDS, 12*(Suppl 1), S3–S14

18. Nunn, A. J., Mulder, D. W., Kamali, A., Ruberantwari, A., Kengeya-Kayondo, J. F. & Whitworth, J. (1997). Mortality associated with HIV-1 infection over five years in a rural Uganda population: Cohort study. *British Medical Journal*, (7111), 767–771

19. Timæus, I. M. & Nunn, A. J. (1997). Measurement of adult mortality in populations affected by AIDS: an assessment of the orphanhood method. *Health Transition Review, 7*(Suppl 2), 23–43

20. Urassa, M., Boerma, J., Isingo, R., Ngalula, J. & Ng'weshemi, J. (2001). The impact of HIV/AIDS on mortality and household mobility in rural Tanzania. *AIDS, 15*(15), 2017–2023

21. Sewankambo, N., Gray, R., Ahmad, S., Serwadda, D. & Wabwire-Mangen, F. (2000). Mortality associated with HIV infection in rural Rakai district, Uganda. *AIDS, 14*(15), 2391–2400

22. Todd, J., Glynn, J. & Zaba, B. (2003). *Age patterns and trends in HIV +ve and HIV –ve mortality rate ratios.* (Paper presented at the scientific meeting on The Empirical Evidence for the Demographic and Socio-Economic Impact of AIDS, Durban, South Africa, March 26–28)

23. Morgan, D., Mahe, C., Mayanja, B., Okongo, J. & Lubega, R. (2002). HIV-1 infection in rural Africa: Is there a difference in median time to AIDS and survival compared with that in industrialized countries? *AIDS, 16*(4), 597–603

24. Timæus, I. M., Dorrington, R., Bradshaw, D., Nannan, N. & Bourne, D. (2001). *Adult Mortality in South Africa, 1980-2000: From Apartheid to AIDS.* (Paper presented at the Population Association of America Annual Meeting, Washington, DC, March 29–31)

25. Schönteich, M. (2001). Crime trends: A turning point? *SA Crime Quarterly*, *1*, 1–6

26. Statistics South Africa (2002). *Causes of death in South Africa, 1997–2001: Advance release of recorded causes of death*. P0309.2. (Pretoria: Statistics South Africa)

27. Bah, S. (2004). Unnoticed decline in the number of unnatural deaths in South Africa. *South African Medical Journal*, *94*(6), 442–443

28. Solarsh, G., Benzler, J., Hosegood, V., Tanser, F., Vanneste, A., Hlabisa, D. S. S., (2002). South Africa. (In INDEPTH Network (Ed.), *Population and health in developing countries. Population, health and survival at INDEPTH sites* (pp. 213–220). Ottawa: International Development Research Centre)

29. Hosegood, V., Vanneste, A.-M. & Timæus, I. M. (2004). Levels and causes of adult mortality in rural South Africa: the impact of AIDS. *AIDS*, *18*(4), 663–671

30. Tollman, S. M., Herbst, K., Garenne, M., Gear, J. & Kahn, K. (1999). The Agincourt demographic and health study: Site description, baseline findings and implications. *South African Medical Journal*, *89*(8), 858–864

31. Notkola, V., Timæus, I. M. & Siiskonen, H. (2004). Impact on mortality of the AIDS epidemic in Northern Namibia assessed using parish registers. *AIDS*, *18*(7), 1061–1065

32. Notkola, V., Timæus, I. M. & Siiskonen, H. (2000). Mortality transition in the Ovamboland region of Namibia, 1930–1990. *Population Studies*, *54*(2), 153–167

33. Timæus, I. M. (1993). Adult mortality. In K. A. Foote, K. H. Hill & L. G. Martin (Eds.),*Demographic change in sub-Saharan Africa* (pp. 218–255). Washington, DC: National Academy Press)

34. Ministry of Health and Social Services [Namibia] (2003). *Namibia demographic and health survey 2000*. (Windhoek, Namibia: MOHSS)

CHAPTER 13. THE ECONOMIC IMPACT OF HIV/AIDS IN DEVELOPING COUNTRIES: AN END TO SYSTEMATIC UNDER-ESTIMATION

JEAN-PAUL MOATTI
INSERM Research Unit 379, University of the Mediterranean, Marseille, France

BRUNO VENTELOU
GREQAM-CNRS and Regional Centre for Disease Control (ORS-PACA), INSERM Research Unit 379, University of the Mediterranean, Marseille, France

Abstract. Public health experts and economists share a common dissatisfaction towards previous economic analyses of the impacts of HIV/AIDS. A growing body of evidence now allows a better understanding of the full economic and societal dimensions of the epidemic. It is now certain that poverty contributes to HIV/AIDS epidemics and that AIDS contributes to poverty, although we still do not know enough about the complex pathways of this relationship. To illustrate this idea, an "endogenous" growth model—which takes into account the evolution of society's human capital—is used in order to re-assess the macroeconomic impact of HIV/AIDS. A fairly wide range of epidemic effects modify the economy's long-term growth regime, creating the risk of what we might call an epidemic or "regressive trap" of rapidly falling GDP. Government action should be designed in view of this risk, with health and educational interventions.

Introduction

This is the third decade of the global HIV/AIDS pandemic. The magnitude and long-term nature of the pandemic and its severe impact on societies and economies are indisputable. In many developing countries and a growing number of countries of Eastern Europe in "transition", the epidemic is now generalised with seroprevalence rates already exceeding 1% of the adult population. The 2006 UNAIDS report on the global AIDS epidemic suggests that 10 out of 42 African countries had a prevalence in the adult population of 10% or more. As the World Bank put it, "AIDS has already reversed 30 years of hard-won social progress in some countries" [1]. It is now at the very centre of a global "development crisis", and one that is hitting the world's poorest countries the hardest.

However, public health experts, as well as economists themselves, share a common dissatisfaction towards previous economic analyses of the impacts of HIV/AIDS.

M. Caraël and J.R. Glynn (eds.), HIV, Resurgent Infections and Population Change in Africa, 245–261.

These analyses are increasingly viewed as only reflecting a limited part of the picture, as underestimating the actual impact of the epidemic on economic and human development, and consequently as leading to a systematic underinvestment in the national and international resources that are devoted to the fight against the epidemic [2,3,4]. A growing body of evidence now allows a better understanding of the full economic and societal dimensions of the epidemic that urgently needs to inform public policies at both national and international levels.

Within the global pandemic of HIV infection there are many different epidemics, each with its own dynamics and each influenced by many factors including time of introduction of the virus, population density, and cultural and social issues. Even within each region the HIV epidemic consists of a multitude of smaller ongoing epidemics, which although related, pursue their own course with different velocities. Spread of the epidemic has varied considerably between developed and developing countries, depending on the existing cultural social and behavioural patterns as well as on the risk environment. This latter concept, recently introduced by some social scientists [4], puts the emphasis on the economic and social characteristics that make individuals and groups more or less vulnerable to the risk of contracting the virus. Higher educational attainment and social status, because they provide greater economic resources, which may facilitate behaviours and opportunities that put individuals at greater risk [5,6], were often associated with a greater risk of HIV infection in Africa at the early phases of diffusion of the epidemic [7]. The recent pattern of new infections is, however, changing towards a greater burden among the less educated and poorest groups. There is increasing evidence that HIV/AIDS spreads more rapidly where there is poverty, grossly unequal distribution of income and wealth, unequal gender relations, unsustainable livelihoods, large scale population movement and civil disorder [8]. It is now certain that poverty contributes to HIV/AIDS epidemics and that AIDS contributes to poverty although we still do not know enough about the complex pathways of this relationship [9].

Until recently, economic research on HIV/AIDS had failed to capture many important aspects of its impact on development because it de facto considered the disease as a sharp exogenous shock to the economy. Indeed, the epidemic installs a continuum between a sharp short term shock and long term structural changes that in the absence of an appropriate response will jeopardise the whole process of development. It is a long wave event which is superimposed on other long wave trends, like endemic poverty, poor governance and market and public sector failures to provide basic services in Africa and other regions, as well as the social costs of rapid transition to market economies and industrialization in many others, which already affected development. The combination of these long term trends often creates dramatic short term situations, as illustrated by the way the HIV/AIDS epidemic fuels the current famines and food crisis in Southern Africa by having increased the vulnerability of small-scale farmers to production shocks [10,11].

The Demographic Impact

The most obvious impact of the epidemic is on demography. Through its direct contribution to the global burden of disease [12], as well as its strong link with the burgeoning of other infectious diseases like tuberculosis [13,14], HIV/AIDS has undermined the optimistic views of the early 1990s about the "epidemiologic transition" that were predicting that communicable diseases will account for only a minor part of morbidity and mortality in developing countries as chronic diseases become more pronounced at the beginning of the 21st century [15]. There is no doubt that the most direct demographic consequence of AIDS is an increase in mortality [16]. AIDS has been shown to be the leading cause of adult death in Abidjan, Kinshasa, and rural communities in Uganda and Tanzania [17]. In two community-based rural studies in Masaka and Rakai districts of Uganda, mortality among HIV-infected adults was over 130 per 1000 person-years of observation, nineteen times higher than among adults not infected with HIV [18]. In South Africa, without interventions to reduce HIV-related mortality, it can be predicted that by the year 2010, AIDS deaths will account for double all other causes of death combined [19].

Hardest hit by excess HIV-related deaths are those aged 25–45 years, usually a group with low mortality. In addition, mother-to-child transmission means that HIV increases infant and more particularly child mortality: when corrected for competing causes of mortality, HIV infection caused 7.7% of under-5 deaths in Sub-Saharan Africa in 1999, a significant rise from 2% in 1990, and 21 out of the 39 countries of the region had HIV-specific under-five mortality rates above 10 per 1000 [20]. Because AIDS deaths are concentrated in childhood and young adulthood, their effects on life expectancy have already been substantial, life expectancy at birth being currently three to more than fifteen years lower in 16 African countries when compared with the 1970–1975 period [21]. Population projections suggest that AIDS mortality will lead to further declines in a growing number of countries [22,23,24]. In addition, AIDS impacts population size and growth rates through the related decline in fertility rates. Although no negative population growth has yet been documented due to the HIV AIDS epidemic, figures suggest that population growth may indeed turn negative in the near future for some African countries or regions [25, 26].

The Economic Impact

The economic consequences of the major demographic changes related to AIDS have however remained rather more uncertain [27]. The current evidence on the implications of HIV/AIDS on the economy has been based on three different approaches.

1. First, *micro studies* have described the consequences of the epidemic on a certain social structure or on specific agents typically private firms, households, orphans, women, communities, etc.

A recent review of the published literature about the impact of HIV/AIDS on households identified a total of 28 studies in developing countries, mostly in Africa but also in Haiti, India, the Philippines, Sri Lanka and Thailand [28]. Most of these studies focus on "affected households", i.e. households that experience illness or death of one (or more) of their members due to HIV/AIDS, and on the impact of illness and death on household finances. These impacts commonly include "direct costs" due to medical and funeral expenditures, and "indirect costs" due to the impact of the illness on productivity [29, 30].

In low and middle income countries out-of-pocket spending represents a large share of health spending even in countries with well-functioning public health delivery systems. In low income countries, on average 4.0% of GDP is spent on health, 2.8% from public spending and 1.2% from private sources, but these figures are respectively 1.5% public and 1.8% private in Africa. Therefore, health costs can represent a significant proportion of the affected households' income: in a survey carried out in South Africa, the households with at least one HIV-infected member spent on average a third of their income in medical related expenses, whereas the national average household expenditure on health care is 4% per year [31]. Deaths are also costly; the funeral rites can last for several days, necessitating a prolonged interruption of work for the entire family concerned.[1] In some studies in Africa, the cost of a funeral may represent four times the total monthly household income. In a longitudinal community study in a rural area in north-west Tanzania, expenditures associated with AIDS terminal illness were higher than for other causes of death, direct medical costs were about 1.5 times higher than the funeral costs, and the sum of both costs exceeded the estimated annual household income per capita in this population [32]. In addition, a person who develops AIDS experiences a reduction in his productive capacity, as he regularly falls ill. The reduction in his work capacity signifies a reduction in household resources. In a survey carried out in Côte d'Ivoire among a sample of HIV-infected patients aware of their serostatus and consulting for HIV care, 30% had lost their job since their HIV diagnosis and 81% had no health insurance coverage [33]. In the study in South Africa already mentioned [31], two thirds of the affected households experienced a fall in their income, and in 40% of households, caregivers had to take time off work and other income generating activities or school. HIV/AIDS does not only push poor households deeper into poverty, it also pushes households that were relatively wealthy into poverty: that was the case in Zambia in two thirds of affected households because monthly disposable income fell by more than 80% when the father died [34].

It is also widely acknowledged that HIV/AIDS has a devastating impact on children. According to UNICEF [35], 13.4 million children have already lost one or both parents to AIDS, including 11 million in sub-Saharan Africa, half of whom being between the ages of 10 and 14. The projected total number of children orphaned by the disease will nearly double to 25 million by 2010. At that point, anywhere from 15% to 25% of the children in a dozen sub-Saharan countries will be orphans, the vast majority of them having been orphaned by HIV/AIDS. Even in countries where HIV prevalence has stabilized or fallen, like Uganda, the numbers of orphans will stay high or rise as parents already infected continue to die from the disease.

Most African businesses that have more than ten employees have already seen at least one employee dying of HIV/AIDS or currently employ infected workers [36]. HIV/AIDS has been shown to have a major impact on African business in terms of reduced labour supply, especially the loss of experienced workers in their most

---

[1] Funeral costs do not refer just to the cost of the funeral in itself: HIV/AIDS does not change this value, given that everyone will die one day. The implicit cost of HIV/AIDS relates on the one hand to the repetition of funeral costs or participation in funeral costs and on the other hand to the fact that the deceased passed away sooner than in the absence of the epidemic: the sooner the death occurs, the less time to save for funeral costs, the bigger the relative cost of funeral.

productive years, increased absenteeism, reduced profitability, loss of international competitiveness, and other financial impacts [37].

2. *Sectorial approaches* have therefore tried to assess the global costs of the epidemic for a whole industry like mining, or the agriculture commercial sector, as well as for private and public delivery of certain services.

These approaches were often carried out in order to assess the potential benefits of alternative policies to mitigate this impact. Indeed, this impact can vary in different productive sectors mainly for two reasons. First, the prevalence is different in each productive sector. Second, the importance of the incapacity due to AIDS varies according to the precise nature of the work.

The public sector, with a concentration of skilled workers, could be particularly affected, especially the education and health sectors. Education and the international effort to enrol all children in school by 2015 are being undermined, since teachers die of AIDS nearly as rapidly as nations can train them [29]. The impact on human resources is increasingly affecting the health sector especially in low-income countries where the rate per 100,000 population is lower than 10 for physicians and 100 for nurses. Existing healthcare systems are already overburdened by the HIV epidemic. In Côte d'Ivoire and Uganda, 50% to 80% of adult hospital beds are occupied by patients with HIV-related conditions [29]; in Swaziland, the average length of stay in hospitals is 6.0 days, but increases to 30.4 days for patients with tuberculosis, associated with HIV in 80% of cases [38]. In hospital services in Nairobi, Kenya, the impact of the escalating demand for HIV/AIDS-related care was accompanied by deteriorating conditions for both HIV-positive and HIV-negative patients and increased mortality during hospital stay in the two groups [39]. In both the public and private sector, the premature death of an employee leads to the disappearance of know-how, which can no longer serve production or be transmitted and may represent a higher loss for the firm than the direct loss due to absenteeism [40].

3. Finally, *macro models* have tried to measure the overall impact of the epidemic on economic development.

Different studies have been conducted to attempt to measure, in terms of GDP points lost, the macroeconomic consequences of HIV/AIDS. The main studies supply comparable figures for the African economies (**Table 1** [41]). On average, the authors forecast a one-point reduction in the rate of growth of national wealth. An estimate of the impact on the national economy of India also gave a similar 1% reduction [42]. These studies are based on an ad hoc modelling of the economy which is supposed to permit a comparative evolution to be derived, with or without the AIDS pandemic.

Why Has the Economic Impact Been Under-estimated ?

Of course, even a loss of around 1% growth matters in developing countries, which desperately need very high rates of growth to catch up with international competition. However, when confronted with the sectorial impacts described above, they

Table 1. Reduction in GDP attributable to HIV/AIDS.

Country	Average reduction in GDP (in annual growth points)	Period	Sources/authors
30 sub-Saharan African countries	[0.8; 1.4]	1990–2025	Over (1992)
Cameroon	2	1987–1991	Kambou et al. (1992)
Zambia	[1; 2]	1993–2000	Forgy (1993)
Tanzania	[0.8; 1.4]	1991–2010	Cuddington (1992)
Kenya	1.5	1996–2005	Hancock et al. (1996)
Mozambique	1	1997–2020	Wils et al. (2001)

Source: Estimations collected by Touzé and Ventelou [41] using the quoted articles, the intervals relate to the size of the impact according to the scenarios studied.

may look quite modest, and policy makers may believe that a 1% loss is similar to exogenous shocks, such as the economic consequences of the terrorist attacks in the United States on September 11, 2002, that are more or less easily absorbed by most countries. The reason why these estimations were modest is precisely that the models used considered AIDS as a traditional shock on labour supply.

These projections consider that HIV-related deaths tend to reduce both total income and the number of people this income must be divided between. The resultant smaller population tends to mean that there is more capital per worker for those that remain[43]. If a country loses 10% of its workforce in the short term, production and consequently GDP may decrease but in a more limited proportion (for example 5% or 8%) which means that mechanically GDP per capita will increase.[2] Similarly if there is scarcity of land or capital, the productivity per worker may increase as a result of the shock. Even if macroeconomic models predicted a decline in savings and investment, which will be partly due to reallocation of resources toward medical care for the HIV-infected, the negative impact on GDP growth was limited by this supposed countervailing effect of increased labour productivity [44].

This quite simplistic view of how the economy functions clearly ignores some phenomena that have been notably highlighted, in recent years, by the theory of endogenous growth [45, 46]. On the one hand, these phenomena, which have been shown to play a major role in the accomplishment of sustained high rates of economic growth, concern the influence of information and subjective expectations on the individuals' long term economic behaviours. On the other hand, they

---

[2] This argument is similar to the one used by Cantor who concludes that the bubonic plague in England in 1450 led to a rise in living standards for those who survived who had higher levels of land for cultivation per capita. However, such comparison leads to misinterpretation because the two epidemics are quite different. The "Black Death" was a very short-term epidemic that only lasted for three years and only produced a short-term one-off reduction in the size of the population.

concern the "complementarities" in the accumulation of the productive factors of the national economy, i.e. the interactions between the different forms of physical capital and human capital entering the production function.

As an example of the first dimension regarding long term trends in adaptative economic behaviours, one key element in the economic "success stories" of some countries in East Asia has been their very high rates of savings and investment, often in excess of 30% of income being saved. It has been shown that this savings boom in East Asia is related to the rapid increase in life expectancy and is dependent on the working population being able to foresee their retirement and engaging in saving to pay for it [47]. The HIV/AIDS epidemic definitely alters the long term economic behaviours in a number of ways that have hardly been quantified in previous studies.

Individuals who know their serostatus will not behave the same way as individuals who ignore it. Similarly, individuals who know they can be treated are likely to make different economic decisions from individuals who ignore the existence of this treatment or whose access to treatment has been denied. Beyond the immediate consequences of income loss and diversion of the remaining income to health expenditures, affected households may develop various "coping" strategies to deal with the long term persistence of the disease, including migration [48], child labour, sale of assets, and use of savings. The coping strategy to face health expenditures could be punctually to sell assets, but the anticipation of future costs may lead to permanent restrictions in consumption in order to pay for those potential expenditures.

The long term impact may also affect households who do not include any HIV-infected member. Non-directly affected households who provide care to a sick person or take care of the family of a deceased incur costs and experience interactions with HIV/AIDS related diseases which may alter their visions of the future. It has been shown that families fostering children, who lost their parents because of AIDS, have a significant reduction of their consumption but also their capital accumulation [49]. New empirical evidence about the impact of being orphaned in the context of AIDS [50, 51] also stresses the importance of taking into account a longer time horizon and the related evolution of economic behaviours to accurately measure impact. The reduction in children's human capital following the loss of parents' presence seems less due to the direct associated loss in income from parental deaths than a product of associated behavioural changes. In particular, the impact of orphanhood on living arrangements and school enrolment seems to depend on the degree of relatedness of the orphans to the head of the household which takes care of them [52, 53].

Moreover, in countries where the epidemic is generalized and the impacts are publicly known, it is likely that a significant portion of the population will turn objective variables—such as life expectancy or future productivity—into subjective ones, due to the presence of HIV/AIDS in their environment. In South Africa, under highly plausible hypotheses about the way consumption decisions will be affected by the fall in the average national life expectancy due to HIV/AIDS, a microsimulation revealed that the saving rate in 2015 would be at minimum 5% lower than the rate that would have prevailed in the absence of the epidemic [54].

The threats to regional security due to the generalisation of the epidemic, that have been highlighted by a series of reports [55], are another example of "indirect deferred costs" whose impact may be considerable on economic activities like tourism [56] or decisions of foreign investors [57].

A second dimension that has been grossly underestimated in most studies and has even been totally neglected in previous macroeconomic models, is the dynamic impact of the epidemic on transmission of human capital and its interaction with physical capital. This relationship must be understood in the current context of the change of paradigm concerning the relationship between health improvements and economic growth. In recent years, there has been a growing awareness that health is not only a consumption good that adds to wellbeing but also an investment good that increases the future productive power of workers and employees. The traditional interpretation of the strong observed correlation between income and health—i.e. that higher income leads to better health—has been increasingly challenged: health, as measured by life expectancy at the beginning of the period, has significant effects on subsequent growth. The landmark report on macroeconomics and health commissioned by WHO has provided compelling evidence that investment in global health spurs economic development [3]. Together with the moral argument, the direct effect of health on workers' productivity is the main mechanism put forward by this report to justify increased transfers of resources to developing countries for health spending.

However, there are also more indirect mechanisms through which health can influence productivity, because health is a complementary input in the formation of human capital. Ill health and premature death lead to wasted investment in human capital and globally reduces the incentives to invest in the future of people. In the absence of an adequate policy response, the reduction in resources linked to HIV/AIDS can have a major impact in decreasing the productivity of education, significantly reducing human capital and its transmission and contributing to a long term decline in savings and investment.

All these considerations, to which may be added the deformation of the age-pyramid of the population due to AIDS [58], lead to the understanding that the impact of the epidemic on growth of GDP is likely to be a lot larger than previously estimated by models that did not take these effects into account. By killing mostly young adults, AIDS does more than destroy the human capital embodied in them. It weakens the whole mechanism through which human capital is accumulated and transmitted across generations, it reduces the incentives to invest in education and weakens the precious informal educational mechanisms through which savoir-faire are transmitted from parents to children.

The conclusions of a recent study by the World Bank [59], which has tried for the first time to fully integrate the effect on human capital on macroeconomic predictions for South Africa state that "in the absence of AIDS, the counterfactual benchmark, there would have been modest growth with universal education attained with three generations. But if nothing is done to combat the epidemic, a complete economic collapse will occur within four generations" with the risk of South Africa being taken back to the level of GDP per capita of Kenya.

The Introduction of *Human Capital* into Macroeconomic Analysis of the Impact of AIDS

In a recent study [60] (see also appendix), we proposed a macro-economic model based on the basic idea that the differential impact of AIDS on the economic growth of different countries depends largely on the level of development already attained. Our model is characterised by a production function with 4 variables (capital K, labour L, human capital H and public productive spending D) and 3 types of agent (firms, households and the State). In this type of macro modelling, *human capital* could be defined very generally as "the ability of people to be economically productive: education, training, and health care can help increase human capital".

Households provide the production factor L, receive wages, and choose between consumption of current goods and consumption of health goods. Health demand is influenced by family morbidity. When morbidity increases, households offer less work, receive fewer wages, and demand more health goods. At the same time, the household's human capital, H, is reduced (deferred indirect cost). The level of public spending is fixed by the State, which also decides its composition, between D, productive spending, and direct transfers to households (healthcare allowances for example). Such a model implies two paths for the economy (**Fig. 1**). For a given population health status and a given level of health expenditure, a threshold exists below which the balanced-growth rate of per capita national income is negative: the

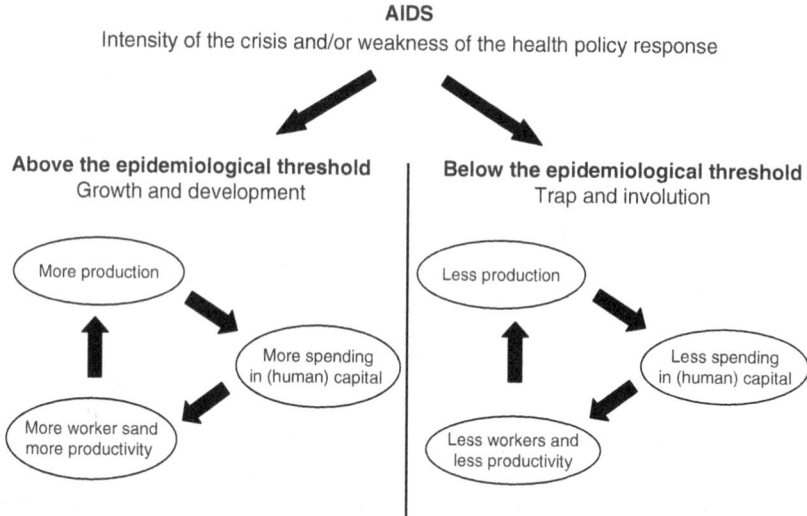

Fig. 1. Two paths for the impact of AIDS on the economy. The basic idea underlying the Figure is that of a differential impact of AIDS on economic growth, crucially depending on the level of development already attained and of the adequacy of the response. For a reasonable range of epidemiological predictions, an *involution trap* may occur, corresponding to a modification of the long-term growth regime of the economy

long-run economic outcome is no-development, a case we will call an "epidemic trap". In this case, the withdrawal resulting from the disease and poor health on the economy's productive factors is too large to allow its development to continue. Above this threshold, however, the economy provides sufficient resources to maintain its cumulative growth (benefiting from the regular provision of human capital at the same time as physical capital accumulates). The existence of the trap is closely linked to the structure of the macroeconomic model: multiple growth engines and productive complementarities. In this view, accumulation of *human capital* turns out to be the essential force that generates economic growth. A large AIDS epidemic brutally disrupts the transmission of knowledge and abilities from one generation to the next and may thus result in deep economic collapse: a "bifurcation".

We evaluated the possibility of an epidemic trap under "plausible" hypotheses. Our model is calibrated with data for Angola, Benin, Cameroon, Central African Republic and Côte d'Ivoire for GNP, population, capital stock, gross domestic investment, fiscal policy, etc., up to 2001. We also set parameters and elasticities (for healthcare demand) from microeconomic and statistical studies. The principal unobservable constant is the human capital at the beginning of the calibration period (1985), and it will be determined as the best fit with the real macroeconomic course of events. **Table 2** reports HIV prevalence[3] and simulated GNP for five countries according to our economic model. The average reduction in GNP is estimated by the difference between the simulated GNP "without AIDS" (that is, prevalence rate set at zero) and with AIDS. The main result of this calibration exercise matches the predictions of our theoretical model. The average reduction of GNP exceeds 10% in four countries, and an epidemic trap appears in Cameroon. Of course, our results are dependent on HIV the prevalence rates estimated by UNAIDS (an input of the macro-modelling), and it is possible that new revisions of data drive Cameroon out of the sample of countries which endure a bifurcation process. But the finding remains that countries with great economic vulnerability could radically shift their growth path when experiencing high HIV prevalence rates.

The introduction of human capital into macroeconomic analysis and the interaction between multiple agents' decisions about production factors create potential "bifurcations" along the balanced-growth pathway of fragile economies. Using a realistic set of parameters and elasticities, we find a *trap phenomenon* to be plausible in face of an epidemic shock such as AIDS. Together households (for healthcare decisions) and firms (for physical capital formation) have essentially been knocked into reverse and are together entering a process named "coordination failure" by certain economists [61]. The example of Cameroon—if HIV prevalence rises—is particularly interesting and dramatic: the growth process may be blocked by the shock and the net GDP-loss may be far higher than anticipated by previous macroeconomic studies: more than 15% in this special case.

---

[3] Source : UNAIDS epidemic projections (by its SPECTRUM software) in 2003 mainly. These figures have been revised regularly by UNAIDS since 2003, knowing that new prevalence studies have been implemented. In 2005, Cameroon encounters a drastic revision, which we have taken into account in this paper (which is why the present figures differ from our earlier forecasts in Oxford Development Studies). We did not integrate the new revisions of 2006.

Table 2. AIDS and economic growth in five African countries.

Years	1995	2000	2005 (f)	2010 (f)
Angola				
Adult HIV prevalence (%)	2.5	5.3	5.1	5.1
GNP (PPP, constant 1987 international US$)	8,617	11,137	9,642	9,975
Average reduction in GNP	5%	7%	8%	9%
Benin				
Adult HIV prevalence (%)	1.5	3.3	2.9	2.6
GNP (PPP, constant 1987 international US$)	4,982	5,955	7,162	8,388
Average reduction in GNP	1%	3%	5%	6%
Cameroon				
Adult HIV prevalence (%) (see Note 3 for the special case of Cameroon HIV prevalence rate)	5	7.2	10.8	13.6
GNP (PPP, constant 1987 international US$)	17,008	19,654	20,314	20,597
Average reduction in GNP	5%	8%	9%	17%
Central African Republic				
Adult HIV prevalence (%)	5.2	9	9.7	9.3
GNP (PPP, constant 1987 international US$)	3,766	3,924	4,093	4,220
Average reduction in GNP	9%	11%	13%	14%
Côte d'Ivoire				
Adult HIV prevalence (%)	2.5	6.5	10	12.3
GNP (PPP, constant 1987 international US$)	16,214	19,680	19,922	20,386
Average reduction in GNP	2%	5%	9%	13%

f = forecasts
Source: [60]

Why Has the Impact on Human Development Been Under-estimated?

While it should now be understandable that the impact of HIV/AIDS on economic growth has been underestimated through its consequences on human capital, it should also be acknowledged that an emphasis on GDP to the exclusion of other aspects of human development does not capture the actual consequences of the epidemic [2]. The morbidity and mortality associated with an HIV/AIDS epidemic also affects the unpaid, non-market economic activities—what may be called non-traded socially reproductive labour and goods—that are of prime importance in the societies of the developing world in proportions that are not anymore the case in high income countries. These activities—child rearing, community participation, self-provisioning through agricultural or pastoral work—do not enter into usual economic calculations. As conceptualised by economists who call attention to the fact that certain social relations may facilitate co-operation and trust and can be a source of value in themselves [62, 63], loss of these activities may strongly affect the whole process of development.

The modern idea of human development characteristic of the United Nations Development Programme (UNDP) has tried to go beyond GDP alone to arrive at a more pragmatic balance between the growths of income, environmental sustainability and people's needs to be full participants in the lives of their societies. It tries to recognise that these goals should be achieved in relation to widely varying cultural and national traditions. It also tries to incorporate the important notion of capabilities, a perspective focusing on the opportunities for choice that their economic and social environment practically offers to people [64].

Human development has four components (UNDP, 1995): the creation of human capabilities (including improved health, knowledge and skills to fully participate in income generation); the elimination of barriers to economic and political opportunities, enabling people to have equal access to and benefit from opportunities; people's full participation in decisions and processes affecting their lives; and intergenerational sustainability of the development process. The Human Development Index (HDI), a composite index measuring average achievement in three basic dimensions (a long and healthy life, knowledge and a decent standard of living) is an attempt, although imperfect, to better capture progress on all its major dimensions. In the 1980s, reversals in HDI were highly unusual and limited to exceptional political or war situations. Unfortunately, the 2003 edition of the Human Development Report shows that 21 countries[4] have exhibited a decline in the value of their HDI and such decline is mainly related to a fall in life expectancy due to the HIV/AIDS epidemic. Even countries which are able to pursue progress in their absolute level of human development are affected in that process because of HIV/AIDS: for example, Thailand in spite of successful efforts to bring the epidemic under control has fallen from 52nd in 1995 to 74th place in 2001 in HDI rankings.

Some Policy Recommendations for Responding to the Economic Impact of AIDS

The recent literature on the economic impact of AIDS in developing countries strongly supports the need for governmental action in three principal policy directions:

---

[4] Between 1980 and 1990, only four countries (Democratic Republic of Congo, Guyana, Rwanda and Zambia) saw a drop in their HDI. Between 1990 and 2000, Armenia, Belarus, Botswana, Burundi, Cameroon, Central African Republic, Côte d'Ivoire, Congo, Dem. Rep. of Congo, Kazakhstan, Kenya, Lesotho, Moldova, Russian Federation, South Africa, Swaziland, Tajikistan, Tanzania, Ukraine, Zambia, Zimbabwe exhibited a decline.

1. Governments must take into account the long-range effects on *human capital*. Policy should prefer *social* intervention, with an increase in health and educational spending. Social support systems must be improved and redesigned, to fight against the "imminent" social consequences of HIV/AIDS, but at the same time to fight against its "deferred" economic consequences.

2. Scaling-up access to antiretroviral treatment for a large part of the working population who already HIV-infected may be much more cost-effective than initially evaluated, in view of the risk of an epidemic underdevelopment trap. In some cases, rapid access to ARV treatments could prevent these countries from experiencing a macroeconomic catastrophic "bifurcation".

3. For countries threatened by such an epidemic trap, internal resources are by definition insufficient to reverse the tendency to collapse. Any policy must therefore be accompanied by increased aid from the international community (by more funds given to the most fragile African countries, or by an agreement on "subsidized" treatment prices for them), because the longer the delay in this policy, the more costly and less efficient it will be.

Mathematical Appendix

The model used for this research is a Computable General Equilibrium Model (CGE-Model), including an endogenous growth property. **Table 3** presents the various channels through which the AIDS pandemic may affect economic growth as well as the list of variables used in the model to capture these effects.

The model assumes the following macroeconomic production function:

$$Y(\varepsilon) = (K(y,\varepsilon))^{\alpha} \times (L \times H(y,\varepsilon))^{\beta} \times (D(y,\varepsilon))^{\chi}$$

with ε, population's epidemiological status (HIV prevalence rate) and $\alpha + \beta + \chi = 1$.

Table 3. Economic variables and AIDS impact on growth.

Channel	Variable of the model	Horizon
Rate of participation (quantitative effect of AIDS on the work supply)	L/N, share of the total labour force effectively capable of working	Short
Productivity of workers (qualitative effects of AIDS on the work supply)	H, "human capital"	Long
Rate of public investment	D, public productive spending	Short/long
Private investment	K, physical capital (possible financial imbalance of the national economy)	Short/long

The complete formal version of the model and detailed results are provided in Couderc and Ventelou (2005) [60].

This equation will serve to analyse the effect of the epidemic on the macroeconomic income Y of a country. Any increase in ε represents a deterioration of the population's health status and affects the accumulation process of each production factor (K, L, H and D, as defined in **Table 3**). A specificity of the model (its "endogenous growth" property) is that these cumulative factors, and consequently the total growth rate of the economy, are an increasing function of the per capita national income level Y/N (= y), with a critical value threshold y that has to be reached in order to obtain positive growth (growth rate $G > 0$ for $y > y_c$). The exact threshold level and the calculation of the macroeconomic rate of growth are based on microeconomic foundations which take into account agents' behaviours including those at the household level. At this level, two health effects are assumed:

AIDS → ill health → reduction in labour participation.

AIDS → Alteration of the long-sight choices of the agents (households and firms) → lower 'human capital' (education, savoir-faire), lower 'physical capital'.

Thus, the model calculates a double effect, both quantitative (short-term) and qualitative (long-term), of AIDS on African economies. When the country is fragile (near a critical value threshold y_c), the epidemic shock may result in deep economic collapse: a "bifurcation".

References

1. World Bank (1999). *Intensifying action against HIV/AIDS in Africa: responding to a development crisis*. (Washington: World Bank)

2. Wehrwein, P. (2000). The economic impact of AIDS in Africa. *Harvard AIDS Review*, (Winter Issue), 12–14

3. Sachs, J. D. (Ed.) (2001). *Macroeconomics and health: Investing in health for economic development*. Report of the Commission on Macroeconomics and Health (CMH) of the World Health Organization. (Geneva, WHO)

4. Barnett, T. & Whiteside, A. (2002). *AIDS in the twenty-first century. Disease and globalization*. (New York: Palgrave Macmillan)

5. Smith, J., Nalagoda, F., Wawer, M. J., et al. (1999). Education attainment as a predictor of HIV risk in rural Uganda: Results from a population-based study. *International Journal of STD & AIDS*, *10*, 452–459

6. Bloom, S. S., Urassa, M., Isingo, R., Ng'weshemi, J. & Boerma, J. T. (2002). Community effects on the risk of HIV infection in rural Tanzania. *Sexually Transmitted Infections*, *78*, 261–266

7. Hargreaves, J. R. & Glynn, J. R. (2002). Educational attainment and HIV-1 infection in developing countries: A systematic review. *Tropical Medicine and International Health*, *7*, 489–498

8. Stillwaggon, E. (2000). HIV transmission in Latin America: Comparison with Africa and policy implications. *Journal South African Ecology*, *68*, 985–1011

9. Loewenson, R. & Whiteside, A. (2001). *HIV/AIDS implications for poverty reduction*. United Nations Development Programme background paper for the UN General Assembly Special Session on HIV/AIDS, New York, June 25–27

10. Haddad, L. & Gillespie, S. (2001). Effective food and nutrition policy responses to HIV/AIDS: What we know and what we need to know. *Journal of International Development, 13*, 487–511

11. Lambrechts, K. & Barry, G. (2003). *Why is Southern Africa hungry? The roots of Southern Africa's food crisis.* A Christian Aid Policy Briefing, London, June

12. Murray, C. J. L. & Lopez, A. D. (1997). Mortality by cause in eight regions of the world: Global burden of disease study. *The Lancet, 349*, 1269–1276

13. Frieden, T. R., Sterling, T. R., Munsiff, S. S., Watt, C. J. & Dye, C. (2003). Tuberculosis. *The Lancet, 362*, 887–899

14. Davies, P. D.O. (2003). The world-wide increase in tuberculosis: How demographic changes, HIV infection and increasing numbers in poverty are increasing tuberculosis. *Annals of Medicine, 35*, 235–243

15. Jamison, D. T. & Mosley, W. H. (1991). Disease control priorities in developing countries: Health policy responses to epidemiological change. *American Journal of Public Health, 81*, 15–22

16. Caraël, M., Schwartländer, B. & Zewdie, D. (1998). Demographic impact of AIDS. Introduction. *AIDS, 12*, S1–S2

17. Boerma, J. T., Nunn, A. J. & Whitworth, J. A. (1998). Mortality impact of the AIDS epidemic: Evidence from community studies in less developed countries. *AIDS, 12*, S3–S14

18. Sewankambo, N. K., Gray, R. H, Ahmad, S., et al. (2000). Mortality associated with HIV infection in rural Rakai District, Uganda. *AIDS, 14*, 2391–2400

19. Bradshaw, D., Schneider, M., Dorrington, R., Bourne, D. E. & Laubscher, R. (2002). South African cause-of-death profile in transition–1996 and future trends. *South African Medical Journal, 92*, 618–623

20. Walker, N., Schwartländer, B. & Bryce, J. (2002). Meeting international goals in child survival and HIV/AIDS. *The Lancet, 360*, 284–289

21. United Nations Development Programme (2003). *Human Development Report 2003.* (Oxford: Oxford University Press)

22. US Bureau of the Census (2000). World population profile 2000. Washington, DC

23. Stover, J. (2003). Modelling the demographic impact of AIDS. *Journal of Hleath Population and Nutrition, 20*, 102–103

24. Heuveline, P. (2003). HIV and population dynamics: A general model and maximum-likelihood standards for East Africa. *Demography, 40*, 217–245

25. US Bureau of the Census (2000). *Monitoring the AIDS Pandemic Network. The Status and Trends of the HIV/AIDS Epidemics in the World, 2000.* Washington, DC

26. Mekonnen, Y., Jegou, R., Coutinho, R. A, Nokes, J. & Fontanet, A. (2002). Demographic impact of AIDS in a low-fertility urban African setting: Projection for Addis Ababa, Ethiopia. *Journal of Health Population and Nutrition, 20*, 120–129

27. Whiteside, A. (2001). Demography and economics of HIV/AIDS. *British Medical Bulletin, 58*, 73–88

28. Booysen, F. le R. & Arntz, T. (2003). The methodology of HIV/AIDS impact studies: A review of current practices. *Social Science and Medicine, 56*, 2391–2405

29. Mutangadura, G., Mukurazita, D. & Jackson, H. (2000). A review of household and community responses to the HIV/AIDS epidemic in the rural areas of sub-Saharan Africa. (Geneva: UNAIDS)

30. Over, M. (1998). Coping with the impact of AIDS. *Finance and Development*, (March), 22–24

31. Steinberg, M., Johnson, S., Schierhout, G., et al. (2002). *Hitting home: How households cope with the impact of the HIV/AIDS epidemic. A survey of households affected by HIV/AIDS in South Africa.* (Washington, DC: The Henry J. Kaiser Family Foundation)

32. Ngalula, J., Urassa, M., Mwaluko, G., Isingo, R. & Boerma, T. J. (2002). Health service use and household expenditure during terminal illness due to AIDS in rural Tanzania. *Tropical Medicine and International Health*, 7, 873–877

33. Msellati, P., Juillet-Amar, A., Prudhomme, J., et al. (2003). Socio-economic and health characteristics of HIV-infected patients seeking care in relation to access to the drug access initiative and to antiretroviral treatment in Côte d'Ivoire. *AIDS*, 17, S63–S68

34. Grassly, N. C., Desai, K., Pegurri, E. et al. (2003). The economic impact of HIV/AIDS on the education sector in Zambia. *AIDS*, 17, 1039–1044

35. UNICEF (2003). *Africa's orphaned generations.* Report issued in November 2003, New York

36. Forsythe, S. (2002). How does HIV/AIDS affect African businesses? In Forsythe, S. (Ed.), *State of the art: AIDS and economics* (pp. 30–37). (Washington, DC: International AIDS and Economics Network (IAEN)). Retrieved from: www.iaen.org

37. Rosen, S., Simon, J., Vincent, J. R., MacLeod, W., Fox, M., Thea, D. M. (2003). AIDS is your business. *Harvard Business Review*, 81, 80–87

38. Kingdom of Swaziland. Ministry of Health and Social Welfare (2000). *Accelerating access to HIV/ AIDS care in Swaziland. A partnership between the Kingdom of Swaziland, the United Nations System, and the Private sector.* Project Document, September 2000

39. Gilks, C. F., Floyd, K., Otieno, L. S., Adam, A. M., Bhatt, S. M. & Warrell, D. A. (1998). Some effects of the rising case load of adult HIV-related disease on a hospital in Nairobi. *Journal of Acquired Immune Deficiency Syndromes*, 18, 234–240

40. Aventin, L. & Huard, P. (2000). The cost of AIDS to three manufacturing firms in Cote d'Ivoire. *Journal of African Ecology*, 9, 161–188

41. Touzé, V. & Ventelou, B. (2002). AIDS and development, a global challenge. *Revue de L'OFCE*, 0, S153–S174

42. Anand, K., Pandav, C. S. & Nath, L. M. (1999). Impact of HIV/AIDS on the national economy of India. *Health Policy*, 47, 195–205

43. Bloom, D. & Canning, D. (2003). Health as human capital and its impact on economic performance. *Geneva Papers on Risk and Insurance*, 28, 304–315

44. Cantor, N. F. (2001). *In the wake of the plague: The Black Death and the world it made.* (New York: The Free Press)

45. Lucas, R. E. Jr. (2000). Some macroeconomics for the 21st century. *Journal of Economic Perspectives*, 14, 159–168

46. Lloyd-Ellis, H. & Roberts, J. (2002). Twin engines of growth: Skills and technology as equal partners in balanced growth. *Journal of Economic Growth*, 7, 87–115

47. Bloom, D. E., Canning, D. & Malaney, P. N. (2000). Demographic change and economic growth in Asia. *Population and Development Review*, 26, S257–S290

48. Bronfman, M. N., Leyva, R., Negroni, M. J. & Rueda, C. M. (2002). Mobile populations and HIV/ AIDS in Central America and Mexico: Research for action. *AIDS*, 16, S42–S49

49. Deininger, K., Garcia, M. & Subbarao, K. (2003). AIDS-induced orphanhood as a systemic shock: Magnitude, impact, and program interventions in Africa. *World Development, 31*, 1201–1220

50. Nyambedha, E. O., Wandibba, S. & Aagaard-Hansen, J. (2003). Changing patterns of orphan care due to the HIV epidemic in western Kenya. *Social Science and Medicine, 57*, 301–311

51. Bicego, G., Rutstein, S. & Johnson, K. (2003). Dimensions of the emerging orphan crisis in sub-Saharan Africa. *Social Science and Medicine, 56*, 1235–1247

52. Case, A., Paxson, P. & Ableidinger, J. (2003). *Orphans in Africa.* (Paper presented at the UNAIDS Reference Group on Economics Meeting, World Bank, Washington DC, April 22–23)

53. Gertler, P., Levine, D. & Martinez, S. (2003). *The presence and presents of parents: Do parents matter for more than money?* (Paper presented at the UNAIDS Reference Group on Economics Meeting, World Bank, Washington, DC, April 22–23)

54. Freire, S. (2002). *The impact of HIV/AIDS on saving behaviour in South Africa.* (Paper presented at the International AIDS Economic Network Symposium on Economics of HIV/AIDS in developing countries, Barcelona, July). Retrieved from www.iaen.org

55. Eberstadt, N. (2002). The future of AIDS: Grim toll in Russia, China, and India. *Foreign Affairs, 81*, 22–45

56. Forsythe, S. (1999). HIV/AIDS and tourism. *AIDS Analysis Africa, 9*, 4–6

57. Hemrich, G. & Topouzis, D. (2000). Multi-sectoral responses to HIV/AIDS: Constraints and opportunities for technical co-operation. *Journal of International Development, 12*, 85–99

58. Easterly, W. & Levine, R. (1997). Africa's growth tragedy: Policies ad ethnic divisions. *Quarterly Journal of Economics, 112*, 1203–1250

59. Bell, C., Devarajan, S. & Gersbach, H. (2003). *The long-run economic costs of AIDS: Theory and an application to South Africa.* (Paper presented at the UNAIDS Reference Group on Economics Meeting, World Bank, Washington, DC, April 22–23). Retreived from www.iaen.org

60. Couderc, N. & Ventelou, B. (2005). AIDS, economic growth and epidemic trap in Africa. *Oxford Development Studies, 33*, 417–426

61. Cooper, R. (2000). *Coordination games, complementarities and macroeconomics.* (Cambridge: Cambridge University Press)

62. Gui, B. (2000). Beyond transactions: On the interpersonal dimension of economic reality. *Annals of Public and Cooperative Economy, 71*, 139–169

63. Bruni, L. & Sugden, R. (2000). Moral canals: Trust and social capital in the work of Hume, Smith and Genovesi. *Ecology and Philosophy, 16*, 21–45

64. Sen, A. (1999). *Development as freedom.* (New York: Albert Knopf)

INDEX